Dermato

Therapeutics

A Pocket Guide

Notice

Dermatologic Therapeutics

A Pocket Guide

FRANCISCO A. KERDEL, B.Sc., M.B.B.S.
Chief of Dermatology and Director of Inpatient Services
Cedars Medical Center
Miami, Florida

PAOLO ROMANELLI, M.D.
Assistant Professor of Dermatology and Dermatopathology
Department of Dermatology and Cutaneous Surgery
University of Miami
Miami, Florida

JENNIFER T. TRENT, M.D.
Department of Dermatology and Cutaneous Surgery
University of Miami
Miami, Florida

McGraw-Hill
Medical Publishing Division

New York Chicago San Francisco Lisbon London Madrid Mexico City
Milan New Delhi San Juan Seoul Singapore Sydney Toronto

Dermatologic Therapeutics: A Pocket Guide

1 2 3 4 5 6 7 8 9 0   DOC/DOC   0 9 8 7 6 5

ISBN: 0-07-143889-0

This book was set in Minion by Circle Graphics.
The editors were Andrea L. Seils, Robert Pancotti, and Mary E. Bele.
The production supervisor was Richard Ruzycka.
The cover designer was Jeannet Leendertse.
The indexer was Andover Publishing Services.
RR Donnelley was printer and binder.

This book is printed on acid-free paper.

Library of Congress Cataloging-in-Publication Data
Kerdel, Francisco A.
    Dermatologic therapeutics : a pocket guide / Francisco A. Kerdel, Paolo Romanelli,
Jennifer T. Trent.
        p. ; cm.
    Includes bibliographical references and index.
    ISBN 0-07-143889-0 (alk. paper)
      1. Dermatology–Handbooks, manuals, etc. 2. Skin–Diseases–Treatment–Handbooks,
manuals, etc. I. Romanelli, Paolo. II. Trent, Jennifer T. III. Title.
    [DNLM: 1. Skin Diseases–therapy–Handbooks. WR 39 K39d 2005]
RL74.K47 2005
616.5′06–dc22
                                                                    2004061045

Contents

Preface .... *ix*

SECTION 1 Dermatologic Medications 1

Appendix I Treatments for Fungal Infections 327

Appendix II Treatments for Bacterial Infections 334

Appendix III Treatments for Mycobacterial Infections 340

General References 344

SECTION 2 Dermatologic Conditions 345

Index 409

Preface

For a long time, dermatologic therapy was based on only a handful of medications. Over the past several decades, however, more specific therapies have been created, which has made a great impact on the practice of dermatology. The field is still expanding, especially with the advent of the use of biologics in our field.

The goal of this book is to provide a concise, evidence-based pocket manual that includes not only dermatologic therapy but also treatment options for certain common dermatologic conditions. Although the disease-descriptive component cannot replace a reference textbook, we hope that this manual will complement such textbooks and will serve as both an introduction to certain topics and a quick reference guide.

The book is organized into two alphabetized sections: a dermatologic therapy section and a dermatologic conditions section. The reader may easily refer to and find pertinent information on either a specific medication or a disease. We hope that this format makes it easy to navigate through the book and to quickly extract the information necessary to care for patients successfully.

There are two features unique to this book, which set it apart from other dermatology pocket guides. One feature is the use of symbols (*, ^, $, +) that are placed after each drug or therapeutic intervention. These symbols denote the following: *, U.S. Food and Drug Administration approval; ^, randomized controlled trials; $, case series; and +, case reports. We believe that this evidence-based approach to understanding different therapies sets this book apart from other pocket manuals. In addition, in a concise and easy-to-read manner, the description of each drug is included, with information on indications, dose, interactions, side effects, laboratory tests to monitor, contraindications, and pregnancy class.

The second unique feature of this book is in the dermatologic conditions section. This section consists of approximately 75 of the most frequently encountered dermatologic conditions. For each entity, there is a brief description of the pathogenesis, followed by different treatment options reported in the literature. The list of therapies also carries the evidence-based symbols previously used in the therapy section.

We hope that this pocket manual serves as a survival guide for residents and medical students learning dermatology and as a quick reference manual for established practicing dermatologists.

Francisco A. Kerdel, B.Sc., M.B.B.S.
Paolo Romanelli, M.D.
Jennifer T. Trent, M.D.

Dermatologic Therapeutics

A Pocket Guide

Section 1

Dermatologic Medications

ACITRETIN

(Soriatane® 10, 25 mg tab)

▓ INDICATIONS

- Actinic keratosis^
- Cutaneous malignancies/chemoprevention^
- Darier's disease$ (see pg. 359)
- Ichthyosis$ (see pg. 369)
- Keratodermas^
- Lichen planus^ (see pg. 371)
- Lichen sclerosus et atrophicus^ (see pg. 372)
- Lupus, cutaneous $ (see pg. 375)
- Pityriasis rubra pilaris$ (see pg. 387)
- Psoriasis* (see pg. 392)
- Squamous cell carcinoma (SCC), the risk of development is lowered in psoriasis patients receiving psoralen-ultraviolet A (PUVA)$ (see pg. 400)

▓ MECHANISM OF ACTION

It induces cellular differentiation and possesses antiproliferative, anti-inflammatory, and antikeratinizing properties. It also inhibits neutrophil function through the activation of retinoic acid receptors in the nucleus of cells.

▓ DOSAGE

Start at 0.5 mg/kg/d. May increase to 1 mg/kg/d as tolerated.

ACTINIC KERATOSIS: 0.2 mg/kg/d PO

SCC RISK LOWERED IN PSORIASIS PATIENTS RECEIVING PUVA: 25–50 mg PO qd

▓ DRUG INTERACTIONS

INCREASED SERUM LEVELS OF ACITRETIN: azole antifungals, macrolides, tetracyclines, vitamin A

DECREASED SERUM LEVELS OF ACITRETIN: anticonvulsants, antituberculosis drugs

INCREASED DRUG LEVELS OF: cyclosporin

DECREASED DRUG LEVELS OF: progestin-only contraceptives

PROLONGED TERATOGENIC POTENTIAL OF ACITRETIN: alcohol (alcohol converts acitretin to etretinate)

INCREASED RISK OF HEPATOTOXICITY: methotrexate

SIDE EFFECTS

COMMON: dry eyes and lips, stickiness and desquamation of the palms and soles, decreased mucus secretion in the nose, headache, nausea/diarrhea/abdominal pain, retinoid dermatitis, telogen effluvium, fragility and onycholysis of the nails, hypercholesterolemia, hypertriglyceridemia, elevated liver function test results

RARE: teratogenicity, reduced night vision, photophobia, diffuse interstitial skeletal hyperostosis, osteophyte formation, osteoporotic changes, premature epiphyseal closure, pancreatitis, flare of inflammatory bowel disease, hepatitis, pseudotumor cerebri (when given in combination with tetracycline, doxycycline, or minocycline), depression/suicide, myopathy/myalgias/arthralgias, stroke, myocardial infarction

MONITORING

BASELINE: serum/urine pregnancy test, complete blood count, liver function test, fasting lipid profile, renal function, urinalysis

MONTHLY FOR FIRST 3–6 MONTHS, THEN EVERY 3 MONTHS: liver function test, fasting lipid profile

MONTHLY FOR WOMEN OF CHILDBEARING POTENTIAL: serum/urine pregnancy test

CONTRAINDICATIONS

Pregnancy, hypersensitivity to retinoids, liver dysfunction

PREGNANCY CLASS

X

ACYCLOVIR

(Zovirax® 200, 400, 800 mg tab; 200 mg/5 mL PO suspension)

INDICATIONS

- Erythema multiforme^ (see pg. 364)
- Herpes simplex virus*
- Herpes zoster*
- Stevens-Johnson syndrome+ (see pg. 400)
- Varicella*

MECHANISM OF ACTION

Activated through phosphorylation by viral thymidine kinase. Inhibits viral DNA polymerase. Activated acyclovir is mistaken for deoxyguanosine triphosphate and becomes incorporated into newly synthesized viral DNA, which results in chain termination. Thus, viral DNA synthesis is completely and irreversible inhibited.

DOSAGE

HERPES SIMPLEX PRIMARY
Immunocompetent: 200 mg PO 5 times a day for 10 days
Immunodeficient: 200–400 mg PO 5 times a day for 10 days or 5 mg/kg IV q8h for 7–10 days

HERPES SIMPLEX RECURRENCES
Immunocompetent: 400 mg PO tid for 5 days
Immunodeficient: 400 mg PO 5 times a day for 7–10 days or 5 mg/kg IV q8h for 7 days

HERPES SIMPLEX SUPPRESSION
Immunocompetent: 400 mg PO bid
Immunodeficient: 400 mg PO bid

VARICELLA
Immunocompetent: 20 mg/kg PO 5 times a day up to 800 mg/dose PO 5 times a day for 5–7 days
Immunodeficient: 10 mg/kg IV q8h for 7–10 days

HERPES ZOSTER
   Immunocompetent: 800 mg PO 5 times a day for 7–10 days
   Immunodeficient: 10 mg/kg IV q8h for 7–10 days

RENAL DOSING IV
   Creatinine clearance (CrCl) 50–90 mL/min: 5–12.4 mg/kg IV q8h
   CrCl 10–50 mL/min: 5–12.4 mg/kg IV q12h–q24h
   CrCl < 10 mL/min: 2.5 mg/kg IV q24h
   Hemodialysis: 2.5 mg/kg IV after dialysis
   Chronic ambulatory peritoneal dialysis: 2.5 mg/kg IV q24h
   Continuous arteriovenous hemofiltration: 3.5 mg/kg/d IV

■ DRUG INTERACTIONS

INCREASED LEVELS OF ACYCLOVIR: probenecid, zidovudine

■ SIDE EFFECTS

COMMON: nausea, vomiting, diarrhea, headache, malaise, dizziness, rash, lethargy, confusion, phlebitis and infusion site reactions with IV form

RARE: seizures, coma, leukopenia, thrombocytopenia, renal dysfunction, reversible renal impairment due to crystalline nephropathy and elevated creatinine with IV form

■ MONITORING

None

■ CONTRAINDICATIONS

Hypersensitivity to drug/class, pregnancy

■ PREGNANCY CLASS

C

ADALIMUMAB

(Humira® 40 mg vials)

▓ INDICATIONS

- Psoriasis^ (see pg. 392)
- Psoriatic arthritis⁺
- Rheumatoid arthritis*

▓ MECHANISM OF ACTION

Fully human recombinant immunoglobulin G1 (IgG1) monoclonal antibody specific for anti–tumor necrosis factor alpha (TNF-α).

▓ DOSAGE

40 mg SC every other week

▓ DRUG INTERACTIONS

DECREASED CLEARANCE OF ADALIMUMAB: methotrexate

INCREASED RISK OF SERIOUS INFECTIONS: immunosuppressants

▓ SIDE EFFECTS

COMMON: injection site reaction, upper respiratory infection symptoms, headache, rash, sinusitis, nausea, urinary tract infection, abdominal pain, headache, back pain

RARE: malignancy/lymphoma, demyelinating disorders, serious infections/sepsis, induction of autoantibodies/anaphylaxis, tuberculosis reactivation, hematuria, elevated liver function test results, hypertension, hyperlipidemia, rheumatoid arthritis flare, lupus-like syndrome

▓ MONITORING

BASELINE: Purified protein derivative (PPD) and chest x-ray

▨ CONTRAINDICATIONS

Malignancy, demyelinating disorders, infections, tuberculosis, hypersensitivity to drug/class, no live vaccines

▨ PREGNANCY CLASS

B

ADAPALENE

(Differin® 0.1% gel in 45 g tubes, solution in 30 mL bottles, 60 pledgets per box, cream in 45 g tubes)

▨ INDICATIONS

- Acne* (see pg. 347), with clindamycin lotion*
- Actinic keratoses^ (see pg. 348)
- Darier's disease+ (see pg. 359)
- Dowling-Degos disease+
- Melasma$
- Solar lentigines^

▨ MECHANISM OF ACTION

Third-generation retinoid that binds to RAR receptor to modulate cellular differentiation, keratinization, and inflammation. May normalize the differentiation of follicular epithelial cells, resulting in decreased microcomedone formation.

▨ DOSAGE

Use small amount qhs.

▨ DRUG INTERACTIONS

None

■ SIDE EFFECTS

COMMON: erythema, scaling, dryness, pruritus, burning, and acne flaring at
treated sites

RARE: none

■ MONITORING

None

■ CONTRAINDICATIONS

Hypersensitivity to drug/class, pregnancy, use of other topical products containing sulfur or alcohols, which can dry the skin

■ PREGNANCY CLASS

C

ALBENDAZOLE

(Albenza® 200 mg tab)

■ INDICATIONS

- Hydatid disease (larval form of *Echinococcus granulosus*)*
- Nematodes (*Ascaris lumbricoides, Capillaria philippinensis, Enterobius
  vermicularis, Necator americanus, Ancylostoma duodenale, Tricho-
  strongylus orientalis, Trichuris trichura, Ancylostoma braziliensis,
  Wuchereria bancrofti, Brugia malayi* and *timori, Mansonella perstans,
  Toxocara, Trichinella spiralis*)§
- Neurocysticercosis (larval form of *Taenia solium*)*
- Protozoa (*Giardia lamblia, Microspora*)§
- Trematodes (*Clonorchis sinensis*)§

■ MECHANISM OF ACTION

Inhibition of tubulin polymerization, which results in loss of cytoplasmic microtubules.

■ DOSAGE

NEUROCYSTICERCOSIS
   ≥60 kg: 400 mg PO bid with meals for 8–30 days
   <60 kg: 15 mg/kg/d divided bid with meals for 8–30 days

HYDATID DISEASE
   ≥60 kg: 400 mg PO bid with meals for 28 day cycle, followed by 14 days free of albendazole, for total of 3 cycles
   <60 kg: 15 mg/kg/d divided bid with meals for 28 day cycle, followed by 14 days free of albendazole, for total of 3 cycles

ASCARIS LUMBRICOIDES: 400 mg PO one time

CAPILLARIA PHILIPPINENSIS: 200 mg PO bid for 20 days

ENTEROBIUS VERMICULARIS: 400 mg PO one time, repeat in 2 weeks

NECATOR AMERICANUS: 400 mg PO one time

ANCYLOSTOMA DUODENALE: 400 mg PO one time

TRICHOSTRONGYLUS ORIENTALIS: 400 mg PO one time

TRICHURIS TRICHURA: 400 mg PO one time

ANCYLOSTOMA BRAZILIENSIS: 200 mg PO bid for 3 days

WUCHERERIA BANCROFTI: 400 mg PO one time

MANSONELLA PERSTANS: 400 mg PO bid for 10 days

TOXOCARA: 400 mg PO bid for 5 days

TRICHINELLA SPIRALIS: 400 mg PO bid for 14 days

BRUGIA MALAYI AND TIMORI: 400 mg PO one time

CLONORCHIS SINENSIS: 10 mg/kg/d for 7 days

GIARDIA LAMBLIA: 400 mg PO qd for 5 days

MICROSPORA: 400 mg PO bid for 3 weeks

DRUG INTERACTIONS

INCREASED LEVELS OF ALBENDAZOLE: dexamethasone, cimetidine, praziquantel

MAY INCREASE LEVELS OF: theophylline

SIDE EFFECTS

COMMON: abnormal liver function, abdominal pain, nausea, vomiting, headache, alopecia, fever, raised intracranial pressure and meningeal signs (in hydatid disease only), dizziness, headache

RARE: leukopenia, pancytopenia, thrombocytopenia, rash, urticaria, acute renal failure

MONITORING

BASELINE: complete blood count, liver function tests

EVERY 2 WEEKS WHILE RECEIVING ALBENDAZOLE: complete blood count, liver function tests

CONTRAINDICATIONS

Hypersensitivity to drug/class, pregnancy

PREGNANCY CLASS

C

ALEFACEPT

(Amevive® 15 mg vials for IM)

▨ INDICATIONS

- Psoriasis, moderate to severe chronic plaque-stage* (see pg. 392)

▨ MECHANISM OF ACTION

Recombinant human dimeric fusion protein composed of the binding portion of LFA3 linked to the Fc portion of IgG1. It binds to the CD2 molecule of the T cell and inhibits co-stimulatory signals. It also causes apoptosis of memory (CD45RO) T cells.

▨ DOSAGE

15 mg IM every week for 12 weeks (further courses optional)

▨ DRUG INTERACTIONS

INCREASED INFECTION/IMMUNOSUPPRESSION: immunosuppressant therapies

▨ SIDE EFFECTS

COMMON: injection site reactions, fever, chills, cough, nausea, pruritus, myalgia, headache, pharyngitis, dizziness

RARE: lymphopenia, malignancy, infection, hypersensitivity reaction with antibody formation/anaphylaxis, elevated liver function test results, cardiovascular events/myocardial infarction, anaphylaxis, angioedema, severe infections

▨ MONITORING

BASELINE: CD4 T lymphocyte levels should be >250 cells/mm³

EVERY WEEK PRIOR TO TREATMENT: CD4 T lymphocyte levels should be >250 cells/mm³ (if CD4 < 250 cells/mm³, hold treatment for that week and recheck next week; if CD4 < 250 cells/mm³ continuously for 1 month, discontinue treatment permanently)

CONTRAINDICATIONS

Hypersensitivity to drug/class, malignancy, infection, CD4 < 250 cells/mm³, no live vaccines

PREGNANCY CLASS

B

ALITRETINOIN

(Panretin® 0.1% gel in 60 g tubes)

INDICATIONS

- Cutaneous T-cell lymphoma$ (see pg. 358)
- Kaposi's sarcoma* (see pg. 370)
- Pyogenic granuloma+

MECHANISM OF ACTION

Binds and activates all known intracellular retinoid receptor subtypes (retinoid X receptors more than retinoid A receptors). When activated, it functions as a transcription factor that regulates expression of genes that control cellular differentiation and proliferation.

DOSAGE

Apply topically bid up to qid.

DRUG INTERACTIONS

INCREASED LEVELS OF: DEET (*N,N*-diethyl-*m*-toluamide), (component in some insect repellents)

SIDE EFFECTS

COMMON: erythema, burning pain, exfoliation, pruritus, rash

RARE: edema, paresthesias

MONITORING

None

CONTRAINDICATIONS

Pregnancy, hypersensitivity to drug/class

PREGNANCY CLASS

D

ALUMINUM CHLORIDE

(Drysol® 20% solution in 35 and 60 mL bottles; Certain-Dri® 12% solution/roll-on [pads over the counter]; Xerac AC® 6.25% solution in 35 and 60 mL bottles)

INDICATIONS

- Acne vulgaris^ (see pg. 347)
- Epidermolysis bullosa+ (see pg. 362)
- Hemostasis*
- Hyperhidrosis*
- Prevention of foot blisters when walking great distances^

MECHANISM OF ACTION

Reversibly inhibits eccrine gland secretion; however, the exact mechanism is unknown.

▓ DOSAGE

HYPERHIDROSIS: daily application at bedtime to dry skin; then occluded if needed

HEMOSTASIS: one application immediately after shave biopsy/minor procedure

EPIDERMOLYSIS BULLOSA: apply 20% solution bid

▓ DRUG INTERACTIONS

None

▓ SIDE EFFECTS

COMMON: irritant dermatitis, burning sensation, pruritus

RARE: none

▓ MONITORING

None

▓ CONTRAINDICATIONS

No electric cautery immediately after use because the solution is flammable, not to be applied to irritated skin, hypersensitivity to drug/class

▓ PREGNANCY CLASS

Not applicable, since it is not an FDA-approved drug. It is not absorbed systemically.

AMINOGLYCOSIDES

Amikacin (Amikin® IV), gentamicin (Garamycin®, Cidomycin®, Genta-mytrex® IV), tobramycin (Nebcin®, TOBI® IV)

■ INDICATIONS

See Appendix II.

- *Acinetobacter baumannii* (amikacin*)
- *Actinomyces* sp. (gentamicin*)
- *Brucella* sp. (gentamicin*)
- *Calymmobacterium* sp. (gentamicin*)
- *Campylobacter* sp. (gentamicin*)
- *Citrobacter* sp. (tobramycin*, gentamicin*)
- *Enterobacter cloaca**
- *Escherichia coli**
- *Francisella* sp. (gentamicin*)
- *Klebsiella pneumoniae**
- *Listeria* sp. (gentamicin*)
- *Proteus vulgaris**
- *Providentia stuartii**
- *Pseudomonas aeruginosa**
- *Serratia marcescens**
- *Staphylococcus aureus*, methicillin-sensitive (tobramycin*, gentamicin*)
- *Staphylococcus epidermidis* (gentamicin*)
- *Vibrio* sp. (gentamicin*)
- *Yersinia* sp. (gentamicin*)

Usually effective:

- *Haemophilus influenzae*
- *Moraxella catarrhalis*
- *Mycobacterium avium* (amikacin)
- *Shigella* sp.
- *Yersenia enterocolitica* (amikacin, tobramycin)

Clinical trials lacking:

- *Staphylococcus epidermidis* (amikacin, tobramycin)
- *Vibrio vulnificus* (amikacin, tobramycin)

■ MECHANISM OF ACTION

They are bactericidal agents that bind to the 30S bacterial ribosomal subunit to inhibit protein synthesis.

■ DOSAGE

GENTAMICIN

1–1.7 mg/kg IM/IV q8h (peak 5–10 µg/mL; trough <2 µg/mL)

RENAL DOSING
   Creatinine clearance (CrCl) 50–90 mL/min: 60–90% q12h
   CrCl 10–50 mL/min: 30–70% q12h
   CrCl <10 mL/min: 20–30% q24–48h
   Hemodialysis: extra $1/2$ of normal dose after dialysis
   Continuous arteriovenous hemofiltration: 30–70% q12h
   Chronic ambulatory peritoneal dialysis (CAPD): 3–4 mg lost/L dialysate qd. (Normally with CAPD dialysis, 2 L of dialysate fluid placed qid or 8 L qd, so 8 × 4 mg = 32 mg of antibiotic supplemented daily.)

AMIKACIN

15 mg/kg IM/IV qd, divide dose q8h–q24h, max of 1.5 g/d (peak <35 µg/mL; trough <10 µg/mL)

RENAL DOSING: same as gentamicin except CAPD dose is 15–20 mg lost/L dialysate qd

TOBRAMYCIN

1–2 mg/kg IM/IV q8h (peak 4–12 µ/mL; trough 0.5–2 µg/mL)

RENAL DOSING: same as gentamicin

■ DRUG INTERACTIONS

INCREASED RISK OF NEPHROTOXICITY: adefovir, aminoglycosides, bisphosphonates, cephalosporins, carboplatin, cidofovir, cisplatin, nephrotoxic agents, tenofovir, vancomycin, lasix, fludarabine, ethacrynic acid

HYPOCALCEMIA: bisphosphonates

INCREASED NEUROMUSCULAR EFFECTS: botulinum toxin, inhaled anesthetics, succinylcholine

DECREASED NEUROMUSCULAR EFFECTS: edrophonium, neostigmine, nondepolarizing neuromuscular blockers, pyridostigmine

OTOTOXICITY: carboplatin, aminoglycosides, cisplatin, loop diuretics

ENHANCED EFFICACY: penicillins

RESPIRATORY DEPRESSION: neuromuscular blockers

ELEVATED LEVELS OF: zalcitabine

■ SIDE EFFECTS

COMMON: nausea, vomiting, pruritus, rash, weakness, tremor, muscle cramps, anorexia, increased salivation, edema, headache, diarrhea, dyspnea, tinnitus, vertigo, elevated blood urea nitrogen/creatinine levels, fever, paresthesias (amikacin), eosinophilia (amikacin), anemia (amikacin), arthralgia (amikacin), hypotension (amikacin)

RARE: nephrotoxicity, ototoxicity, agranulocytosis (not amikacin), thrombocytopenia (not amikacin), neurotoxicity, pseudotumor cerebri (not amikacin), enterocolitis (not amikacin), elevated liver function test results, elevated bilirubin level, decreased calcium/magnesium/sodium/ potassium levels, leukopenia, eosinophilia, anemia, exfoliative dermatitis, Stevens-Johnson syndrome, toxic epidermal necrolysis, urticaria, hypocalcemia, hypomagnesemia, hypokalemia, hyponatremia, elevated renal function test results, confusion, lethargy

■ MONITORING

AFTER 3 DOSES, THEN Q3–4D: peak (draw 30 min after IV infusion or 1 h after IM injection), trough (draw just before giving next dose or 8 h after last dose)

FREQUENTLY: renal function, magnesium, calcium, electrolytes

CONTRAINDICATIONS

Hypersensitivity to drug/class, myasthenia gravis (not amikacin), vestibular/cochlear implants (not amikacin), nephrotoxic agents, impaired renal function, sulfite sensitivity, pregnancy.

PREGNANCY CLASS

D

AMITRIPTYLINE

(Elavil® 10, 25, 50, 75, 100, 150 mg tabs; 10 mg/mL solution for IM injection)

INDICATIONS

- Chronic pain*
- Depression*
- Neuropathic pain^
- Postherpetic neuralgia^ (PHN) (see pg. 389)

MECHANISM OF ACTION

Inhibits serotonin and norepinephrine uptake at the nerve endings.

DOSAGE

POSTHERPETIC NEURALGIA: Start 25 mg PO qhs and titrate to 75 mg PO qhs.

DRUG INTERACTIONS

INCREASED CENTRAL NERVOUS SYSTEM DEPRESSION: opiates, propoxyphene, tramadol, antidepressants, antihistamine ± decongestant, barbiturates, benzodiazepines, carbamazepine, clozapine, alcohol, haloperidol, lithium, loxapine, meperidine, metoclopramide, molindone, olanzapine, phenothiazines, protease inhibitors, quetiapine, risperidone, sedatives, muscle relaxants, thalidomide, thiothixene, ziprasidone

INCREASED ARRHYTHMIAS: class Ia and III antiarrhythmics, carbonic anhydrase inhibitors, cisapride, beta-2 agonists, flumazenil, haloperidol, halothane, mefloquine, quinolones, risperidone, ziprasidone

INCREASED EFFECTS OF AMITRIPTYLINE: bupropion, cimetidine, imatinib, methylphenidate, modafinil, protease inhibitors, selective serotonin reuptake inhibitors, terbinafine

DECREASED EFFECTS OF AMITRIPTYLINE: rifampin

DECREASED EFFICACY OF: alpha-2 agonists, cholinergics, nitrates

INCREASED EFFICACY OF: anticholinergics

INCREASED SEIZURES: bupropion, monoamine oxidase inhibitors, phenytoin

SEROTONIN SYNDROME: linezolid

INCREASED HYPERTENSION: epinephrine, sympathomimetics, reserpine

INCREASED ADVERSE CARDIOVASCULAR EFFECTS: amphetamines

▓ SIDE EFFECTS

COMMON: dry mouth, drowsiness, dizziness, constipation, urinary retention, tachycardia, blurred vision, increased appetite, confusion, disorientation, syncope, fatigue, headache, paresthesias, dysarthria, urticaria, rash, edema, dry mouth, nausea, vomiting, diarrhea, abdominal pain

RARE: seizures, myocardial infarction, stroke, agranulocytosis, thrombocytopenia, heart block, arrhythmias, hypo/hyperthyroidism, photosensitization, paralytic ileus, hepatitis, stomatitis, black tongue, testicular swelling, gynecomastia, purpura, eosinophilia, decreased libido, alopecia, lupuslike syndrome

▓ MONITORING

None

CONTRAINDICATIONS

Hypersensitivity to drug/class, already taking monoamine oxidase inhibitors, acute recovery phase of myocardial infarction. Use with caution in patients with urinary retention, increased intraocular pressure/glaucoma, hyperthyroid, seizures, pregnancy.

PREGNANCY CLASS

C

AMMONIUM LACTATE

(Lac Hydrin® 12% cream 280 g tube, and lotion in 225 g and 400 g bottles; AmLactin® 12% cream in 4.9 oz tube, and lotion in 8 oz and 14 oz bottles, [over the counter])

INDICATIONS

- Ichthyosis* (see pg. 369)
- Nevoid hyperkeratosis of areola+
- Seborrheic keratosis^
- Xerosis* (see pg. 408)

MECHANISM OF ACTION

Binds to stratum corneum and makes it more flexible and less likely to crack. Induces increased thickness of viable epidermis and dermis.

DOSAGE

Apply qd to bid.

DRUG INTERACTIONS

None

▨ SIDE EFFECTS

COMMON: erythema, stinging, burning, peeling, irritation, hyperpigmentation

RARE: none

▨ MONITORING

None

▨ CONTRAINDICATIONS

Hypersensitivity to drug/class, do not apply to abraded/irritated skin, pregnancy

▨ PREGNANCY CLASS

C

AMPHOTERICIN B

(Amphocin® IV; Fungizone® 100 mg/mL IV, PO, can use topically; Abelcet® lipid complex IV injection 100 mg/20 mL and 50 mg/10 mL; AmBisome® liposomal IV injection; Amphotec® cholesteryl complex IV injection)

▨ INDICATIONS

- Aspergillosis*
- Blastomycosis$
- Candidiasis, blood, and endocarditis*
- Candidiasis, peritonitis, and cystitis*
- Coccidioidomycosis, disseminated, and meningitis$
- Cryptococcosis*
- Histoplasmosis^
- Leischmaniasis, visceral*
- Lobomycosis+
- Mucormycosis^
- Neutropenia, febrile with likely fungal infection*
- Paracoccidioidomycosis$
- Penicilliosis$
- Sporotrichosis, disseminated and meningeal$

■ MECHANISM OF ACTION

It binds to fungal cell membranes and then causes a change in permeability, allowing leakage of intracellular components.

■ DOSAGE

See Appendix I.

■ DRUG INTERACTIONS

INCREASED HYPOKALEMIA: angiotensin receptor blockers, angiotensin-converting enzyme inhibitors, beta blockers, hydrochlorothiazide, budesonide, carbonic anhydrase inhibitors, steroids, loop diuretics, flucytosine

INCREASED NEPHROTOXICITY: adefovir, aminoglycosides, carboplatin, cidofovir, cisplatin, zoledronic acid

INCREASED QT PROLONGATION: class III antiarrhythmics, bepridil, cisapride, dolasetron, droperidol, flucytosine, meperidine, phenothiazines, pimozide, quinolones, risperidone, ziprasidone

INCREASED LEVELS OF: digoxin, tenofovir

INCREASED LACTIC ACIDOSIS: metformin, sulfonylureas

■ SIDE EFFECTS

COMMON: chills, fever, hypotension, tachycardia, elevated creatinine/blood urea nitrogen levels, hypertension, nausea, vomiting, hypokalemia, headache, dyspnea, thrombocytopenia, anorexia, diarrhea, dry mouth, generalized pain, rash

RARE: seizures, arrhythmia, asystole, hemorrhagic gastritis, renal failure, agranulocytosis, hepatic dysfunction, anaphylaxis, anemia, infection, hyperbilirubinemia, leukopenia, respiratory failure, chest pain, bronchospasm, wheezing, asthma, myocardial infarction, pulmonary embolus, arrhythmia, cardiomyopathy, hemoptysis, pleural effusion, malaise, weight loss, deafness, injection site reaction, erythema multiforme, hepatitis, jaundice, melena, hepatomegaly, cholangitis, cholecystitis, myasthenia, tinnitus, visual impairment, vertigo, diplopia, cerebral vascular accident, hypomagnesemia, hypocalcemia, anuria, impotence, acidosis, hyperamylasemia, hyperuricemia, hypophosphatemia, hyperglycemia

▨ MONITORING

BASELINE, THEN WEEKLY: liver and renal function, electrolytes, complete
blood count

▨ CONTRAINDICATIONS

Hypersensitivity to drug/class, impaired renal function

▨ PREGNANCY CLASS

B

ANTHRALIN

(Drithocreme® 0.1%, 0.25%, 0.5%, 1.0% cream in 50 g tubes; Dritho-Scalp®
0.25%, 0.5% cream in 50 g tubes; Micanol® 1% cream in 50 g tubes)

▨ INDICATIONS

- Alopecia areata (see pg. 349)$
- Inflammatory Linear Verrucous Epidermal Nevus (ILVEN)+
- Porokeratosis of Mibelli+
- Psoriasis, chronic plague* (see pg. 392)
- Verruca vulgaris^ (see pg. 406)

▨ MECHANISM OF ACTION

Inhibits T lymphocytes and Langerhans cells. Stimulates monocyte proinflammatory activity and induces extracellular generation of oxygen free
radicals.

▨ DOSAGE

Apply qd to bid.
Begin by leaving on for 10–20 min (short contact), increasing weekly to maximum of 1 hour.

DRUG INTERACTIONS

None

SIDE EFFECTS

COMMON: irritation, contact dermatitis, erythema, discoloration of hair and
   nails

RARE: None.

Micanol® is encapsulated in a matrix of semicrystalline monoglycerides,
   which causes fewer side effects.

Cura-Stain® helps with irritation and staining if sprayed on before removing
   anthralin.

MONITORING

None

CONTRAINDICATIONS

Hypersensitivity to drug/class, use on face/genitals, salicylate allergy, impaired renal function, pregnancy

PREGNANCY CLASS

C

ATORVASTATIN

(Lipitor® 10, 20, 40, 80 mg tabs)

INDICATIONS

- Cutaneous T-cell lymphoma$ (works synergistically with bexarotene)
  (see pg. 358)
- Hypercholesterolemia*
- Hypertriglyceridemia*

■ MECHANISM OF ACTION

It inhibits hydroxymethylglutaryl coenzyme A reductase and may modulate class II major histocompatibility complex on T cells.

■ DOSAGE

10–80 mg PO qhs

■ DRUG INTERACTIONS

INCREASED MYOPATHY: amiodarone, azole antifungals, macrolides, cyclosporin, danazol, delavirdine, diltiazem, fibric acid derivatives, fluvoxamine, imatinib, niacin, nefazodone, protease inhibitors, quinupristin/dalfopristin, verapamil

DECREASED EFFICACY OF ATORVASTATIN: aprepitant, bile acid–binding resins, bosentan, rifampins

DECREASED LEVELS OF ATORVASTATIN: efavirenz, griseofulvin

INCREASED LEVELS OF: clopidogrel

ELEVATED LIVER FUNCTION TEST RESULTS: ezetimibe

■ SIDE EFFECTS

COMMON: headache, sinusitis/rhinitis, myalgia, diarrhea, arthralgia, rash, nausea, abdominal pain, flu-like symptoms, dyspepsia, flatulence, constipation, elevated creatine kinase levels, elevated liver function test results

RARE: myopathy, rhabdomyolysis, hepatotoxicity, pancreatitis, hypersensitivity reaction, anaphylaxis, angioedema, lupus-like syndrome, polymyalgia rheumatica, dermatomyositis, vasculitis, thrombocytopenia, leukopenia, hemolytic anemia, photosensitivity, toxic epidermal necrolysis, erythema multiforme, Stevens-Johnson syndrome, infection, asthenia, pharyngitis, chest pain, insomnia, dizziness, tinnitus, palpitations, migraine, ecchymosis, edema, sweating, acne, urticaria, paresthesia, depression, eczema, skin ulcers, anorexia, gastrointestinal ulcers, cholestatic jaundice

▓ MONITORING

BASELINE: fasting lipids, liver function tests, creatine kinase

MONTHLY: fasting lipids, liver function tests

COMPLAINTS OF MYALGIA: creatine kinase

▓ CONTRAINDICATIONS

Hypersensitivity to drug/class, pregnancy, liver disease, lactation, alcohol abuse

▓ PREGNANCY CLASS

X

AZATHIOPRINE

(Imuran® 50 mg tabs)

▓ INDICATIONS

- Atopic dermatitis^ (see pg. 353)
- Behçet's^ syndrome (see pg. 355)
- Bullous pemphigoid^ (showed no significant difference with use of steroids but showed good results$) (see pg. 355)
- Chronic actinic dermatitis^
- Cicatricial pemphigoid^ (see pg. 356)
- Contact dermatitis$ (see pg. 357)
- Dermatomyositis$ (see pg. 361)
- Erythema multiforme$ (see pg. 364)
- Graft-versus-host disease, chronic$ (see pg. 365)
- Inflammatory bowel disease^
- Leukocytoclastic vasculitis$ (see pg. 404)
- Lichen planus+ (see pg. 371)
- Lupus, systemic $(see pg. 375)
- Pemphigus vulgaris$ (see pg. 385)
- Polyarteritis nodosa$ (see pg. 404)
- Polymorphous light eruption+
- Psoriasis$ (see pg. 392)
- Pyoderma gangrenosum+ (see pg. 394)

- Relapsing polychondritis[$]
- Renal allograft rejection[*]
- Rheumatoid arthritis[*]
- Sarcoidosis[$] (see pg. 396)
- Scleroderma[$] (see pg. 398)
- Sjögren's syndrome[$]
- Weber-Christian syndrome[+]
- Wegener's syndrome[$] (see pg. 404)

MECHANISM OF ACTION

Immunosuppressive and anti-inflammatory. Its active metabolite (6-thioguanine) is a purine analog that inhibits DNA and RNA synthesis by inhibiting purine metabolism and cell division. Inhibits T-cell–mediated immune function, decreases antibody production by B cells, and decreases the number of Langerhans cells and antigen presenting cells. It is metabolized by thiopurine methyltransferase (TPMT), xanthine oxidase, and hypoxanthine guanine phosphoribosyltransferase.

DOSAGE

Begin 1 mg/kg/d divided bid, increase by 25 mg every month to maximum dose of 2.5 mg/kg/d. (If TPMT < 5 U, do not give. If TPMT 5–13.7 U, 0.5 mg/kg maximum dose. If TMPT 13.7–19 U, 1.5 mg/kg maximum dose. If TPMT > 19 U, 2.5 mg/kg maximum dose.)

DRUG INTERACTIONS

LEUKOPENIA: angiotensin-converting enzyme inhibitors, hydrochlorothiazides

IMMUNOSUPPRESSION: alefacept

AZATHIOPRINE TOXICITY: allopurinol

BONE MARROW SUPPRESSION: bone marrow suppressants, cytotoxic chemotherapy, clozapine, interferon alpha and beta, mycophenolate mofetil, rituximab, zidovudine, pancuronium

DECREASES INTERNATIONAL NORMALIZATION RATIO (INR): warfarin

INCREASED RISK OF INFECTION: leflunomide

SIDE EFFECTS

COMMON: leukopenia, thrombocytopenia, anemia, nausea, vomiting, diarrhea, malaise, myalgia, fever, rash, infection, elevated liver function test results, anorexia, fever, rash

RARE: myelosuppression, gastrointestinal upset, pancreatitis, hepatotoxicity, hepatic veno-occlusive disease, lymphoma, malignancy, hypersensitivity syndrome

MONITORING

BASELINE: liver function tests, pregnancy test, complete blood counts, serum chemistry, urinalysis, TPMT (if available)

MONTHLY FOR FIRST 3 MONTHS, THEN EVERY 2 MONTHS: Complete blood counts, liver function tests

CONTRAINDICATIONS

Pregnancy, hypersensitivity to drug/class, active infection, allopurinol use, alkylating agent use

PREGNANCY CLASS

D

AZELAIC ACID

(Azelex® 20% cream in 30 and 50 g tubes, Finacea® 15% gel in 30 g tubes)

INDICATIONS

- Acne vulgaris* (see pg. 347)
- Lentigo maligna$
- Melanoma$ (see pg. 378)
- Melasma^
- Reticulated acropigmentation of Kitamura[+]
- Rosacea^ (see pg. 395)

■ MECHANISM OF ACTION

Antimicrobial. Normalization of keratinization, leading to anti-comedonal effects. Reduction in thickness of stratum corneum, keratohyaline granules, and filaggrin, leading to decreased microcomedone formation.

■ DOSAGE

Apply bid. May need to start qd first if irritation develops.

■ DRUG INTERACTIONS

None

■ SIDE EFFECTS

COMMON: pruritus, burning, stinging, tingling, erythema, peeling, irritation, dermatitis

RARE: asthma exacerbation, vitiligo, hypertrichosis, keratosis pilaris, recurrent herpes labialis

■ MONITORING

None

■ CONTRAINDICATIONS

Hypersensitivity to propylene glycol or drug/class. Not well studied in darkly pigmented patients.

■ PREGNANCY CLASS

B

AZTREONAM

(Azactam® IV)

▓ INDICATIONS

- *Citrobacter freundii**
- *Enterobacter cloacae**
- *Escherichia coli**
- *Haemophilus influenzae**
- *Klebsiella pneumoniae* and *oxytoca**
- *Proteus mirabilis**
- *Pseudomonas aeruginosa**
- *Serratia marcescens**

See Appendix II.

Usually effective:

- *Aeromonas* sp.
- *Haemophilus ducreyi*
- *Moraxella catarrhalis*
- *Morganella* sp.
- *Neisseria gonorrhoeae*
- *Neisseria meningitidis*
- *Proteus vulgaris*
- *Providencia* sp.
- *Shigella* sp.
- *Yersinia enterocolitica*

▓ MECHANISM OF ACTION

It is a bacteriocidal agent that inhibits bacterial cell wall synthesis.

▓ DOSAGE

0.5–2 g IV/IM q6–12h

RENAL DOSING
  Creatinine clearance (CrCl) 50–90 mL/min and continuous arteriovenous hemofiltration: 50–75% of normal dose
  CrCl < 10 mL/min and chronic ambulatory peritoneal dialysis: 25% of normal dose
  Hemodialysis: extra 0.5 g IV after dialysis

■ DRUG INTERACTIONS

None

■ SIDE EFFECTS

COMMON: phlebitis, injection site reactions, diarrhea, nausea, vomiting, rash

RARE: pseudomembranous colitis, seizures, eosinophilia, anaphylaxis, elevated liver function test results, pancytopenia, angioedema, hepatitis, jaundice, hypotension, dyspnea, chest pain, neutropenia, thrombocytopenia, anemia, seizure, confusion, vertigo, myalgias, tinnitus, erythema multiforme, toxic epidermal necrolysis, urticaria, pruritus, vaginitis, headache, fever, malaise, nasal congestion, oral ulcers, halitosis, numb tongue, diplopia, insomnia

■ MONITORING

None

■ CONTRAINDICATIONS

Hypersensitivity to drug/class, impaired renal function, allergy to penicillins, allergy to ceftazidime

■ PREGNANCY CLASS

B

BACITRACIN, TOPICAL

(500 U/g in 1, 15, 30 g tubes; [over the counter])

BACITRACIN, NEOMYCIN, AND POLYMYXIN

(Neosporin® ointment in 15, 30 g tubes; cream in 15 tubes; with bacitracin 400 U/g, neomycin 35 mg/g, and polymyxin 5,000 U/g; [over the counter])

BACITRACIN AND POLYMYXIN

(Polysporin® ointment in 15 and 30 g tubes; powder in 10 g tubes; with bacitracin 500 U/g and polymyxin 10,000 U/g; [over the counter])

▓ INDICATIONS

- Burns$^{\$}$
- Skin bacterial infections* (Bacitracin and neomycin provide good gram-positive bacteria coverage, and polymyxin provides good gram-negative bacteria coverage.)
- Wound healing^ (see pg. 407)

▓ MECHANISM OF ACTION

BACITRACIN

Bacteriocidal agent that inhibits bacterial cell wall synthesis by binding to C55 prenol pyrophosphate carrier protein, which transfers polysaccharides, liposaccharides, and peptidoglycans.

POLYMYXIN

Bacteriocidal agent that increases permeability of bacterial cell walls.

NEOMYCIN

Bacteriocidal agent that inhibits protein synthesis by binding to 30S bacterial ribosomal subunit (aminoglycoside).

▓ DOSAGE

Apply qd to tid.

▓ DRUG INTERACTIONS

None

▓ SIDE EFFECTS (FOR BACITRACIN UNLESS OTHERWISE INDICATED)

COMMON: contact dermatitis, erythema, burning, pruritus, rash, sensitizer in ulcers

RARE: superinfection, anaphylaxis, acute renal failure (polymyxin), ototoxicity (neomycin), nephrotoxicity (neomycin)

▓ MONITORING

None

▓ CONTRAINDICATIONS

Hypersensitivity to drug/class, myasthenia gravis, large wounds, pregnancy

▓ PREGNANCY CLASS

C

BECAPLERMIN

(Regranex® 0.01% gel in 15 g tubes)

▓ INDICATIONS

- Chronic ulcers[$]
- Diabetic neuropathic ulcers[*]
- Hemangioma, ulcerated[+]
- Lichen planus, ulcerated[+] (see pg. 371)
- Necrobiosis lipoidica diabeticorum[^] (see pg. 381)
- Periodontal regeneration[^]
- Post-surgical abdominal wound separation[^]
- Pressure ulcers[^]
- Pyoderma gangrenosum[+] (see pg. 394)
- Scleroderma, ulcers[$] (see pg. 398)

▓ MECHANISM OF ACTION

Recombinant platelet-derived growth factor, which promotes chemotactic recruitment and proliferation of cells for wound repair and granulation tissue formation.

▓ DOSAGE

After debridement, apply thin, continuous $\frac{1}{16}$ inch thick layer qd. Remove in 12 h.

DRUG INTERACTIONS

None

SIDE EFFECTS

Rash

MONITORING

None

CONTRAINDICATIONS

Hypersensitivity to drug/class, neoplasm at treatment site, pregnancy

PREGNANCY CLASS

C

BENZOYL PEROXIDE

(Benzac AC® 2.5%, 5%, 10% gel in 60 and 80 g tubes, and wash in 8 oz bottles; Brevoxyl® 4%, 8% cleansing lotion in 10.5 oz bottles, wash in 6 oz bottles, and gel in 42.5 and 90 g tubes; Triaz® 3%, 6%, 10% cleanser in 6 and 12 oz bottles and gel in 42.5 g tubes; Benzagel® 5%, 10% gel in 42.5 and 85 g tubes; PanOxyl® 5%, 10% gel in 56.7 and 113.4 g tubes; PanOxyl AQ® 2.5%, 5%, 10% gel in 56.7 and 113.4 g tubes)

BENZOYL PEROXIDE AND CLINDAMYCIN

(Duac®, see pg. 86)
(Benzaclin®, see pg. 86)

■ INDICATIONS

- Acne vulgaris* (see pg. 347)
- Acute Mohs surgical wounds+
- Acute surgical wounds^
- Decubitus ulcers+
- Electrical burn on scalp+
- Fox-Fordyce disease+
- Leg ulcers$
- Necrobiosis lipoidica diabeticorum ulcers+ (see pg. 381)
- Pyoderma gangrenosum+ (see pg. 394)
- Rosacea, with clindamycin gel^ (see pg. 395)
- Seborrheic dermatitis^ (see pg. 399)
- Tinea versicolor$

■ MECHANISM OF ACTION

It is an oxidizing agent that possess antibacterial properties (especially against *Propionibacterium acnes*) and acts as a comedolytic and keratolytic agent. Its use results in a decrease of free fatty acids and lipids in the treated skin.

■ DOSAGE

Apply qd to bid.

■ DRUG INTERACTIONS

Use with isotretinoin and tretinoin may increase dryness of skin, and topical tretinoin neutralizes benzoyl peroxide unless specially formulated.

■ SIDE EFFECTS

COMMON: bleach hair/fabric/skin, contact dermatitis, dryness, erythema, peeling

RARE: none

■ MONITORING

None

▩ CONTRAINDICATIONS

Hypersensitivity to drug/class, pregnancy

▩ PREGNANCY CLASS

C

BEXAROTENE

(Targretin® 75 mg tab, 1% gel in 60 g tubes)

▩ INDICATIONS

- CD30+ large-cell lymphoma[+]
- Cutaneous T-cell lymphoma* (gel only for stages Ia and Ib*, 2a[$]), may give with bath psoralens and ultraviolet A light qiw[+] (see pg. 358)
- Hand dermatitis[^]
- Lymphomatoid papulosis[$] (see pg. 377)
- Metastatic breast carcinoma[$]
- Non–small cell lung carcinoma[$]
- Parapsoriasis[$] (see pg. 383)
- Renal cell carcinoma[$]

▩ MECHANISM OF ACTION

Selectively binds and activates retinoid X receptors, which function as transcription factors to regulate gene expression and control cellular differentiation and proliferation.

▩ DOSAGE

GEL: Begin once a day every other day for first week, then every day for one week, increasing every week up to maximum dose of qid.

ORAL: Begin 300 mg/m^2/d, may increase to maximum of 400 mg/m^2/d after 8 weeks of nonresponse.

▓ DRUG INTERACTIONS (ORAL)

INCREASED LEVELS OF: diethyltoluamide (DEET; insect repellent)

INCREASED DRUG LEVELS OF BEXAROTENE: ketoconazole, itraconazole, erythromycin, gemfibrozil, grapefruit juice, inhibitors of cytochrome P450 3A4

DECREASED DRUG LEVELS OF BEXAROTENE: rifampin, phenytoin, phenobarbital, inducers of cytochrome P450 3A4

▓ SIDE EFFECTS

GEL

COMMON: rash, pruritus, pain, contact dermatitis

RARE: none

ORAL

COMMON: hypertriglyceridemia, hypercholesterolemia, central hypothyroidism, headache, asthenia, rash, nausea, diarrhea, infection, edema, abdominal pain, dry skin, fatigue, constipation, cheilitis

RARE: hepatitis, pancreatitis, photosensitivity, leukopenia, muscle spasm, anemia, pneumonia, confusion, subdural hematoma, liver failure, chills, chest pain, candida, hypertension, angina, syncope, hypoproteinemia, hyperglycemia, change in weight, arthralgia, myalgia, bone pain, depression, agitation, ataxia, neuropathy, pharyngitis, rhinitis, dyspnea, cough, hypoxia, acne, alopecia, dry eyes, visual field defects, keratitis, otitis externa, hematuria, urinary incontinence, dysuria, breast pain

▓ MONITORING

GEL

None

ORAL

BASELINE: serum pregnancy test, complete blood count, liver function tests, fasting lipid profile, renal function, thyroid-stimulating hormone, thyroxine, urinalysis (if renal disease, diabetes, proteinuria, hypertension), eye exam (if history of cataracts)

EVERY 1–2 WEEKS FOR 2–4 WEEKS, THEN MONTHLY FOR FIRST 3–6 MONTHS, THEN EVERY 3 MONTHS: fasting lipid profile

MONTHLY FOR FIRST 3–6 MONTHS, THEN EVERY 3 MONTHS: complete blood count, liver function, renal function, thyroid-stimulating hormone, thyroxine

MONTHLY: serum pregnancy test

PERIODICALLY: eye exam if history of abnormal ocular findings

CONTRAINDICATIONS

Pregnancy, hypersensitivity to drug/class, vitamin A supplementation, diabetics on insulin, gemfibrozil

PREGNANCY CLASS

X

BLEOMYCIN

(Blenoxane® 0.1% solution)

INDICATIONS

- Head and neck squamous cell carcinoma*
- Hodgkin's and non-Hodgkin's lymphoma*
- Testicular carcinoma*
- Verruca vulgaris^ (see pg. 406)

MECHANISM OF ACTION

Inhibits DNA synthesis by binding to it and causing single-strand breakage, leading to keratinocyte apoptosis and necrosis.

▨ DOSAGE (IL)

VERRUCA VULGARIS: 0.1 mL of 1 U/mL solution intralesional (IL) to each wart for total of 2 mL per treatment every 2–3 weeks (may require nerve block or topical anesthetics prior to treatment and ice water soaks post-injection)

▪ DRUG INTERACTIONS (IL)

None

▨ SIDE EFFECTS (IL)

COMMON: local pain, burning, erythema, swelling, eschar formation, Raynaud's phenomenon of the fingers, nail dystrophy

RARE: none

▨ MONITORING (IL)

None

▨ CONTRAINDICATIONS

Pregnancy, immunosuppression, vascular compromise, hypersensitivity to drug/class, history of Raynaud's phenomenon

▨ PREGNANCY CLASS

D

BUTENAFINE

(Mentax® 1% cream in 15 and 30 g tubes)

▨ INDICATIONS

- Tinea*

MECHANISM OF ACTION

It is fungistatic and fungicidal. It inhibits squalene epoxidase for ergosterol biosynthesis.

DOSAGE

TINEA PEDIS: Apply bid for 7 days or qd for 4 weeks.

TINEA: Apply qd for 14 days.

DRUG INTERACTIONS

None

SIDE EFFECTS

COMMON: burning, pruritus, erythema

RARE: irritation, contact dermatitis, stinging

MONITORING

None

CONTRAINDICATIONS

Hypersensitivity to drug/class, hypersensitivity to terbinafine

PREGNANCY CLASS

B

CADEXOMER IODINE

(Iodosorb® gel with 0.9% iodine in 10 and 20 g tubes; Iodosorb® powder with 0.9% iodine in 3 g sachet, 7 sachets per carton; Iodoflex® 0.9% paste in gauze backing in box of 5 pads each with 5 g in 6 × 4 size, box of 3 each with 10 g in 8 × 6 size, box of 2 each with 17 g in 10 × 8 size [each 1 g has 600 mg of cadexomer iodine])

■ INDICATIONS

- Decubitus ulcers*
- Infected traumatic and surgical wounds*
- Venous ulcers*
- Exudative ulcers*

■ MECHANISM OF ACTION

As cadexomer polymer beads absorb wound exudates, the pores of each bead swell and slowly release iodine, which is bacteriostatic and bacteriocidal.

■ DOSAGE

IODOSORB®: Use 3 times a week, ⅛ inch thick evenly spread over wound. May need to change more frequently, when brown color changes to yellow-gray. Do not use for more than 3 consecutive months per treatment cycle.

IODOFLEX®: Use 2–3 times a week depending on amount of exudates from the wound. Change when color changes from brown to yellow-gray. Do not use more than 50 g per application or more than 150 g per week. Do not use for more than 3 months per treatment cycle.

■ DRUG INTERACTIONS

INCREASES RISK OF HYPOTHYROIDISM: lithium

INCREASES RISK OF METABOLIC ACIDOSIS: taurolidine

CROSS REACTS WITH: mercurial antiseptics

SIDE EFFECTS

Pain, irritation, erythema, dermatitis, allergy, elevated thyroid-stimulating hormone (TSH) levels

MONITORING

BASELINE: TSH if thyroid disease is suspected

CONTRAINDICATIONS

Hashimoto's thyroiditis, Graves' disease, nontoxic nodular goiter, pregnancy, iodine allergy, children, lactation, renal disease, hypersensitivity to drug/class

PREGNANCY CLASS

Since it was FDA approved as a device and not a medication, it was not given a pregnancy class. However, it does cause thyroid problems in the fetus of women treated during pregnancy.

CALCIPOTRIENE

(Dovonex® 0.005% cream in 60 and 120 g tubes, ointment in 60 and 120 g tubes, solution in 60 mL bottles)

INDICATIONS

- Acanthosis nigricans[+] (see pg. 347)
- Acrodermatitis of Hallopeau[+]
- Confluent and reticulated papillomatosis of Gougerot and Carteaud[+]
- Congenital ichthyosis[^] (see pg. 369)
- Cutaneous T-cell lymphoma[+] (see pg. 358)
- Disseminated superficial actinic porokeratosis[+]
- Dyshidrotic dermatitis[+]
- Erythema annulare centrifugum[+]
- Grover's disease[+] (see pg. 366)
- Inflammatory linear verrucous epidermal nevus[+]
- Keratosis lichenoides chronica[+]

- Lichen planus$^{\$}$ (see pg. 371)
- Lichen sclerosus et atrophicus^{+} (see pg. 372)
- Morphea$^{\$}$ (see pg. 381)
- Nevoid hyperkeratosis of the areola^{+}
- Oral leukoplakia$^{\wedge}$
- Pityriasis rubra pilaris^{+} (see pg. 387)
- Prurigo nodularis$^{\wedge}$
- Psoriasis with Diprolene® ointment* (see pg. 392)
- Seborrheic dermatitis$^{\wedge}$ (see pg. 399)
- Sjögren-Larsson keratoderma$^{\$}$
- Vitiligo$^{\wedge}$, with narrow-band ultraviolet B^{+} (see pg. 405)
- X-linked ichthyosis$^{\wedge}$ (see pg. 369)

MECHANISM OF ACTION

It is a vitamin D analog that acts via vitamin D receptors to regulate growth, differentiation, and immune function by binding to specific DNA binding sites (vitamin D response elements) to regulate genes.

DOSAGE

Apply bid.

DRUG INTERACTIONS

None

SIDE EFFECTS

COMMON: irritation, photosensitivity, contact dermatitis, pruritus, worsening of psoriasis, burning, rash, erythema, dry skin

RARE: hypercalcemia, atrophy

MONITORING

None

CONTRAINDICATIONS

Hypersensitivity to drug/class, hypercalcemia, vitamin D toxicity, pregnancy. Should not be used on the face or intertriginous areas.

PREGNANCY CLASS

C

CANTHARIDIN

(Canthacur® 0.7% solution in 7.5 mL bottles; Canthacur PS® 0.7% solution with podophyllin 2% and salicylic acid 30% in 7.5 mL bottles)

INDICATIONS

- Molluscum contagiosum[$] (see pg. 380)
- Verruca vulgaris[$] (see pg. 406)

MECHANISM OF ACTION

It is a vesicant and also interferes with mitochondrial function, leading to cell death and resultant blister formation. It is derived from *Lytta vesicatoria*, the blister beetle.

DOSAGE

Small amount is applied to the lesion with the wooden end of an applicator stick or toothpick. It may be occluded for 24 h. It may be washed off in 4–6 hours. Blisters may take up to 2 days to form and 1 week to resolve.

DRUG INTERACTIONS

None

■ SIDE EFFECTS

COMMON: blister, pain, erythema, irritation, small satellite warts around the blister, hypo-/hyperpigmentation

RARE: scarring

■ MONITORING

None

■ CONTRAINDICATIONS

Hypersensitivity to drug/class, ingestion results in poisoning

■ PREGNANCY CLASS

Not applicable

CAPSAICIN

(Zostrix® 0.025% cream in 45 g tubes, 0.075% cream in 45 g tubes)

■ INDICATIONS

- Apocrine chromhidrosis[+]
- Burning pain[^]
- Diabetic neuropathy[*]
- Erythromelalgia[+]
- Notalgia paresthetica[^]
- Pain due to tumor infiltration[+]
- Pain from rheumatoid arthritis and osteoarthritis[^]
- Postherpetic neuralgia[^] (see pg. 389)
- Postmastectomy pain[^]
- Prurigo nodularis[$]
- Pruritus of psoriasis[^] (see pg. 392)
- Psoralen ultraviolet A–induced pain[+]
- Reflex sympathetic dystrophy[^]

- Stump pain[+]
- Vulvar vestibulitis[§]

MECHANISM OF ACTION

It stimulates release of substance P from sensory nerve endings, but with prolonged use it depletes substance P, which inhibits pain sensation. It selectively excites unmyelinated peripheral afferent C fibers.

DOSAGE

Apply tid to qid. Wash hands immediately and thoroughly after use.

DRUG INTERACTIONS

None

SIDE EFFECTS

COMMON: burning, erythema, thermal hyperalgesia

RARE: neurotoxicity

MONITORING

None

CONTRAINDICATIONS

Hypersensitivity to drug/class, broken skin, noncompliance

PREGNANCY CLASS

Not applicable

CARBAPENEMS

Imipenem/cilastatin (Primaxin® IV/IM); meropenem (Merrem® IV)

▓ INDICATIONS

- *Acinetobacter calcoaceticus* (imipenem)*
- *Bacteroides fragilis, B. distasonis* (imipenem), *B. intermedius* (imipenem), *B. thetaiotaomicron**
- *Citrobacter* sp. (imipenem)*
- *Enterobacter* sp. (imipenem)*
- *Enterococcus faecalis**
- *Escherichia coli**
- *Fusobacterium* sp. (imipenem)*
- *Haemophilus influenzae**
- *Klebsiella pneumoniae**
- *Morganella* sp. (imipenem)*
- *Neisseria meningitidis* (meropenem)*
- *Peptostreptococcus* sp.*
- *Pseudomonas aeruginosa**
- *Staphylococcus aureus,* methicillin sensitive*
- *Streptococcus pneumoniae**
- *Streptococcus viridans**

See Appendix II.

Usually effective:

- *Acinetobacter* sp. (meropenem)
- *Actinomyces* sp. (imipenem)
- *Aeromonas* sp.
- *Burkholderia cepacia* (meropenem)
- *Citrobacter* sp. (meropenem)
- *Clostridium difficile* and others
- *Enterobacter* sp. (meropenem)
- *Enterococcus faecalis* (imipenem)
- *Listeria monocytogenes*
- *Moraxella catarrhalis*
- *Morganella* sp. (meropenem)
- *Neisseria gonorrhoeae*
- *Prevotella melaninogenica*
- *Proteus mirabilis* and *vulgaris*
- *Providentia* sp.
- *Salmonella* sp.
- *Serratia* sp.

- *Shigella* sp.
- *Staphylococcus epidermidis*
- *Streptococcus milleri*
- *Yersenia enterocolitica* (imipenem)

Clinical trials lacking:

- *Enterococcus faecalis* (meropenem)
- *Enterococcus faecium* (imipenem)

▦ MECHANISM OF ACTION

They are bactericidal agents that inhibit cell wall synthesis.

▦ DOSAGE

IMIPENEM

500–750 mg IM q12h; 250–1000 mg IV q6–8h (maximum of 50 mg/kg/d or 4 g/d)

RENAL DOSING
   Creatinine clearance (CrCL) 50–90 mL/min: 250–500 mg IV q6h
   CrCl 10–50 mL/min and continuous arteriovenous hemofiltration: 250 mg IV q6–12h
   CrCL < 10 mL/min and chronic peritoneal dialysis: 125–250 mg IV q12h
   Hemodialysis: dose after dialysis

MEROPENEM

1 g IV q8h

RENAL DOSING
   CrCl 50–90 mL/min: 1 g IV q8h
   CrCl 10–50 mL/min and continuous arteriovenous hemofiltration: 1 g IV q12h
   CrCl < 10 mL/min and chronic peritoneal dialysis: 500 mg IV q24h
   Hemodialysis: dose after dialysis

▦ DRUG INTERACTIONS

INCREASED SEIZURES: ganciclovir (imipenem)

INCREASED LEVELS OF CARBAPENEMS: probenecid (meropenem)

▨ SIDE EFFECTS

COMMON: thrombocytosis, diarrhea, rash, phlebitis, oliguria, tachycardia, oral candidiasis, injection site reactions, urine discoloration (imipenem), gastroenteritis, nausea, vomiting, elevated blood urea nitrogen/creatinine, vaginitis

RARE: anaphylaxis, seizures (both), agranulocytosis, pseudomembranous colitis, hypotension, urticaria, pruritus, somnolence, dizziness, hemorrhagic colitis (imipenem), jaundice (imipenem), hepatitis (imipenem), glossitis (imipenem), confusion, tremor, hemolytic anemia, hearing loss, tinnitus, dyspnea, palpitations, Stevens-Johnson syndrome (imipenem), erythema multiforme (imipenem), toxic epidermal necrolysis (imipenem), hyperhidrosis (imipenem), cyanosis, flushing, arthralgia, hyponatremia (imipenem), hyperkalemia (imipenem), eosinophilia, proteinuria, pulmonary embolism (meropenem), myocardial infarction (meropenem), congestive heart failure (meropenem), bradycardia (meropenem), hallucinations (meropenem), vertigo, insomnia, urticaria, sweating, confusion, jaundice, hepatic failure, dysuria, hypokalemia, anemia, thrombocytosis, elevated liver function test results, elevated renal function test results, eosinophilia

▨ MONITORING

FREQUENTLY IF LONG-TERM USE: complete blood count, renal function, liver function

▨ CONTRAINDICATIONS

Hypersensitivity to drug/class, impaired renal function, seizures, cephalosporin allergy, pregnancy (imipenem)

▨ PREGNANCY CLASS

C (imipenem), B (meropenem)

CARMUSTINE, TOPICAL

(BCNU® 100 mg in each vial)

▓ INDICATIONS

- Cutaneous T-cell lymphoma[$] (see pg. 358)
- Lymphomatoid papulosis[$] (see pg. 377)
- Parapsoriasis en plaques[+] (see pg. 383)

▓ MECHANISM OF ACTION

It alkylates DNA and RNA which inhibits replication. It is a nitrosourea that inhibits key enzymes in the carbamoylation of amino acids in proteins.

▓ DOSAGE

TOPICAL SOLUTION: 100 mg in 50 mL of 95% ethanol, then mixed with tap water. May use 5 mL of solution with 60 mL of tap water. Apply qd.

TOPICAL OINTMENT: 100 mg in 50 mL of 95% ethanol, then mixed with white petrolatum. May use 20–40 mg of carmustine in 100 g of white petrolatum. Apply qd.

▓ DRUG INTERACTIONS

None

▓ SIDE EFFECTS

COMMON: erythema, pruritus, irritant or contact dermatitis, burning, hyperpigmentation

RARE: telangiectasias, leukopenia

▓ MONITORING

BASELINE AND MONTHLY: complete blood count

CONTRAINDICATIONS

Hypersensitivity to drug or class, pregnancy

PREGNANCY CLASS

D

CASPOFUNGIN

(Cancidas® IV)

INDICATIONS

- Aspergillosis, refractory*
- Candidemia*
- Candidiasis in HIV-positive patients, vaginitis or stomatitis or esophagitis*

MECHANISM OF ACTION

It inhibits synthesis of β-1,3-D-glucan in filamentous fungal cell walls.

DOSAGE

70 mg IV day 1, then 50–70 mg IV qd

HEPATIC DOSING: 70 mg IV day 1, then 35 mg IV qd

DRUG INTERACTIONS

DECREASED LEVELS OF CASPOFUNGIN: carbamazepine, dexamethasone, efavirenz, nevirapine, phenytoin, rifabutin, rifampins

INCREASED LEVELS OF CASPOFUNGIN: cyclosporin

DECREASED LEVELS OF: sirolimus

SIDE EFFECTS

COMMON: fever, infusion site reaction, nausea, vomiting, flushing, headache, chills, diarrhea, anemia, abdominal pain, eosinophilia, hypokalemia, elevated liver function test results

RARE: anaphylaxis, acute respiratory distress syndrome, pulmonary edema, blood dyscrasias, hypercalcemia, hepatotoxicity, tachycardia, vasculitis, anorexia, tremor, paresthesia, insomnia, tachypnea, elevated creatinine, hematuria, proteinuria

MONITORING

PERIODICALLY: renal function, liver function, urinalysis

CONTRAINDICATIONS

Hypersensitivity to drug/class, hepatic dysfunction, pregnancy

PREGNANCY CLASS

C

CEPHALOSPORINS, FIRST GENERATION

Cefadroxil (Duricef® 500 mg caps; 1,000 mg tabs; 125, 250, 500 mg/5 mL suspension); cefazolin (Kefzol® IM/IV, Ancef® IM/IV); cephalexin (Keflex® 250, 500 mg caps; 125, 250 mg/5 mL suspension)

INDICATIONS

- *Enterobacter* sp. (cefazolin*)
- *Enterococcus* sp. (cefazolin*)
- *Escherichia coli**
- *Haemophilus influenzae**
- *Klebsiella* sp.*
- *Moraxella catarrhalis* (cephalexin*)
- *Proteus mirabilis**
- *Staphylococcus aureus*, methicillin sensitive*

- *Staphylococcus epidermidis**
- *Streptococcus pneumoniae**
- *Streptococcus viridans**
- *Streptococcus pyogenes* and others*

See Appendix II.

Usually effective:

- *Neisseria gonorrhoeae* (cefazolin)

MECHANISM OF ACTION

They are bactericidal agents that inhibit cell wall synthesis.

DOSAGE

CEFADROXIL

1–2 g PO qd

RENAL DOSING
Creatinine clearance (CrCl) 10–25: q24h
CrCl < 10: q36h

CEFAZOLIN

0.5–1.5 g IM/IV q6–8h

RENAL DOSING
CrCl 50–90 mL/min: 1–2 g IV q8h
CrCl 10–50 mL/min and continuous arteriovenous hemofiltration: q12h
CrCl < 10 mL/min: q24–48h
Hemodialysis: extra 1 g after dialysis
Chronic ambulatory peritoneal dialysis: 0.5 g q12h

CEPHALEXIN

250–1,000 mg PO q6h

RENAL DOSING
CrCL 10–40 mL/min: q8–12h
CrCl < 10 mL/min: q12–24h

■ DRUG INTERACTIONS

NEPHROTOXICITY: aminoglycosides

INCREASED LEVELS OF CEPHALOSPORINS: probenecid

DECREASED EFFICACY OF CEPHALOSPORINS: oral contraceptives

■ SIDE EFFECTS

COMMON: diarrhea, nausea, vomiting, rash, headache, dizziness, dyspepsia, pruritus, vaginal candidiasis, thrombophlebitis (cefazolin), urticaria

RARE: neutropenia, thrombocytopenia, anaphylaxis, pseudomembranous colitis, seizures (cefadroxil, cefazolin), nephrotoxicity, Stevens-Johnson syndrome (cefadroxil, cefazolin), hemolytic anemia (cefadroxil), thrombocytopenia, elevated liver function test results, toxic epidermal necrolysis, hepatitis, gastritis, interstitial nephritis, confusion, hallucinations, insomnia, fatigue, agitation, arthritis, eosinophilia

■ MONITORING

None

■ CONTRAINDICATIONS

Hypersensitivity to drug/class, penicillin allergy, antibiotic-associated colitis, nephrotoxic agents, impaired renal function, lactation, seizures (cefadroxil), nephrotoxic agents

■ PREGNANCY CLASS

B

CEPHALOSPORINS, SECOND GENERATION

Cefaclor (Ceclor® 250, 500 mg caps; 125, 187, 250, 375 mg/5 mL suspension; Ceclor CD® 375, 500 mg extended-release caps); cefotetan (Cefotan® IV); cefoxitin (Mefoxin® IV); cefprozil (Cefzil® 250, 500 mg tabs; 125, 250 mg/5 mL suspension); cefuroxime (Zinacef® IV/IM; Ceftin® 125, 250, 500 mg tabs; 125, 500 mg/5 mL suspension; Kefurox® IV/IM); loracarbef (Lorabid® 200, 400 mg caps; 100, 200 mg/5 mL suspension)

▩ INDICATIONS

- *Bacteroides fragilis* (cefoxitin*, cefotetan*)
- *Clostridium,* not *difficile* (cefoxitin*, cefotetan*)
- *Enterobacter* sp. (cefuroxime*)
- *Escherichia coli** (not cefprozil)
- *Haemophilus influenzae**
- *Klebsiella pneumoniae** (not cefprozil and loracarbef)
- *Moraxella catarrhalis* (cefprozil*, loracarbef*)
- *Morganella morganii* (cefotetan*, cefoxitin*)
- *Neisseria gonorrhoeae* (cefoxitin*, cefuroxime*, cefotetan*)
- *Neisseria meningitidis* (cefuroxime*)
- *Peptococcus niger* (cefotetan*, cefoxitin*)
- *Peptostreptococcus* sp. (cefotetan*, cefoxitin*)
- *Proteus mirabilis** (not cefprozil, not cefuroxime, not loracarbef)
- *Proteus vulgaris* (cefotetan*, cefoxitin*)
- *Providencia rettgeri* (cefotetan*, cefoxitin*)
- *Serratia marcescens* (cefotetan*)
- *Staphylococcus aureus,* methicillin sensitive*
- *Staphylococcus epidermidis* (not cefprozil, not cefuroxime, not loracarbef)
- *Staphylococcus saprophyticus* (loracarbef*)
- *Streptococcus agalactiae* (cefotetan*)
- *Streptococcus pneumoniae**
- *Streptococcus pyogenes**

See Appendix II.

Usually effective:

- *Aeromonas* sp. (cefotetan, cefuroxime)
- *Clostridium,* not *difficile* (cefuroxime, cefprozil)
- *Haemophilus ducreyi* (cefoxitin)
- *Klebsiella* sp. (cefprozil, loracarbef)
- *Moraxella catarrhalis* (cefotetan, cefoxitin, cefuroxime)
- *Peptostreptococcus* sp. (cefuroxime, cefprozil, cefaclor, loracarbef)

- *Prevotella melaninogenica* (cefotetan, cefoxitin, cefuroxime, cefaclor, cefprozil, loracarbef)
- *Proteus mirabilis* (cefprozil, cefuroxime, loracarbef)
- *Proteus vulgaris* (cefuroxime)
- *Providencia* (cefuroxime)
- *Streptococcus viridans* (cefacolor, loracarbef, cefuroxime, cefoxitin, cefotetan)

Clinical trials lacking:

- *Aeromonas* sp. (cefoxitin)
- *Citrobacter* sp. (cefotetan, cefoxitin, cefuroxime, cefaclor, loracarbef)
- *Enterobacter* sp. (cefotetan, cefuroxime)
- *Moraxella catarrhalis* (cefaclor)
- *Morganella* sp. (cefuroxime)
- *Neisseria gonorrhoeae* (cefaclor, cefprozil, loracarbef)
- *Neisseria meningitidis* (cefprozil, cefaclor, loracarbef, cefotetan, cefoxitin)
- *Staphylococus epidermidis* (cefprozil, cefuroxime, loracarbef)
- *Yersinia enterocolitica* (cefotetan, cefuroxime, cefoxitin)

MECHANISM OF ACTION

They are bactericidal agents that inhibit bacterial cell wall synthesis.

DOSAGE

CEFACLOR

250–500 mg PO tid or 375–500 g PO bid (extended release)

RENAL DOSING
Creatinine clearance (CrCl) < 10 mL/min: decrease dose by 50%

CEFOTETAN

1–2 g IM/IV q12h, maximum of 6 g/d

RENAL DOSING
CrCl 50–90 mL/min: 100%
CrCl 10–50 mL/min: 50%
CrCL < 10 mL/min: 25%
Hemodialysis: extra 1 g after dialysis
Continuous arteriovenous hemofiltration (CAVH): 750 mg IV q12h
Chronic ambulatory peritoneal dialysis (CAPD): 1 g IV qd

CEFOXITIN

1–2 g IM/IV q6–8h, maximum of 12 g/d

RENAL DOSING
   CrCl 50–90 mL/min: 2 g IV q8h
   CrCl 10–50 mL/min: 2 g IV q8–12h
   CrCL < 10 mL/min: 2 g IV q24–48h
   Hemodialysis: extra 1 g after dialysis
   CAVH: 2 g IV q8–12h
   CAPD: 1 g IV qd

CEFPROZIL

250–500 mg PO qd or divided bid

RENAL DOSING
   CrCl < 30 mL/min: 50% of normal dose

CEFUROXIME

750–1,500 mg IM/IV q8h; 250–500 mg PO bid

RENAL DOSING
   CrCl 50–90 mL/min: 0.75–1.5 g IV q8h
   CrCl 10–50 mL/min: 0.75–1.5 g IV q8–12h
   CrCl < 10 mL/min: 0.75–1.5 g IV q24–48h
   Hemodialysis: dose after dialysis
   CAVH: 1.5 g IV, then 0.75 g IV q24h
   CAPD: 0.75–1.5 g IV q24h

LORACARBEF

200–400 mg PO bid

RENAL DOSING
   CrCl 10–50 mL/min: 50% of normal dose
   CrCl < 10 mL/min: 200–400 mg PO q3–5d

■ DRUG INTERACTIONS

NEPHROTOXICITY: aminoglycosides

INCREASED EFFICACY OF CEPHALOSPORINS: aminoglycosides

DECREASED EFFICACY OF CEPHALOSPORINS: antacids, didanosine (cefuroxime), proton pump inhibitors (cefuroxime)

DECREASED EFFICACY OF: oral contraceptives

INCREASED LEVELS OF CEPHALOSPORINS: probenecid

INCREASED BLEEDING: aspirin (cefotetan), heparin (cefotetan), thrombin inhibitors (cefotetan), warfarin (cefotetan)

DISULFIRAM-LIKE REACTION: ethanol (cefotetan)

▥ SIDE EFFECTS

COMMON: diarrhea, nausea, vomiting, vaginitis, pruritus, rash, urticaria, dyspepsia, eosinophilia (cefaclor, cefotetan, cefprozil, cefuroxime), elevated blood urea nitrogen/creatinine levels (cefotetan, cefuroxime), phlebitis (cefotetan, cefoxitin, cefuroxime), injection site reactions (cefotetan, cefuroxime), hypotension (cefoxitin), angioedema (cefuroxime)

RARE: anaphylaxis, thrombocytopenia, pseudomembranous colitis, serum sickness reaction, seizures, nephrotoxicity, neutropenia, hemolytic anemia, exfoliative dermatitis, Stevens-Johnson syndrome, toxic epidermal necrolysis, superinfection, cholestatic jaundice, agranulocytosis (cefotetan, cefuroxime), prolonged international normalized ratio (INR) (cefotetan), renal failure, interstitial nephritis (cefuroxime), anemia, leukopenia, elevated liver function test results, elevated renal function test results (cefaclor, cefotetan, cefprozil, cefuroxime), confusion, psychosis, hallucinations, insomnia, serum sickness reaction

▥ MONITORING

None

▥ CONTRAINDICATIONS

Hypersensitivity to drug/class, penicillin allergy, impaired renal function, antibiotic-associated colitis, seizures (cefaclor, cefotetan, cefprozil, cefuroxime), nephrotoxic agents, use in children (cefotetan, cefuroxime), vitamin K deficiency (cefotetan), impaired liver function (cefotetan), phenylketonuria (cefprozil suspension), lactating (loracarbef)

▥ PREGNANCY CLASS

B

CEPHALOSPORINS, THIRD GENERATION

Cefdinir (Omnicef® 300 mg caps; 125 mg/5 mL suspension); cefixime (Suprax® 200, 400 mg tabs; 100 mg/5 mL suspension); cefoperazone (Cefobid® IV/IM); cefotaxime (Claforan® IM/IV); cefpodoxime (Vantin® 100, 200 mg tabs; 50, 100 mg/5 mL suspension); ceftazidime (Ceptaz®, Fortaz®, Tazidime®, Tazicef® IM/IV); ceftibuten (Cedax® IV); ceftizoxime (Cefizox® IV); ceftriaxone (Rocephin® IM/IV)

▓ INDICATIONS

- *Acinetobacter calcoaceticus* (cefotaxime*, ceftriaxone*)
- *Bacteroides fragilis* (ceftazidime*, cefoperazone*, cefotaxime*, ceftizoxime*, ceftriaxone*)
- *Citrobacter freundii* (cefotaxime*, ceftazidime*)
- *Clostridium,* not *difficile* (cefoperazone*, cefotaxime*, ceftriaxone*)
- *Enterobacter* sp. (cefoperazone*, cefotaxime*, ceftazidime*, ceftizoxime*, ceftriaxone*)
- *Enterococcus faecium* (cefoperazone*, cefotaxime*)
- *Escherichia coli* (cefixime*, cefoperazone*, cefotaxime*, cefpodoxime*, ceftazidime*, ceftizoxime*, ceftriaxone*)
- *Fusobacterium nucleatum* (cefotaxime*)
- *Haemophilus influenzae**
- *Haemophilus parainfluenzae* (cefdinir*, cefotaxime*, ceftriaxone*)
- *Klebsiella pneumoniae* (cefoperazone*, cefotaxime*, cefpodoxime*, ceftazidime*, ceftizoxime*, ceftriaxone*)
- *Moraxella catarrhalis** (not ceftazidime, not cefoperazone, not cefotaxime, not ceftizoxime)
- *Morganella morganii* (cefotaxime*, ceftizoxime*, ceftriaxone*)
- *Neisseria gonorrhoeae* (cefixime*, cefoperazone*, cefotaxime*, cefpodoxime*, ceftizoxime*, ceftriaxone*)
- *Neisseria meningitidis* (cefotaxime*, ceftazidime*, ceftriaxone*)
- *Peptococcus* sp. (cefotaxime*, ceftizoxime*)
- *Peptostreptococcus* sp. (cefotaxime*, ceftizoxime*, ceftriaxone*)
- *Proteus mirabilis* (cefixime*, cefoperazone*, cefotaxime*, cefpodoxime*, ceftazidime*, ceftizoxime*, ceftriaxone*)
- *Proteus vulgaris* (cefotaxime*, ceftizoxime*)
- *Providencia stuartii* and *rettgeri* (cefotaxime*, ceftizoxime*)
- *Pseudomonas aeruginosa* (cefoperazone*, cefotaxime*, ceftazidime*, ceftizoxime*, ceftriaxone*)
- *Serratia marcescens* (cefotaxime*, ceftazidime*, ceftizoxime*, ceftriaxone*)
- *Staphylococcus aureus,* methicillin sensitive* (not ceftibuten and cefixime)

- *Staphylococcus epidermidis* (cefoperazone*, cefotaxime*, ceftizoxime*, ceftriaxone*)
- *Staphylococcus saprophyticus* (cefpodoxime*)
- *Streptococcus agalactiae* (cefoperazone*, ceftizoxime*)
- *Streptococcus pneumoniae*
- *Streptococcus viridans* (ceftriaxone*)
- *Streptococcus pyogenes*

See Appendix II.

Usually effective:

- *Acinetobacter* sp. (cefotaxime, ceftizoxime, ceftriaxone, ceftazidime)
- *Actinomyces* sp. (ceftizoxime, ceftriaxone)
- *Aeromonas* sp. (cefotaxime, ceftizoxime, ceftriaxone, cefoperazone, ceftazidime, cefixime, ceftibuten)
- *Burkholderia cepacia* (ceftazidime, ceftibuten)
- *Citrobacter* sp. (ceftizoxime, ceftriaxone, cefoperazone, cefixime, ceftibuten, cepodoxime, cefdinir)
- *Clostridium,* not *difficile* (ceftazidime, ceftizoxime)
- *Escherichia coli* (cefdinir, ceftibuten)
- *Haemophilus ducreyi* (cefotaxime, ceftizoxime, ceftriaxone, ceftazidime, cefixime)
- *Klebsiella* sp. (cefixime, ceftibuten)
- *Moraxella catarrhalis* (ceftazidime, cefoperazone, cefotaxime, ceftizoxime)
- *Morganella* sp. (cefperazone, ceftazidime)
- *Neisseria gonorrhoeae* (cefpodoxime, cefdinir)
- *Pasteurella multocida* (ceftizoxime, ceftriaxone, cefoperazone, cefixime, cefpodoxime, cefdinir)
- *Peptostreptococcus* sp. (cefoperazone, ceftazidime, cefixime)
- *Prevotella melaninogenica* (cefotaxime, ceftizoxime, cefoperazone, ceftazidime, cefixime)
- *Proteus mirabilis* (ceftibuten, cefdinir)
- *Proteus vulgaris* (ceftriaxone, cefperazone, ceftazidime, cefixime, ceftibuten)
- *Providencia* sp. (ceftriaxone, cefperazone, ceftazidime, cefixime, ceftibuten)
- *Salmonella* sp. (cefotaxime, ceftriaxone, cefoperazone)
- *Serratia* sp. (cefperazone)
- *Streptococcus viridans* (cefotaxime, ceftizoxime, cefoperazone, cefixime, cepodoxime, cefdinir)
- *Yersinia entercolitica* (cefotaxime, ceftizoxime, ceftriaxone, cefixime, ceftibuten)

Clinical trials lacking:

- *Burkholderia cepacia* (cefotaxime, ceftriaxone, ceftixozime, cefoperazone)
- *Enterobacter* sp. (ceftibuten)
- *Neisseria gonorrhoeae* (ceftazidime, ceftibuten)
- *Neisseria meningitidis* (ceftizoxime, cefoperazone, cefixime, ceftibuten)
- *Prevotella melaninogenica* (ceftriaxone)
- *Proteus vulgaris* (cefpodoxime, cefdinir)
- *Serratia* sp. (cefixime, ceftibuten)
- *Staphylococcus epidermidis* (ceftazidime, cefpodoxime, cefdinir)
- *Stenotrophomonas maltophilia* (cefoperazone, ceftazidime)
- *Streptococcus viridans* (ceftazidime)
- *Yersinia enterocolitica* (cefoperazone, ceftazidime)

MECHANISM OF ACTION

They are bactericidal agents, which inhibit bacterial cell wall synthesis.

DOSAGE

CEFDINIR

600 mg PO qd

RENAL DOSING
Creatinine clearance (CrCl) < 30 mL/min: 300 mg PO qd

CEFIXIME

400 mg PO qd

RENAL DOSING
CrCl 20–60 mL/min: decrease dose by 25%
CrCl < 20 mL/min: decrease dose by 50%

CEFOPERAZONE

2–4 g IV/IM q12h

RENAL DOSING
Hemodialysis: dose after dialysis

CEFOTAXIME

1–2 g IV/IM q6–8h, maximum of 12 g/d

RENAL DOSING
  CrCl 50–90 mL/min: 2 g IV q8–12h
  CrCl 10–50 mL/min: 2 g IV q12–24h
  CrCl < 10 mL/min: 2 g IV q24h
  Hemodialysis: extra 1 g after dialysis
  Chronic ambulatory peritoneal dialysis (CAPD): 0.5–1 g IV qd
  Continuous arteriovenous hemofiltration (CAVH): 2 g IV q12–24h

CEFPODOXIME

100–400 mg PO bid

RENAL DOSING
  CrCl < 30 mL/min: dose q12h

CEFTAZIDIME

1 g IV/IM q8–12h; 2 g IV q8–12h

RENAL DOSING
  CrCl 50–90 mL/min: 2 g IV q8–12h
  CrCl 10–50 mL/min: 2 g IV q24–48h
  CrCl < 10 mL/min: 2 g IV q48h
  Hemodialysis: extra 1 g after dialysis
  CAPD: 1 g IV qd
  CAVH: 2 g IV q24–48h

CEFTIBUTEN

400 mg PO qd

RENAL DOSING
  CrCl 30–50 mL/min: 200 mg PO qd
  CrCl < 30 mL/min: 100 mg PO qd

CEFTIZOXIME

1–2 g IV q8–12h

RENAL DOSING
  CrCl 50–90 mL/min: 2 g IV q8–12h
  CrCl 10–50 mL/min: 2 g IV q12–24h

CrCl < 10 mL/min: 2 g IV q24h
Hemodialysis: extra 1 g after dialysis
CAPD: 0.5–1 g IV qd
CAVH: 2 g IV q12–24h

CEFTRIAXONE

1–2 g IV/IM qd

■ DRUG INTERACTIONS

NEPHROTOXICITY: aminoglycosides

INCREASED EFFICACY OF CEPHALOSPORINS: aminoglycosides

DECREASED EFFICACY OF CEPHALOSPORINS: antacids, iron salts (cefdinir), multivitamins with minerals (cefdinir), didanosine (cefpodoxime)

DECREASED LEVELS OF CEPHALOSPORINS: H2 blockers (cefpodoxime), proton pump inhibitors (cefpodoxime)

DECREASED EFFICACY OF: oral contraceptives

INCREASED LEVELS OF CEPHALOSPORINS: probenecid

INCREASED BLEEDING: aspirin (cefoperazone), warfarin (cefoperazone), thrombin inhibitors (cefoperazone), heparin (cefoperazone)

DISULFIRAM-LIKE REACTION: ethanol (cefoperazone)

■ SIDE EFFECTS

COMMON: diarrhea, nausea, vomiting, abdominal pain, headache, rash, vaginitis, pruritus, eosinophilia, urticaria, elevated blood urea nirogen/creatinine levels, thrombophlebitis (cefoperazone), anemia (cefoperazone), injection site reaction, (cefoperazone, cefotaxime, ceftazidime, ceftizoxime, ceftriaxone), fever (cefotaxime), decreased hemoglobin (ceftibuten), elevated bilirubin levels (ceftibuten), thrombocytosis (ceftizoxime, ceftriaxone), leukopenia (ceftriaxone)

RARE: hepatotoxicity, thrombocytopenia, anaphylaxis, hemolytic anemia, seizures, neutropenia, pseudomembranous colitis, serum sickness (cefoperazone, ceftibuten), disulfiram-like reaction (cefoperazone), agranulocytosis (cefotaxime), interstitial nephritis (cefotaxime, ceftibuten), toxic epidermal necrolysis (cefotaxime, cefpodoxime, ceftibuten), Stevens-

Johnson syndrome (cefotaxime, cefpodoxime, ceftibuten), superinfection (cefpodoxime), erythema multiforme (cefotaxime), leukopenia (cefpodoxime), pancytopenia (ceftibuten), hypoprothrombinemia (ceftriaxone), thrombocytosis, vertigo, sweating, flushing, palpitations, fever, chills, elevated renal function test results, elevated liver function test results, flatulence, kidney stones

MONITORING

None

CONTRAINDICATIONS

Hypersensitivity to drug/class, penicillin allergy, antibiotic-associated colitis, nephrotoxic agents, seizures, impaired liver function (cefoperazone), impaired renal function, lactating (cefoperazone, ceftizoxime), hyperbilirubinemia (ceftriaxone)

PREGNANCY CLASS

B

CEPHALOSPORINS, FOURTH GENERATION

Cefepime (Maxipime® IM/IV)

INDICATIONS

- *Bacteroides fragilis**
- *Enterobacter* sp.*
- *Escherichia coli**
- *Klebsiella pneumoniae**
- *Proteus mirabilis**
- *Pseudomonas aeruginosa**
- *Staphylococcus aureus,* methicillin sensitive*
- *Streptococcus pneumoniae**
- *Streptococcus pyogenes**

See Appendix II.

Usually effective:

- *Aeromonas* sp.
- *Citrobacter* sp.
- *Haemophilus influenzae*
- *Moraxella catarrhalis*
- *Morganella* sp.
- *Neisseria gonorrhoeae*
- *Neisseria meningitidis*
- *Peptostreptococcus* sp.
- *Proteus vulgaris*
- *Providencia* sp.
- *Serratia* sp.
- *Streptococcus viridans*
- *Yersinia enterocolitica*

Clinical trials lacking:

- *Acinetobacter* sp.
- *Bulkholderia cepacia*
- *Staphylococcus epidermidis*

■ MECHANISM OF ACTION

It is a bactericidal agent that inhibits bacterial cell wall synthesis.

■ DOSAGE

0.5–2 g IV/IM q12h

RENAL DOSING
  Creatinine clearance (CrCl) 50–90 mL/min: 2 g IV q8h
  CrCl 50–10 mL/min: 2 g IV q12–24h
  CrCl < 10 mL/min: 1 g IV q24h
  Hemodialysis: extra 1 g IV after dialysis
  Chronic ambulatory peritoneal dialysis (CAPD): 1–2 g IV q48h
  Continuous arteriovenous hemofiltration (CAVH): not recommended

■ DRUG INTERACTIONS

NEPHROTOXICITY: aminoglycosides

INCREASED EFFICACY OF CEPHALOSPORINS: aminoglycosides

DECREASED EFFICACY OF: oral contraceptives

INCREASED LEVELS OF CEPHALOSPORINS: probenecid

SIDE EFFECTS

COMMON: diarrhea, nausea, vomiting, pruritus, headache, injection site reactions, rash, fever, vaginitis

RARE: anaphylaxis, encephalopathy, seizures, pseudomembranous colitis,
interstitial nephritis, leukopenia, Stevens-Johnson syndrome, toxic epidermal necrolysis, thrombocytopenia, hemolytic anemia, erythema multiforme, confusion, vertigo, urticaria, elevated liver function test results,
hypoglycemia, anemia, elevated renal function results, hypocalcemia

MONITORING

None

CONTRAINDICATIONS

Hypersensitivity to drug/class, penicillin allergy, impaired renal function,
antibiotic-associated colitis, seizures, nephrotoxic agents

PREGNANCY CLASS

B

CETIRIZINE

(Zyrtec® 5, 10 mg tabs; 5 mL/5 mL liquid in 120 mL bottles)

INDICATIONS

- Allergic rhinitis*
- Atopic dermatitis^ (see pg. 353)
- Dermatographism^
- Eosinophilic cellulitis+

- Eosinophilic pustular folliculitis of HIV[+]
- Erythema gyratum repens[+]
- Pruritus, burn wounds[^] (see pg. 391)
- Pruritus, mosquito bites[^] (see pg. 391)
- Psoriasis[^] (see pg. 392)
- Urticaria (see pg. 403)
  Acute[^]
  Cholinergic[^]
  Chronic[*]
  Cold[^], with zafirlucast 20mg PO qd[^]
  Heat[^]
  Solar[^]
- Urticaria pigmentosa[+]
- Urticarial vasculitis[+] (see pg. 404)

MECHANISM OF ACTION

It is a second-generation H1 histamine receptor blocker that is a carboxylic acid metabolite of the first-generation antihistamine hydroxyzine. It also inhibits eosinophil chemotaxis and accumulation in the skin. It is a long-acting, minimally sedating antihistamine.

DOSAGE

5–10 mg PO qd. May need to use as much as 40 mg PO qd in urticaria and atopic dermatitis.

RENAL DOSING
CrCl < 30: 5 mg PO qd

HEPATIC DOSING: 5 mg PO qd

DRUG INTERACTIONS

INCREASED CENTRAL NERVOUS SYSTEM DEPRESSION: opiates, tramadol, antidepressants, antihistamines, antipsychotics, propoxyphene, barbiturates, benzodiazepines, droperidol, ethanol, meperidine, central alpha-2 agonists, meprobamate, metoclopramide, muscle relaxants, phenothiazines, promethazine, sedatives/hypnotics, thalidomide

INCREASED RISK OF HYPERTENSION: central alpha-2 agonists (eg, methyldopa)

■ SIDE EFFECTS

COMMON: somnolence, fatigue, dry mouth, pharyngitis, dizziness, abdominal pain, nausea, vomiting, diarrhea, headache, coughing, epistaxis, bronchospasm

RARE: hepatitis, hypersensitivity reaction, anorexia, flushing, increased salivation, urinary retention, cardiac failure, hypertension, palpitation, tachycardia, abnormal coordination, ataxia, confusion, dysphonia, hyperesthesia, leg cramps, migraine, myelitis, paralysis, paresthesia, ptosis, syncope, tremor, twitching, vertigo, visual field defect, constipation, dyspepsia, flatulence, gastritis, hemorrhoids, increased appetite, melena, rectal hemorrhage, stomatitis, tongue edema, tongue discoloration, cystitis, dysuria, hematuria, polyuria, urinary incontinence, deafness, ear ache, ototoxicity, tinnitus, dehydration, diabetes, thirst, arthralgia, arthritis, arthrosis, myalgia, muscle weakness, agitation, amnesia, anxiety, decreased libido, depression, emotional lability, euphoria, impaired concentration, insomnia, nervousness, paranoia, bronchitis, dyspnea, pneumonia, increased sputum, sinusitis, upper respiratory tract infection, dysmenorrhea, breast pain, intermenstrual bleeding, leukorrhea, menorrhagia, vaginitis, lymphadenopathy, acne, alopecia, angioedema, bullous eruption, dermatitis, dry skin, eczema, furunculosis, hyperkeratosis, hypertrichosis, rash, photosensitivity, pruritus, purpura, seborrhea, urticaria, parosmia, ageusia, blindness, conjunctivitis, glaucoma, ocular hemorrhage, xeropthalmia, asthenia, back pain, face edema, fever, increased weight, pallor, nasal polyps, edema, rigors

■ MONITORING

None

■ CONTRAINDICATIONS

Hypersensitivity to drug/class, hypersensitivity to hydroxyzine, impaired liver or renal function, concurrent use of central nervous system depressants

■ PREGNANCY CLASS

B

CHLORAMBUCIL

(Leukeran® 2 mg tabs)

▦ INDICATIONS

- Amyloidosis due to rheumatoid arthritis$ (see pg. 350)
- Behçet's disease (cutaneous,^ ocular$) (see pg. 355)
- Benign lymphocytic angiitis+
- Bullous pemphigoid$ (see pg. 355)
- Chronic lymphocytic leukemia*
- Cryofibrinogenemia+
- Cryoglobulinemia$
- Dermatomyositis$ (see pg. 361)
- Disseminated histiocytosis$
- Epidermolysis bullosa acquisita+ (see pg. 363)
- Erythema elevatum diutinum+
- Giant follicular lymphoma*
- Granuloma annulare$ (see pg. 365)
- Histiocytosis X$
- Hodgkin's lymphoma*
- Kaposi's sarcoma$ (see pg. 370)
- Lichen myxedematosus+
- Lupus erythematosus nephritis^ (see pg. 375)
- Lymphosarcoma*
- Mastocytosis$
- Multicentric histiocytosis+
- Mycosis fungoides$ (see pg. 358)
- Necrobiotic xanthogranuloma with paraproteinemia$
- Pemphigus foliaceus$ (see pg. 383)
- Pemphigus vulgaris$ (see pg. 385)
- Polyarteritis nodosa+ (see pg. 404)
- Pyoderma gangrenosum$ (see pg. 394)
- Relapsing polychondritis$
- Sarcoidosis$ (see pg. 396)
- Scleroderma^ (see pg. 398)
- Scleromyxedema+
- Sézary syndrome$ (see pg. 358)
- Sinus histiocytosis with massive lymphadenopathy+
- Sweet's syndrome+ (see pg. 401)
- Waldenström's macroglobulinemia$
- Wegener's granulomatosis+ (see pg. 404)

MECHANISM OF ACTION

It is an alkylating agent, derived from nitrogen mustard, that cross-links DNA.

DOSAGE

2–16 mg PO qd (0.05–0.2 mg/kg/d)

DRUG INTERACTIONS

None

SIDE EFFECTS

COMMON: male sterility, female amenorrhea, chromatid/chromosome damage, myelosuppression, nausea, vomiting, diarrhea, oral ulceration, alopecia

RARE: cough, tremors, confusion, agitation, ataxia, flaccid paresis, hallucinations, pulmonary fibrosis, peripheral neuropathy, interstitial pneumonia, toxic epidermal necrolysis, Stevens-Johnson syndrome, erythema multiforme, leukemia, squamous cell carcinoma, seizures, drug fever, hepatotoxicity, jaundice, cystitis

MONITORING

BASELINE: complete blood counts, serum chemistry, chest x-ray

WEEKLY FOR 3 MONTHS, THEN MONTHLY FOR 3 MONTHS, THEN EVERY 3 MONTHS: complete blood count, serum chemistry

EVERY 6 MONTHS: chest x-ray

CONTRAINDICATIONS

Hypersensitivity to drug or class, prior resistance to chlorambucil, additive immunosuppression with use with other alkylating agents and immunosuppressants, administration of live viral vaccines, pregnancy

PREGNANCY CLASS

D

CHLORAMPHENICOL

(Chloromycetin® IV; Amphicol® 250 mg caps)

▦ INDICATIONS

- *Aeromonas aerogenes**
- *Burkholderia cepecia**
- *Enterobacter* sp.*
- *Escherichia coli**
- *Haemophilus influenzae**
- *Klebsiella* sp.*
- *Moraxella catarrhalis**
- *Neisseria gonorrhoeae**
- *Neisseria meningitidis**
- *Proteus* sp.*
- *Pseudomonas aeruginosa**
- Rickettsial diseases
- *Salmonella* sp.*
- *Staphylococcus aureus*, methicillin sensitive*
- *Streptococcus pneumoniae**
- *Streptococcus pyogenes**

See Appendix II.

Usually effective:

- *Actinomyces* sp.
- *Bacteroides fragilis*
- *Brucella* sp.
- *Chlamydia* sp.
- *Clostridium*, not *difficile*
- *Francisella tularensis*
- *Haemophilus ducreyi*
- *Listeria monocytogenes*
- *Mycoplasma pneumoniae*
- *Peptostreptococcus* sp.
- *Prevotella melaninogenica*
- *Salmonella* sp.
- *Shigella* sp.
- *Stenotrophomonas maltophilia*
- *Vibrio vulnificus*
- *Yersinia enterocolitica*

Clinical trials lacking:

- *Clostridium difficile*
- *Enterococcus faecalis*
- *Enterococcus faecium*

MECHANISM OF ACTION

It is a bacteriostatic agent that binds to the 50S ribosomal subunit to inhibit protein synthesis.

DOSAGE

50–100 mg/kg IV qd

RENAL DOSING
   Hemodialysis: dose after dialysis

HEPATIC DOSING
   Hepatic failure: 1 g loading dose, then 500 mg q6h. Monitor levels.
   Hepatic damage/cirrhosis: 500 mg q6h
   Jaundice: 25 mg/kg/d

DRUG INTERACTIONS

INCREASED LEVELS OF: bosentan, phenytoin, voriconazole, warfarin

DECREASED EFFICACY OF: cyanocobalamin, cyclophosphamide, iron, methotrexate, penicillin

INCREASED TOXICITY: phenobarbital

DECREASED EFFICACY OF CHLORAMPHENICOL: methohexital

HYPOGLYCEMIA: sulfonylureas

INCREASED BONE MARROW SUPPRESSION: cimetidine

SIDE EFFECTS

COMMON: headache, nausea, vomiting, diarrhea, fever, rash, urticaria, pruritus, peripheral neuropathy, optic neuritis, blurred vision

Rare: aplastic anemia, hypoplastic anemia, agranulocytosis, thrombocytopenia, anaphylaxis, gray baby syndrome, pseudomembranous colitis

▨ MONITORING

Frequently If Long-Term Use: complete blood count

▨ CONTRAINDICATIONS

Hypersensitivity to drug/class, pregnancy, infancy, mild infections, impaired liver or renal function, glucose-6-phosphate dehydrogenase deficiency, hematologic disorders, bone marrow suppressants, perforated tympanic membrane

▨ PREGNANCY CLASS

C

CHLOROQUINE

(Aralen® 250, 500 mg tabs; 250 mg/5 mL vials)

▨ INDICATIONS

- Atopic dermatitis[$] (see pg. 353)
- Dermatomyositis[+](see pg. 361)
- Extraintestinal amebiasis (*Entamoeba histolytica* trophozoites)[*]
- Granuloma annulare[+](see pg. 365)
- Idiopathic panniculitis[+]
- Jessner's lymphocytic infiltrate[$]
- Lichen planus, oral[+] (see pg. 371)
- Lupus, cutaneous[*], panniculitis[+] (see pg. 375)
- Lymphocytoma cutis[+]
- Malaria prophylaxis[*]
- Malaria treatment (*Plasmodium vivax* and *malariae* erythrocytic forms, *P. falciparum* except gametocytes)[*]
- Polymorphous light eruption[^]

- Porphyria cutanea tarda^ (see pg. 388)
- Psoriatic arthritis$
- Sarcoidosis, cutaneous$, pulmonary^ (see pg. 396)
- Weber-Christian panniculitis+

MECHANISM OF ACTION

The exact mechanism is unknown. It is thought to inhibit certain enzymes by interacting with DNA to exert its plasmodicidal action. It affects light filtration by altering prostaglandin synthesis and inhibiting superoxide production and binding to DNA. It inhibits antigen-antibody complex formation, decreases lymphocyte responsiveness, and decreases the ability of macrophages to express cell surface antigens, which leads to immunosuppression. It decreases lysosomal size and function, and impairs chemotaxis to exert its antiinflammatory action. It also inhibits platelet aggregation.

DOSAGE

Each 500 mg tab contains 300 mg chloroquine base. Each milliliter of intravenous drug contains 40 mg chloroquine base. Intravenous drug should be given only if oral chloroquine not available. Daily dose should not exceed 4 mg/kg.

DERMATOMYOSITIS, LUPUS PANNICULITIS: 250 mg PO bid

EXTRAINTESTINAL AMEBIASIS: start 1 g PO qd for 2 days then 500 mg PO qd for 2–3 weeks

GRANULOMA ANNULARE: 3 mg/kg/d PO

LUPUS ERYTHEMATOSUS, PSORIATIC ARTHRITIS, WEBER-CHRISTIAN PANNICULITIS: 250 mg PO qd

MALARIA PROPHYLAXIS: 1–2 weeks prior to exposure, 500 mg PO every week. If started after exposure, 500 mg PO q6h twice.

MALARIA TREATMENT: start 1 g PO one time, then 500 mg PO 6 h after, then 500 mg PO qd for 2 days

PORPHYRIA CUTANEA TARDA: 250 mg PO twice a week

PULMONARY SARCOIDOSIS: 750 mg PO qd for 6 months, then 500 mg PO qd for 2 months, then 250 mg PO qd

DRUG INTERACTIONS

INCREASED RISK OF SEIZURES: mefloquine

INCREASED RISK OF GASTROINTESTINAL SIDE EFFECTS: pyridostigmine

SIDE EFFECTS

COMMON: nausea, vomiting, anorexia, diarrhea, abdominal pain, headache, blurred vision, rash, pruritus, fatigue, alopecia, pigmentary changes

RARE: seizures, agranulocytosis, aplastic anemia, thrombocytopenia, retinopathy (>4 mg/kg/d), methemoglobinemia, hearing loss, hypotension, electrocardiographic abnormalities, weakness, personality changes, tinnitus, nyctalopia, scotomas, nerve deafness, abdominal cramps, lichen planus-like eruption

MONITORING

BASELINE: eye exam/visual fields, complete blood count, glucose-6-phosphate dehydrogenase level, liver function, 24 h urine for porphyrin

EVERY 6 MONTHS: eye exam

MONTHLY FOR 3 MONTHS, THEN EVERY 4–6 MONTHS: complete blood counts, liver function

CONTRAINDICATIONS

Hypersensitivity to drug or class, retinal field changes, porphyria, gastrointestinal disorders, neurological disease, psoriasis, impaired liver function, glucose-6-phosphate dehydrogenase deficiency, use of other antimalarials, pregnancy, concomitant use of hydroxychloroquine

PREGNANCY CLASS

C

CHOLESTYRAMINE

(Prevalite® powder 5.5 g packets in cartons of 42 or 60, 231 g cans; Questran®
powder 4 g packets in box of 60, 378 g cans)

▨ INDICATIONS

- Hypercholesterolemia*
- Pruritus associated with: (see pg. 391)
    Cholestasis^
    Cholestasis of pregnancy$
    Dermatitis herpetiformis+
    Hepatic failure^
    Hepatic involvement with porphyrias+
    Polycythemia vera+
    Sickle cell disease+
    Uremia^
- Pseudomembranous colitis*
- Skin irritation secondary to:
    Bilary fistula+
    Diarrhea with elevated bile acids+
    Enterostomy$
    Ileoanal anastomosis$

▨ MECHANISM OF ACTION

It binds intestinal bile acids, preventing their enterohepatic circulation.

▨ DOSAGE

PRURITUS: 2–8 g PO bid. Mix with water and take before meals.

SKIN IRRITATION: May compound 20 g with Aquaphor® to create ointment
to use qd to bid.

▨ DRUG INTERACTIONS

DECREASED EFFICACY OF: angiotensin receptor blockers, angiotensin-
converting enzyme inhibitors, amiodarone, beta blocker/thiazide combinations, digoxin, potassium-sparing diuretics/hydrochlorothiazide
combinations, thiazides, fat-soluble vitamins, fibric acid derivatives,

folic acid, leflunomide, lovastatin/niacin combinations, meloxicam, multivitamin with minerals, mycophenolate mofetil, niacin, statins, thyroid hormones, ursodial, valproic acid, warfarin

▓ SIDE EFFECTS

COMMON: constipation, flatulence, nausea, dyspepsia, abdominal pain, anorexia, sour taste, headache, urticaria, rash, fatigue, weight loss

RARE: fecal impaction, bleeding gums, hematuria

▓ MONITORING

None

▓ CONTRAINDICATIONS

Hypersensitivity to drug/class, biliary obstruction, coronary artery disease, constipation, pregnancy

▓ PREGNANCY CLASS

C

CICLOPIROX

(Penlac® 8% nail lacquer solution in 3.3, 6.6 mL bottles)

▓ INDICATIONS

- Onychomycosis*

▓ MECHANISM OF ACTION

It inhibits fungal transmembrane transport, altering fungal cell membrane permeability.

DOSAGE

Apply to nails qhs. Clean with alcohol q8d. Use for maximum of 48 weeks.

DRUG INTERACTIONS

None

SIDE EFFECTS

COMMON: erythema, irritation

RARE: nail shape change, ingrown nails, discoloration of nails

MONITORING

None

CONTRAINDICATIONS

Hypersensitivity to drug/class, immunosuppressed, diabetic

PREGNANCY CLASS

B

CIDOFOVIR

(Vistide® 375 mg vials)

INDICATIONS

- Basal cell carcinoma$ (see pg. 354)
- Cervical intraepithelial neoplasia$
- Condylomata acuminata^ (see pg. 406)
- Cytomegalovirus retinitis in HIV-positive patients*
- Herpes simplex^

- Laryngeal papillomatosis$
- Molluscum contagiosum$ (see pg. 380)
- Squamous cell carcinoma+ (see pg. 400)
- Verruca vulgaris in HIV-positive patients+ (see pg. 406)

▥ MECHANISM OF ACTION

It is a nucleoside analog of deoxycytidine monophosphate that becomes incorporated in viral DNA by viral DNA polymerases and blocks further DNA synthesis. It does not depend on viral thymidine kinase for phosphorylation.

▥ DOSAGE

CYTOMEGALOVIRUS RETINITIS

5 mg/kg IV every week for 2 weeks, then po every week. Give saline prehydration and probenecid.

RENAL DOSING INDUCTION
   Creatinine clearance (CrCl) 50–90 mL/min: 5 mg/kg IV every week
   CrCl 10–50 mL/min: 0.5–2 mg/kg IV every week
   CrCl < 10 mL/min: 0.5 mg/kg IV every week
   Hemodialysis: no data

RENAL DOSING MAINTENANCE
   CrCl 50–90 mL/min: 5 mg/kg IV every 2 weeks
   CrCl 10–50 mL/min: 0.5–2 mg/kg IV every 2 weeks
   CrCl < 10 mL/min: 0.5 mg/kg IV
   Hemodialysis: no data

VERRUCA VULGARIS IN HIV-POSITIVE PATIENTS

375 mg IV every 2 weeks

OTHER DOSAGES

May compound into cream or gel, which can be used qd to bid. Add 15 mg of cidofovir (75 mg/mL) to 22.5 g of Dermovan® vehicle to make 3% cidofovir cream.

▓ DRUG INTERACTIONS

HYPOKALEMIA: angiotensin receptor blockers/hydrochlorothiazide combinations, carbonic anhydrase inhibitors

INCREASED NEPHROTOXICITY: adefovir, aminoglycosides, cyclooxygenase-2 inhibitors, nephrotoxic agents, nonsteroidal anti-inflammatory drugs, tenofovir

INCREASED QT PROLONGATION: class III antiarrhythmics, bepridil, cisapride, meperidine/promethazine, phenothiazines, pimozide, quinolones

INCREASED BONE MARROW SUPPRESSION: bone marrow suppressants, carboplatin, cisplatin, clozapine, cytotoxic chemotherapy, interferon alpha and beta, oxaliplatin, rituximab, zidovudine

INCREASED LACTIC ACIDOSIS: metformin/sulfonylureas

▓ SIDE EFFECTS

TOPICAL

COMMON: headache, nausea, pharyngitis, pruritus, rash, paresthesias, ulceration, pain

RARE: none

SYSTEMIC

COMMON: proteinuria, nausea, vomiting, asthenia, rash, headache, diarrhea, alopecia, infection, chills, fever, anorexia, dyspnea, anemia, abdominal pain, elevated creatinine

RARE: nephrotoxicity, neutropenia, anterior uveitis, decreased intraocular pressure, metabolic acidosis

▓ MONITORING

BASELINE AND 48 H PRIOR TO EACH DOSE: creatinine, absolute neutrophil count, urine protein

▦ CONTRAINDICATIONS

Hypersensitivity to drug or class of drug, hypersensitivity to probenecid, creatinine > 1.5 mg/dL, creatinine clearance ≤ 55 mL/min, urine protein ≥100 mg/dL (proteinuria), pregnancy.

Do not administer nephrotoxic agents within 7 days of using cidofovir.

▦ PREGNANCY CLASS

C

CIMETIDINE

(Tagamet® 200, 300, 400, 800 mg tabs; 300 mg/5 ML in 8 oz bottles; 300 mg/ 5 mL single-use bottles; 300 mg/2 mL in 2, 8 mL vials)

▦ INDICATIONS

- Acne[+] (see pg. 347)
- Androgenic alopecia[$] (see pg. 351)
- Candidiasis, cutaneous[$]
- Duodenal ulcers, active and maintenance[*]
- Erythema multiforme[+] (see pg. 364)
- Gastric ulcers, benign active[*]
- Gastroesophageal reflux[*]
- Gastrointestinal bleed, prophylaxis[*]
- Herpes simplex[+]
- Hirsutism[+]
- Hypersecretory syndromes[*]
- Mastocytosis/urticaria pigmentosa[+]
- Molluscum contagiosum[$] (see pg. 380)
- Prevention of hemolysis with dapsone use[$]
- Scleroderma, esophagitis[+] (see pg. 398)
- Urticaria[^] (see pg. 403)
- Verruca vulgaris[^] (see pg. 406)

▦ MECHANISM OF ACTION

It competitively inhibits histamine at H2 receptors of the parietal cells and inhibits gastric acid secretion. It also exerts antiandrogenic effects by binding to androgen receptors. There are also H2 receptors on T suppressor cells that, when blocked by cimetidine, stimulate the cell-mediated immune system.

■ DOSAGE

20–40 mg/kg PO qd or 800–1,600 mg PO qd

■ DRUG INTERACTIONS

INCREASED LEVELS OF: albendazole, amiodarone, aripiprazole, caffeine, atamoxetine, bupivacaine, bupropion, buspirone, benzodiazepines, carbamazepine, citalopram, clozapine, cyclosporin, dolasetron, escitalopram, alcohol, fluvastatin, galantamine, metformin, mifepristone, moricizine, nevirapine, olanzapine, paroxetine, phenytoin, procainamide, quetiapine, quinidine, sertraline, sildenafil, sirolimus, tacrine, tacrolimus, terbinafine, theophylline, valproic acid, warfarin, zolmitriptan

DECREASED LEVELS OF: atazanavir, cefpodoxime, delavirdine, gefitinib, iron, itraconazole, ketoconazole

INCREASED CENTRAL NERVOUS SYSTEM AND RESPIRATORY DEPRESSION: alfentanil, fentanyl, tricyclic antidepressants

INCREASED RISK OF HYPOTENSION: bepridil, beta blockers, calcium channel blockers

INCREASED CARDIAC ARRHYTHMIAS: cisapride, flecainide, lidocaine, mepivacaine, thioridazine

INCREASED RISK OF MYOPATHY: lovastatin, simvastatin

■ SIDE EFFECTS

COMMON: headaches, diarrhea, gynecomastia, nausea, vomiting, dizziness, drowsiness, rash

RARE: neutropenia, thrombocytopenia, agranulocytosis, aplastic anemia, confusion, agitation, drowsiness, elevated liver function test results, hypotension, cardiac arrhythmias, impotence, pancytopenia, interstitial nephritis, urinary retention, anaphylaxis, arthralgia, myalgia, erythema multiforme, erythema nodosum, Stevens-Johnson syndrome, toxic epidermal necrolysis

■ MONITORING

None

CONTRAINDICATIONS

Hypersensitivity to drug or class.

PREGNANCY CLASS

B

CLINDAMYCIN

(Cleocin® 75, 150, 300 mg caps; IV/IM; 75 mg/5 mL suspension)

INDICATIONS

- *Actinomyces* sp.*
- *Bacteroides fragilis**
- *Clostridium perfringens**
- *Eubacterium* sp.*
- *Fusobacterium* sp.*
- *Peptococcus* sp.*
- *Peptostreptococcus* sp.*
- *Propionibacterium* sp.*
- *Staphylococcus aureus,* methicillin sensitive*
- *Streptococcus pneumoniae**
- *Streptococcus pyogenes**

See Appendix II.

Usually effective:

- *Prevotella melaninogenica*

Clinical trials lacking:

- *Chlamydia* sp.

MECHANISM OF ACTION

It binds to the 50S ribosomal subunit, which inhibits bacterial protein synthesis.

▓ DOSAGE

150–450 mg PO qid, 300–600 mg IM q6–12h, 300–900 mg IV q6–12h

▓ DRUG INTERACTIONS

INCREASED NEUROMUSCULAR EFFECTS OF: botulinum toxin

PROLONGED NEUROMUSCULAR BLOCKADE: nondepolarizing neuromuscular blockers

DECREASED EFFICACY OF: oral contraceptives

▓ SIDE EFFECTS

COMMON: diarrhea, nausea, vomiting, abdominal pain, rash, pruritus, jaundice, urticaria, hypotension, thrombophlebitis (IV)

RARE: pseudomembranous colitis, thrombocytopenia, anaphylaxis, Stevens-Johnson syndrome, granulocytopenia, esophagitis

▓ MONITORING

FREQUENTLY IF LONG-TERM USE: complete blood count, renal function, liver function

▓ CONTRAINDICATIONS

Hypersensitivity to drug/class, ulcerative colitis, antibiotic-associated colitis, impaired liver or renal function

▓ PREGNANCY CLASS

B

CLINDAMYCIN, TOPICAL

(Clindets® 1% clindamycin in pledgets, 69 pledgets per box; Cleocin T® 1% gel in 30, 60 g tubes; lotion in 60 mL bottles; solution in 30, 60 mL bottles; pledgets); clindamycin 1% and benzoyl peroxide 5% (Duac® gel in 45 g tubes); clindamycin 1% and benzoyl peroxide 5% (BenzaClin® gel in 20, 50 g tubes)

▩ INDICATIONS

- Acne vulgaris (clindamycin*, clindamycin with benzoyl peroxide*) (broad spectrum: gram positive, gram negative, and anaerobic bacteria), with adapalene gel* (see pg. 347)
- Erythrasma (clindamycin$)
- Fox-Fordyce disease (clindamycin+)
- Hidradenitis suppurativa (clindamycin^)
- Rosacea (clindamycin,^ clindamycin with benzoyl peroxide^) (see pg. 395)
- Tufted folliculitis (clindamycin+)

▩ MECHANISM OF ACTION

It binds to the bacterial 50S ribosomal subunit, which interferes with protein synthesis by preventing the elongation of peptide chains by inhibiting peptidyl transfer.

▩ DOSAGE

Apply bid (qd for Duac®).

▩ DRUG INTERACTIONS

DECREASED EFFICACY/ANTAGONISM: erythromycin topical

INCREASED IRRITATION/DRYNESS: isotretinoin, tretinoin topical

▩ SIDE EFFECTS

COMMON: burning, pruritus, dryness, erythema, peeling, oily skin

RARE: pseudomembranous colitis, gram-negative folliculitis

▥ MONITORING

None

▥ CONTRAINDICATIONS

Hypersensitivity to drug/class, pseudomembranous colitis, ulcerative colitis, pregnancy (benzoyl peroxide)

▥ PREGNANCY CLASS

B (clindamycin), C (clindamycin with benzoyl peroxide)

CLOFAZIMINE

(Lamprene® 50 mg tabs)

▥ INDICATIONS

- Acne conglobata[+] (see pg. 347)
- Acne fulminans[+] (see pg. 347)
- Annular elastolytic giant-cell granuloma[+]
- Atypical mycobacterial infections[^]
- Erythema dyschromicum perstans[$]
- Erythema elevatum diutinum[+]
- Graft-versus-host disease, chronic[$] (see pg. 365)
- Granuloma annulare[+] (see pg. 365)
- Granuloma faciale[+]
- Histiocytosis, ulcerative[+]
- Leischmaniasis[$]
- Lepromatous leprosy[*]
- Lobomycosis[+]
- Lupus, cutaneous[$] (see pg. 375)
- Lupus vulgaris[+] (see pg. 396)
- Malakoplakia[+]
- Melkersson-Rosenthal syndrome[$]
- Miescher's cheilitis[+]
- Necrobiosis lipoidica diabeticorum[+] (see pg. 381)
- Prurigo nodularis[+]
- Psoriasis, pustular[$] (see pg. 392)

- Pyoderma gangrenosum$ (see pg. 394)
- Rhinoscleroma$
- Rothmann-Makai syndrome+
- Sarcoidosis, laryngeal+ (see pg. 396)
- Sweet's syndrome+ (see pg. 401)
- Tuberculosis^
- Vitiligo+ (see pg. 405)

MECHANISM OF ACTION

It binds to DNA guanine residues. It inhibits mitochondrial respiratory chain and free-radical formation. It alters function of monocytes and neutrophils. It exerts anti-inflammatory and antimicrobial effects with selective immunomodulation.

DOSAGE

50–400 mg PO qd

DRUG INTERACTIONS

INCREASED LEVELS OF CLOFAZIMINE: isoniazid

ALTERED PHARMACODYNAMICS OF: rifampin

SIDE EFFECTS

COMMON: orange-brown hyperpigmentation of skin, xerosis, abdominal cramping, nausea, vomiting, diarrhea

RARE: hyperpigmentation of tears/sweat/milk/urine/feces/hair/sputum, ichthyosis, crystal deposition in viscera, fatal enteropathy, splenic infarction, eosinophilic enteritis, cardiac arrhythmias, edema, worsening of vitiligo, electrolyte disturbances, nail changes

MONITORING

BASELINE, THEN MONTHLY: liver function, electrolytes, bilirubin

CONTRAINDICATIONS

Hypersensitivity to drug or class, pregnancy, gastrointestinal disease, electrolyte disturbances

PREGNANCY CLASS

C

CLOTRIMAZOLE

(Mycelex® 10 mg troches, 70 and 100 troches per bottle; Mycelex® 1% cream 15, 30 and 90 g tubes; Mycelex® 1% vaginal cream—[over the counter]; Lotrimin® 1% cream in 15, 30 and 45 g tubes; Lotrimin AF® 1% cream, lotion, solution—[over the counter])

INDICATIONS

- Candidiasis, cutaneous* (topical)
- Candidiasis, oropharyngeal* (troche)
- Tinea* (topical)

MECHANISM OF ACTION

It alters fungal cell membrane permeability by inhibiting 14-alpha demethylase in ergosterol biosynthesis, which leads to cessation of cell growth.

DOSAGE

CANDIDIASIS, CUTANEOUS: Apply bid for 2–4 weeks.

CANDIDIASIS, OROPHARYNGEAL: 1 troche PO 5 times a day for 14 days

TINEA: Apply bid for 2–4 weeks.

DRUG INTERACTIONS

None

■ SIDE EFFECTS

TROCHE

COMMON: nausea

RARE: vomiting, abdominal cramps, elevated liver function test results

TOPICAL

COMMON: irritation, burning, stinging, pruritus, erythema

RARE: edema, urticaria, peeling, blistering

■ MONITORING

None

■ CONTRAINDICATIONS

Hypersensitivity to drug/class, impaired liver function, pregnancy (troche)

■ PREGNANCY CLASS

C (troche), B (topical)

COAL TAR

(Polytar® soap 3.2%—[over the counter]; Polytar® shampoo 4.5%—[over the counter]; Zetar® 30% emulsion and 1% shampoo in 180 mL bottles; Betatar® 1% shampoo in 240 mL bottles; Denorex extra strength® 2.5% shampoo in 120, 240, 360 mL bottles; Denorex® 1.8% shampoo in 120, 240, 360 mL bottles; DHS® 0.5% shampoo in 120, 240, 480 mL bottles; Duplex T® 2% shampoo in 480, 3,840 mL bottles; Doak Tar shampoo® 3% in 240 mL bottles; coal tar 20% solution® in 120, 480, 3,840 mL bottles; LCD® ointment; Elta Tar® 2% cream in 114, 480 g tubes; Balnetar® 2.5% liquid in 225 mL bottles; Medotar® 1% ointment in 454 g tubes; Estar® 5% gel in 90 g tubes). May compound in 5–20% concentrations, in creams or ointments. This is only a partial list of all the products.

INDICATIONS

- Atopic dermatitis^ (see pg. 353)
- Psoriasis* (see pg. 392)
- Seborrheic dermatitis* (see pg. 399)
- Tinea versicolor$
- Vitiligo$ (see pg. 405)

MECHANISM OF ACTION

It suppresses DNA synthesis and reduces mitotic activity of the epidermis. It acts as a keratolytic.

DOSAGE

CREAMS, OINTMENT: Use once a week to three times a week, 2 h prior to ultraviolet light exposure. Then remove with mineral oil immediately before exposure. The Goeckerman regimen can be used for inpatient hospitalization. In such cases, the steps delineated above may be performed bid to tid.

SHAMPOO: Use qd to once a week, then rinse.

DRUG INTERACTIONS

None

SIDE EFFECTS

COMMON: phototoxicity, contact dermatitis, irritant dermatitis, pruritus, folliculitis, comedones/acneiform eruption, keratoses

RARE: skin cancers

MONITORING

None

▨ CONTRAINDICATIONS

Hypersensitivity to drug or class

▨ PREGNANCY CLASS

Not applicable

COLCHICINE

(Colchicine® 0.5, 0.6 mg tabs)

▨ INDICATIONS

- Amyloidosis$ (see pg. 350)
- Anetoderma+
- Behçet's syndrome^ (see pg. 355)
- Dermatitis herpetiformis+ (see pg. 360)
- Dermatomyositis+ (see pg. 361)
- Epidermolysis bullosa acquisita+ (see pg. 363)
- Erythema elevatum diutinum+
- Familial Mediterranean fever^
- Gout, acute and maintenance*
- Henoch-Schönlein purpura+ (see pg. 404)
- Leukocytoclastic vasculitis$ (see pg. 404)
- Linear IgA dermatosis+ (see pg. 374)
- Pachydermoperiostosis+
- Palmoplantar pustulosis$
- Polyarteritis nodosa+ (see pg. 404)
- Psoriasis, plaque$, pustular+ (see pg. 392)
- Psoriatic arthritis$
- Purpura annularis telangiectoides+
- Pyoderma gangrenosum+ (see pg. 394)
- Relapsing polychondritis+
- Scleroderma$ (see pg. 398)
- Subcorneal pustular dermatosis$
- Sweet's syndrome$ (see pg. 401)
- Type II lepra reaction$
- Urticarial vasculitis+ (see pg. 404)

█ MECHANISM OF ACTION

It inhibits tubulin dimer assembly, which arrests cells in metaphase to inhibit cell motility. It also decreases polymorphonuclear mobility, adhesiveness, and chemotaxis. It interferes with lysosomal degranulation, histamine release, and melanosome movement.

█ DOSAGE

1–2.4 mg PO qd

█ DRUG INTERACTIONS

INCREASED RISK OF HEPATIC AND RENAL SIDE EFFECTS: cyclosporine

█ SIDE EFFECTS

COMMON: diarrhea, headache, nausea, vomiting, abdominal pain, neutropenia, alopecia, rash, anemia

RARE: aplastic anemia, thrombocytopenia, agranulocytosis, cellulitis, myoneuropathy, thrombophlebitis, dehydration, hypokalemia, hypocalcemia, hyponatremia, metabolic acidosis, stomatitis, porphyria cutanea tarda, disseminated intravascular coagulation, respiratory distress

█ MONITORING

BASELINE, THEN MONTHLY: complete blood count, serum chemistry, urinalysis

█ CONTRAINDICATIONS

Hypersensitivity to drug or class, blood dyscrasias, cardiovascular disease, pregnancy, gastrointestinal dysfunction, impaired renal function, impaired liver function

█ PREGNANCY CLASS

C

CYCLOPHOSPHAMIDE

(Cytoxan® 25, 50 mg tabs; 100, 200, 500, 1000, 2000 mg vials)

INDICATIONS

- Acute lymphoblastic leukemia*
- Acute monocytic leukemia*
- Acute myelogenous leukemia*
- Behçet's disease[§] (see pg. 355)
- B-cell lymphoma, primary with rituximab[§]
- Breast carcinoma*
- Bullous pemphigoid[§] (see pg. 355)
- Chronic granulocytic leukemia*
- Chronic lymphocytic leukemia*
- Cicatricial pemphigoid[^] (see pg. 356)
- Cryofibrinogenemia[+]
- Cryoglobulinemia[§]
- Cytophagic histiocytic panniculitis[+]
- Dermatomyositis, lung[§] (see pg. 361)
- Eczematous dermatitis[^]
- Erythema elevatum diutinum[+]
- Histiocytic lymphoma*
- Histiocytosis X[§]
- Hodgkin's lymphoma*
- Ichthyosis linearis circumflexa[+]
- Leukocytoclastic vasculitis[^] (see pg. 404)
- Lichen myxedematosus[+]
- Lupus, renal[^], lung/eye/cerebral[§] (see pg. 375)
- Lymphocytic lymphoma*
- Lymphomatoid granulomatosis[§]
- Malignant lymphoma Ann Arbor stage III and IV*
- Minimal change nephrotic syndrome in children*
- Mixed cell–type lymphoma*
- Multicentric reticulohistiocytosis[§]
- Multiple myeloma*
- Mycosis fungoides* (see pg. 358)
- Neuroblastoma*
- Ovarian adenocarcinoma*
- Pemphigus foliaceus[§] with prednisone (see pg. 383)
- Pemphigus vulgaris[§] with prednisone (see pg. 385)
- Polyarteritis nodosa[^] (see pg. 404)
- Pyoderma gangrenosum[§] (see pg. 394)
- Relapsing polychondritis[§]

- Retinoblastoma*
- Scleroderma$ (see pg. 398)
- Scleromyxedema⁺
- Stevens-Johnson syndrome⁺ (see pg. 400)
- Toxic epidermal necrolysis⁺ (see pg. 402)
- Wegener's granulomatosis^ (see pg. 404)

MECHANISM OF ACTION

It is an alkylating agent that cross-links DNA.

DOSAGE

BULLOUS DERMATOSES, CONNECTIVE TISSUE DISEASES, MYCOSIS FUN-GOIDES: 1–5 mg/kg/PO qd (may give with prednisone 1 mg/kg/d PO for bullous diseases)

VASCULITIS, MALIGNANCIES: 5–9 mg/kg IV qd for 1–2 weeks every month

LUPUS NEPHROPATHY, LUPUS VASCULITIS: 0.5–1 g/m^2 pulse IV once a month

PRIMARY B-CELL LYMPHOMA: 1.5 g/m^2 IV 1 week prior to rituximab, 375 mg/m^2 IV every week for 4 weeks total

DRUG INTERACTIONS

INCREASED LEVELS OF CYCLOPHOSPHAMIDE: allopurinol, cimetidine, chloramphenicol

INCREASED LEVELS OF: succinylcholine

DECREASED LEVELS OF CYCLOPHOSPHAMIDE: barbiturates

DECREASED LEVELS OF: digoxin

INCREASED CARDIAC TOXICITY: doxorubicin

INCREASED RISK OF IMMUNOSUPPRESSION: alefacept

INCREASED RISK OF BONE MARROW SUPPRESSION: rituximab, zidovudine

■ SIDE EFFECTS

COMMON: sterility, amenorrhea, hemorrhagic cystitis, infections, nausea, vomiting, alopecia, leukopenia, diarrhea, anorexia, rash, malaise, stomatitis, darkened skin/teeth/nails

RARE: abdominal pain, hemorrhagic colitis, mucosal erosions, jaundice, Stevens-Johnson syndrome, toxic epidermal necrolysis, thrombocytopenia, anemia, renal tubular necrosis, interstitial pneumonia, pulmonary fibrosis, asthenia, syndrome of inappropriate antidiuretic hormone (ADH) secretion, congestive heart failure, pericarditis, anaphylaxis, inhibit wound healing, bladder fibrosis, dysuria, acral erythema, urticaria, hepatotoxicity, cardiomyopathy, seizures, malignancies (bladder, leukemia, lymphoma, squamous cell carcinoma)

■ MONITORING

BASELINE: complete blood count, serum chemistry, urinalysis, chest x-ray

WEEKLY FOR 3 MONTHS, THEN MONTHLY FOR 3 MONTHS, THEN EVERY 6 MONTHS: complete blood count, serum chemistry, urinalysis

EVERY 6 MONTHS: chest x-ray, urine cytology

■ CONTRAINDICATIONS

Hypersensitivity to drug or class, severe bone marrow suppression, use with other alkylating agents or immunosuppressants, use of live viral vaccines, pregnancy

■ PREGNANCY CLASS

D

CYCLOSPORIN

(Neoral® 25, 50, 100 mg tab, 100 mg/mL PO solution, 50 mg/mL IV solution; Sandimmune® 25, 100 mg tab, 100 mg/mL PO solution)

▪ INDICATIONS

- Alopecia areata[$] (see pg. 349)
- Aphthous stomatitis[^] (see pg. 352)
- Atopic dermatitis[^] (see pg. 353)
- Behçet's disease (oral),[^] (topical)[+] (see pg. 355)
- Bullous pemphigoid[$] (see pg. 355)
- Cicatricial pemphigoid[+] (see pg. 356)
- Cutaneous T-cell lymphoma, subcutaneous childhood[+] (see pg. 358)
- Darier's disease[+] (see pg. 359)
- Dermatomyositis[$] (see pg. 361)
- Epidermolysis bullosa acquisita[+] (see pg. 363)
- Graft-versus-host disease[^] (see pg. 365)
- Granuloma annulare[+] (see pg. 365)
- Hailey-Hailey disease[+] (see pg. 367)
- Herpes gestationis[+] (see pg. 368)
- Hypereosinophlic syndrome[+] (see pg. 368)
- Lichen planopilaris[+] (see pg. 371)
- Lichen planus[+] (see pg. 371)
- Linear IgA Dermatosis[+] (see pg. 374)
- Lupus, bullous[+], panniculitis[+], systemic[$] (see pg. 375)
- Necrobiosis lipoidica diabeticorum[+] (see pg. 381)
- Paraneoplastic pemphigus[+] (see pg. 382)
- Pemphigus erythematosus[+]
- Pemphigus vulgaris[^] (see pg. 385)
- Photodermatitis[+]
- Pityriasis lichenoides chronica[+] (see pg. 386)
- Pityriasis rubra pilaris[+] (see pg. 387)
- Prurigo nodularis[+]
- Psoriasis, plaque[*], pustular[$] (see pg. 392)
- Pyoderma gangrenosum[$] (see pg. 394)
- Reiter's disease[+] (see pg. 395)
- Scleroderma, systemic[^], linear[+] (see pg. 398)
- Sweet's syndrome[+] (see pg. 401)
- Toxic epidermal necrolysis[+] (see pg. 402)

▪ MECHANISM OF ACTION

Binds to cyclophilin to inhibit calcineurin and decrease activity of NFAT1 transciption factor, which reduces the transcription of proinflammatory cytokines, such as interleukin-2, interferon-gamma, and neutrophilic chemoattractant cytokines.

■ DOSAGE

3–5 mg/kg/d divided into 2 BID

SUBCUTANEOUS CHILDHOOD CUTANEOUS T-CELL LYMPHOMA: 5–12 mg/kg/d PO with cyclophosphamide/doxorubicin/vincristine/predisone

■ DRUG INTERACTIONS

INCREASED RISK OF HYPERKALEMIA: angiotensin-converting enzyme inhibitors, potassium-sparing diuretics, potassium

INCREASED RISK OF NEPHROTOXICITY: angiotensin-converting enzyme inhibitors, adefovir, aminoglycosides, carboplatin, cidofovir, cisplatin, colchicine, nonsteroidal anti-inflammatory drugs, nephrotoxic agents, sirolimus, tacrolimus, zoledronic acid

INCREASED RISK OF IMMUNOSUPPRESSION: alefacept

INCREASED RISK OF CENTRAL NERVOUS SYSTEM DEPRESSION: alfentanil, benzodiazepines, fentanyl

INCREASED LEVELS OF CYCLOSPORIN: amiodarone, androgens, aprepitant, azoles, antifungals, bromocriptine, cimetidine, ciprofloxacin, macrolide antibiotics, oral contraceptives, steroids, delavirdine, diltiazem, efavirenz, fluvoxamine, griseofulvin, metoclopramide, metronidazole, nefazodone, nicardipine, protease inhibitors, quinupristin/dalfopristin, verapamil

INCREASED LEVELS OF: aripiprazole, bosentan, buprenorphine, caspofungin, digoxin, eletriptan, etoposide, ezetimibe, paclitaxel, sildenafil, tadalafil, tenofovir, tolteradine, vinca alkaloids

INCREASED RISK OF MYOPATHY: statins

DECREASED LEVELS OF CYCLOSPORIN: barbiturates, carbamazepine, imatinib, modafinil, nafcillin, octreotide, orlistat, phenytoin, rifabutin, rifampin, rifapentine, terbinafine

INCREASED RISK OF HYPOTENSION: calcium channel blockers

INCREASED QT INTERVAL: cisapride, pimozide

SEIZURES: doxorubicin

INCREASED RISK OF ERGOT TOXICITY: ergots

INCREASED RISK OF INFECTION: leflunomide, tumor necrosis factor–blocking agents

INCREASED RISK OF LACTIC ACIDOSIS: metformin

SIDE EFFECTS

COMMON: hypertension, acne, leg cramps, diarrhea, paresthesias, headache, abdominal pain, sinusitis, nausea, vomiting, hirsutism, gingival hyperplasia, myalgias, lethargy, infection, elevated blood urea nitrogen/creatinine levels, hypomagnesemia, hyperkalemia, hyperuricemia, hyperglycemia

RARE: seizures, leukopenia, thrombocytopenia, hepatotoxicity, anaphylaxis, nephrotoxicity, malignancy, infection, glomerular capillary thrombosis, diabetes

MONITORING

BASELINE: blood pressure, creatinine, blood urea nitrogen, magnesium

AFTER 2 WEEKS: blood pressure, creatinine, blood urea nitrogen, magnesium

MONTHLY THEREAFTER: blood pressure, creatinine, blood urea nitrogen, magnesium

CONTRAINDICATIONS

HIV or cancer, liver or renal problems, hypersensitivity to drug/class, hypersensitivity to castor oil, nephrotoxic agents, use of live vaccines, pregnancy

PREGNANCY CLASS

C

CYPROHEPTADINE

(Periactin® 4 mg tabs, 2 mg/5 mL liquid)

INDICATIONS

- Acanthosis nigricans[+] (see pg. 347)
- Allergic reactions in blood products[*]
- Allergic rhinitis[*]
- Anaphylaxis[*]
- Angioedema[*] (see pg. 351)
- Atopic dermatitis[^] (see pg. 353)
- Dermatographism[*]
- Epidermolysis bullosa simplex[^] (see pg. 362)
- Mastocytosis[+]
- Pruritus, histamine induced[^] (see pg. 391)
- Urticaria, chronic[*], aquagenic[+] (see pg. 403)
- Urticaria pigmentosa[+]

MECHANISM OF ACTION

It is a first-generation H1 histamine receptor blocker with anticholinergic, sedative, and antiserotonergic activity.

DOSAGE

4 mg PO tid

DRUG INTERACTIONS

INCREASED CENTRAL NERVOUS SYSTEM DEPRESSION: opiates, tramadol, propoxyphene, antidepressants, antihistamines, antipsychotics, barbiturates, benzodiazepines, central alpha-2 agonists, dexmedetomidine, dronabinol, droperidol, ethanol, meperidine, meprobamate, metoclopramide, muscle relaxants, phenothiazines, promethazine, codeine, sedative/hypnotics, thalidomide

INCREASED ANTICHOLINERGIC EFFECTS: anticholinergics, central alpha-2 agonists, cyclopentolate/phenylephrine, disopyramide, monoamine oxidase inhibitors

DECREASED EFFICACY OF CYPROHEPTADINE: cholinergics

SIDE EFFECTS

COMMON: dry mouth, nausea, vomiting, abdominal pain, dizziness, headache, fatigue, urinary retention, rash, urticaria, weight gain, diarrhea, sedation, drowsiness

RARE: agranulocytosis, thrombocytopenia, confusion, disturbed coordination, restlessness, nervousness, tremor, irritability, insomnia, paresthesias, neuritis, seizures, euphoria, hallucinations, faintness, hysteria, edema, photosensitivity, hypotension, palpitations, labyrinthitis, blurred vision, diplopia, vertigo, tinnitus, tachycardia, shock, hemolytic anemia, leukopenia, cholestasis, hepatic failure, hepatitis, anorexia, constipation, jaundice, urinary frequency/retention, early menses, thickened bronchial secretions, nasal congestion, chest tightness, wheezing, fatigue, chills, headache, fever, weight gain

MONITORING

None

CONTRAINDICATIONS

Hypersensitivity to drug/class, peptic ulcer disease, glaucoma, newborn/premature, lactation, monoamine oxidase inhibitors, bladder neck obstruction, prostatic hypertrophy, elderly, asthma, hyperthyroidism, cardiovascular disease/hypertension

PREGNANCY CLASS

B

DANAZOL

(Danocrine® 50, 100, 200 mg caps)

▨ INDICATIONS

- Angioedema, hereditary* (see pg. 351)
- Endometriosis*
- Fibrocystic breast disease*
- Immune thrombocytopenia of systemic lupus$ (see pg. 375)
- Livedoid vasculitis$ (see pg. 404)
- Lupus, discoid+ (see pg. 375)
- Pruritus of myelodysplastic disease$ (see pg. 391)
- Urticaria, cholinergic^, chronic^ (see pg. 403)

▨ MECHANISM OF ACTION

It suppresses luteinizing hormone and follicle-stimulating hormone, inhibits pituitary-ovarian axis, exhibits weak androgenic activity, and decreases immunoglobulin G, M, and A.

▨ DOSAGE

ENDOMETRIOSIS
  Mild: 100–200 mg PO bid for 3–6 months, then adjust
  Severe: 400 mg PO bid for 3–6 months, then adjust

FIBROCYSTIC BREAST DISEASE: 50–200 mg PO bid for 2–6 months, then adjust

HEREDITARY ANGIOEDEMA, URTICARIA (CHOLINERGIC AND CHRONIC):
  200 mg PO bid to tid until response, then half dose q1–3 months

LIVEDOID VASCULITIS: 200 mg PO qd

PRURITUS OF MYELOPROLIFERATIVE DISEASE: 400–800 mg PO qd

THROMBOCYTOPENIA OF SYSTEMIC LUPUS: 1 mg/kg/d PO

▨ DRUG INTERACTIONS

INCREASED RISK OF CENTRAL NERVOUS SYSTEM DEPRESSION: alfentanil, fentanyl

INCREASED LEVELS OF: aprepitant, aripiprazole, buprenorphine, cyclosporin, eletriptan, eplerenone, gefitinib, paclitaxel, sirolimus, tacrolimus, tolterodine

INCREASED RISK OF HYPERCALCEMIA: systemic steroids

INCREASED RISK OF HYPOGLYCEMIA: hypoglycemics, insulin, thizolidinediones

INCREASED RISK OF MYOPATHY: statins

INCREASED INTERNATIONAL NORMALIZED RATIO (INR): warfarin

▦ SIDE EFFECTS

COMMON: acne, vaginitis, menstrual irregularities, emotional lability, weight gain, hirsutism, deepened voice, increased spermatogenesis, elevated liver function test results

RARE: hepatic dysfunction, thromboembolism, contraception failure, virilization, pseudotumor cerebri, hepatic adenoma, hemorrhagic cystitis, microscopic hematuria, exacerbation of prostatic hypertrophy, exacerbation of migraines, anxiety, exacerbation of hypertension, exacerbation of congestive heart failure, increased low-density lipoprotein levels, cholestatic jaundice

▦ MONITORING

BASELINE: prostate-specific antigen in men, liver function tests

MONTHLY: liver function tests

▦ CONTRAINDICATIONS

Hypersensitivity to drug/class, porphyria, pregnancy, lactation, undiagnosed vaginal bleeding, migraines, liver dysfunction, congestive heart failure, seizures, prostatic carcinoma, hypertension, prostatic hypertrophy

▦ PREGNANCY CLASS

X

DAPSONE

(Dapsone® 25, 100 mg tabs)

▨ INDICATIONS

- Behçet's syndrome^ (see pg. 355)
- Brown recluse spider bites^
- Bullous pemphigoid$ (see pg. 355)
- Cicatricial pemphigoid$ (see pg. 356)
- Dermatitis herpetiformis* (see pg. 360)
- Dermatomyositis+ (see pg. 361)
- Erythema dyschromicum perstans+
- Erythema elevatum diutinum$
- Giant elastolytic giant-cell granuloma+
- Granuloma annulare+ (see pg. 365)
- Henoch-Schönlein purpura+ (see pg. 404)
- Leprosy*
- Leukocytoclastic vasculitis+ (see pg. 404)
- Linear IgA dermatosis$, with mycophenolate mofetil 155 mg/m² PO qd+ (see pg. 374)
- Lupus, bullous$, subacute cutaneous+ (see pg. 375)
- Pemphigus foliaceus$ (see pg. 383)
- Pemphigus vulgaris$ (see pg. 385)
- Polyarteritis nodosa+ (see pg. 404)
- Pyoderma gangrenosum$ (see pg. 394)
- Relapsing polychondritis$
- Subcorneal pustular dermatosis+
- Sweet's syndrome+ (see pg. 401)
- Urticarial vasculitis+ (see pg. 404)

▨ MECHANISM OF ACTION

It is a sulfone with bactericidal and bacteriostatic activity against *Mycobacterium leprae*. It also inhibits neutrophil chemotaxis and tissue damage.

▨ DOSAGE

25–300 mg PO qd

▨ DRUG INTERACTIONS

INCREASED LEVELS OF DAPSONE: trimethoprim, probenecid, folic acid antagonists

DECREASED LEVELS OF DAPSONE: activated charcoal, PABA, rifampin, rifabutin, rifapentine, antacids, didanosine

INCREASED HEMOLYSIS OF RED BLOOD CELLS: sulfonamides, hydroxychloroquine

INCREASED BONE MARROW SUPPRESSION: clozapine, bone marrow suppressants, interferon alpha and beta, rituximab, zidovudine

SIDE EFFECTS

COMMON: sore throat, fever, pallor, purpura, jaundice, hemolysis, fatigue, nausea, vomiting, myalgia, chills, malaise, dizziness, rash, abdominal pain, headache, anemia

RARE: agranulocytosis, aplastic anemia, methemoglobinemia, erythema multiforme, Stevens-Johnson syndrome, toxic epidermal necrolysis, urticaria, erythema nodosum, acute tubular necrosis, peripheral neuropathy, hepatotoxicity, anorexia, blurred vision, tinnitus, albuminuria, arthralgias, pancreatitis, photosensitivity, pulmonary eosinophilia, nephrotic syndrome, vertigo, tachycardia, psychosis, hypoalbuminuria, renal papillary necrosis, male infertility, drug-induced lupus erythematosus

MONITORING

BASELINE: complete blood count, glucose-6-phosphate dehydrogenase, liver function tests

WEEKLY FOR FIRST MONTH, THEN MONTHLY FOR 6 MONTHS, THEN EVERY 6 MONTHS: complete blood count, liver function tests

CONTRAINDICATIONS

Hypersensitivity to drug/class, glucose-6-phosphate dehydrogenase deficiency, liver dysfunction, renal dysfunction, cardiovascular dysfunction, pregnancy

PREGNANCY CLASS

C

DAPTOMYCIN

(Cubicin® IV)

▨ INDICATIONS

- *Enterococcus faecalis**
- *Staphylococcus aureus*, methicillin resistant*
- *Staphylococcus aureus*, methicillin sensitive*
- *Streptococcus agalactiae**
- *Streptococcus dysgalactiae**
- *Streptococcus pyogenes**

See Appendix II.

Usually effective:

- *Enterococcus faecium*
- *Listeria monocytogenes*
- *Staphylococcus epidermidis*
- *Streptococcus pneumoniae*

▨ MECHANISM OF ACTION

It is a cyclic lipoprotein that binds bacterial membranes and causes rapid depolarization of membranes, leading to inhibition of DNA, RNA, and protein synthesis and ultimately death.

▨ DOSAGE

4 mg/kg IV q24h

RENAL DOSING
Creatinine clearance < 30 mL/min, peritoneal dialysis, hemodialysis: 4 mg/kg IV q48h

▨ DRUG INTERACTIONS

INCREASED LEVELS OF DAPTOMYCIN: tobramycin

POTENTIAL RHABDOMYOLYSIS: statins

■ SIDE EFFECTS

COMMON: nausea, vomiting, diarrhea, constipation, injection site reaction, headache, pruritus, insomnia, renal failure, elevated creatine kinase levels

RARE: dizziness, limb pain, anemia, thrombocytopenia, leukocytosis, hypotension, hypertension, elevated liver function test results, dyspepsia, fever, arthralgia, fatigue, weakness, flushing, supraventricular arrhythmia, eosinophilia, vertigo, change in taste, jaundice, elevated lactate dehydrogenase levels, hypomagnesemia, elevated bicarbonate levels

■ MONITORING

BASELINE AND WEEKLY: creatine kinase

■ CONTRAINDICATIONS

Hypersensitivity to drug/class

■ PREGNANCY CLASS

B

DENILEUKIN DIFTITOX

(Ontak® 300 μg vials)

■ INDICATIONS

- Cutaneous T-cell lymphoma with CD25+ expression* (see pg. 358)
- Psoriasis$ (see pg. 392)

■ MECHANISM OF ACTION

It is a fusion protein consisting of diphtheria toxin and interleukin 2 (IL-2), which directs the cytotoxic activity of the diphtheria toxin to cells expressing the IL-2 receptor (CD25).

DOSAGE

9–18 μg/kg/d IV for 5 consecutive days, given every 21 days

DRUG INTERACTIONS

None

SIDE EFFECTS

COMMON: hypersensitivity reaction, capillary leak syndrome, fever, chills, asthenia, infection, pain, headache, chest pain, flu-like symptoms, injection site reactions, hypotension, vasodilation, tachycardia, thrombotic events, hypertension, arrhythmia, nausea, vomiting, diarrhea, constipation, dyspepsia, dysphagia, anemia, thrombocytopenia, leukopenia, hypoalbuminemia, elevated transaminase levels, edema, hypocalcemia, weight loss, dehydration, hypokalemia, myalgia, arthralgia, dizziness, paresthesias, confusion, insomnia, dyspnea, cough, pharyngitis, rhinitis, rash, pruritus, sweating, hematuria, albuminuria, pyuria, elevated creatinine levels

RARE: pancreatitis, acute renal insufficiency, microscopic hematuria, hyperthyroidism, hypothyroidism

MONITORING

BASELINE: skin biopsy with immunohistochemistry for CD25+, complete blood count, liver function, renal function, albumin

PRIOR TO INFUSION: complete blood count, liver function, renal function, albumin (Do not administer if albumin <3.)

CONTRAINDICATIONS

Hypersensitivity to drug/class, diphtheria toxin or interleukin-2, serum albumin <2 g/dL, pregnancy

PREGNANCY CLASS

C

DESLORATADINE

(Clarinex® 5 mg tabs; Clarinex Reditabs® 5 mg tabs, which dissolve in mouth)

▓ INDICATIONS

- Allergic rhinitis*
- Atopic dermatitis^ (see pg. 353)
- Urticaria, chronic* (see pg. 403)

▓ MECHANISM OF ACTION

It is a long-acting H1 histamine receptor blocker with minimal sedation and anticholinergic effects.

▓ DOSAGE

5 mg PO qd

RENAL DOSING: 5 mg PO qod

HEPATIC DOSING: 5 mg PO qod

▓ DRUG INTERACTIONS

None

▓ SIDE EFFECTS

COMMON: headache, nausea, fatigue, pharyngitis, dry mouth, dizziness, dyspepsia, myalgia, somnolence, dysmenorrhea

RARE: hypersensitivity reaction, hepatotoxicity

▓ MONITORING

None

▨ CONTRAINDICATIONS

Hypersensitivity to drug/class, hypersensitivity to loratadine, impaired liver or renal function, phenylketonuria, pregnancy

▨ PREGNANCY CLASS

C

DIPHENHYDRAMINE

(Benadryl® 25, 50 mg tabs; 12.5 mg/5 mL liquid; 50 mg/mL for IV/IM in 10 mL vials, 1 mL syringes, 1 mL ampules)

▨ INDICATIONS

- Anaphylaxis*
- Antihistaminic*
- Antiparkinsonian*
- Antitussive*
- Atopic dermatitis^ (see pg. 353)
- Dystonic reactions*
- Insomnia*
- Motion sickness*
- Pruritus, due to morphine^, histaminic^ (see pg. 391)
- Sedation*
- Urticaria^ (see pg. 403)

▨ MECHANISM OF ACTION

It is a first-generation central and peripheral H1 histamine receptor blocker with sedative and anticholinergic effects.

▨ DOSAGE

25–50 mg PO/IM/IV q4h, maximum of 400 mg qd, 100 mg dose

▦ DRUG INTERACTIONS

INCREASED CENTRAL NERVOUS SYSTEM DEPRESSION: opiates, propoxyphene, tramadol, antidepressants, antihistamines, antipsychotics, barbiturates, benzodiazepines, central alpha-2 agonists, dexmedetomidine, dronabinol, droperidol, ethanol, meperidine, meprobamate, metoclopramide, muscle relaxants, phenothiazines, codeine, sedative/hypnotics, thalidomide

INCREASED ANTICHOLINERGIC EFFECTS: anticholinergics, central alpha-2 agonists, cyclopentolate/phenylephrine, disopyramide

DECREASED EFFICACY OF DIPHENHYDRAMINE: cholinergics

▦ SIDE EFFECTS

COMMON: sedation, dizziness, coordination problems, thickened bronchial secretions, dry mucosa, blurred vision, central nervous system stimulation, nasal congestion, constipation, palpitations, urinary retention, epigastric pain, anorexia, confusion, increased sweating, tremor, chest tightness, tinnitus, rash/urticaria, photosensitivity, hypotension, wheezing, anticholinergic effects, convulsions, labyrinthitis, neuritis

RARE: hemolytic anemia, thrombocytopenia, agranulocytosis, anaphylaxis

▦ MONITORING

None

▦ CONTRAINDICATIONS

Hypersensitivity to drug/class, lactation, subcutaneous/intradermal injection, newborn/premature, narrow-angle glaucoma, increased intraocular pressure, gastrointestinal obstruction, prostatic hypertrophy, bladder neck obstruction, asthma, pulmonary disease, pediatric patients, elderly patients , cardiovascular disease, hypertension, peptic ulcer, concurrent central nervous system depressant use

▦ PREGNANCY CLASS

B

DOXEPIN

(Sinequan® 10, 25, 50, 75, 100, 150 mg tabs; 10 mg/mL liquid in 120 mL bottles; Zonalon® cream 5% in 30, 45 g tubes; Prudoxin® cream 5% in 45 g tubes)

▓ INDICATIONS

- Anxiety*
- Atopic dermatitis (oral,^ topical*) (see pg. 353)
- Depression*
- Lichen simplex chronicus (topical*) (see pg. 373)
- Neurotic excoriations+
- Pruritus, allergic cutaneous reaction^, HIV^, (see pg. 391)
- Scalp dysesthesia$ (see pg. 362)
- Urticaria, chronic^, cold^ (see pg. 403)

▓ MECHANISM OF ACTION

Its exact mechanism of action is unknown. It exhibits anticholinergic and antihistaminic effects. It influences adrenergic activity at the synapses so that deactivation of norepinephrine by reuptake into the nerve terminals is prevented. It also inhibits serotonin reuptake.

▓ DOSAGE

ORAL
   Depression/Anxiety: 150–300 mg PO qd
   Cutaneous: 10–15 mg PO q6h
Maximum 300 mg qd

TOPICAL
   Cream: Use bid to qid.

▓ DRUG INTERACTIONS

INCREASED CENTRAL NERVOUS SYSTEM DEPRESSION: opiates, propoxyphene, tramadol, alpha-2 agonists, antidepressants, antihistamines, barbiturates, benzodiazepines, carbamazepine, cimetidine, clozapine, dexmedetomidine, dronabinol, droperidol, ethanol, haloperidol, loxapine, meperidine, meprobamate, metoclopramide, molindone, muscle relaxants, antipsychotics, phenothiazines, promethazine/codeine, protease inhibitors, quetiapine, sedative/hypnotics, thalidomide, thiothixene

INCREASED CARDIOVASCULAR ADVERSE EVENTS: amphetamines

INCREASED QT PROLONGATION: class Ia and III antiarrhythmics, beta-2 agonists, carbonic anhydrase inhibitors, cisapride, flumazenil, halothane, mefloquine, pimozide, quinolones

INCREASED ANTICHOLINERGIC EFFECTS: alpha-2 agonists, anticholinergics, cyclopentolate/phenylephrine

HYPOKALEMIA: carbonic anhydrase inhibitors

DECREASED EFFICACY OF DOXEPIN: cholinergics

HYPERTENSION: epinephrine, reserpine, sympathomimetics

INCREASED TRICYCLIC ANTIDEPRESSANT (TCA) LEVELS: imatinib, linezolid, monoamine oxidase inhibitors, methylphenidate, modafinil, protease inhibitors, terbinafine, bupropion, cimetidine, flumazenil

DECREASED TCA LEVELS: rifampins, barbiturates, carbamazepine

CENTRAL NERVOUS SYSTEM TOXICITY: lithium

DECREASED ABSORPTION OF DOXEPIN: nitrates

DECREASED SEIZURE THRESHOLD: phenytoin

▨ SIDE EFFECTS

COMMON: dry mouth, blurred vision, constipation, hypotension, tachycardia, drowsiness, dizziness, diaphoresis, urinary retention, nausea, vomiting, tinnitus, confusion, hallucinations, ataxia, weakness, rash, urticaria, anorexia

RARE: paresthesia, ataxia, tardive dyskinesia, extrapyramidal symptoms, tremor, rash, edema, photosensitivity, pruritus, eosinophilia, bone marrow suppression, seizures, purpura, taste disturbances, diarrhea, stomatitis, change in libido, testicular swelling, gynecomastia, change in blood sugar, sweating, chills, flushing, jaundice, headache, asthma, fever

▨ MONITORING

None

▨ CONTRAINDICATIONS

Hypersensitivity to drug/class, glaucoma, urinary retention, pregnancy

▨ PREGNANCY CLASS

C

ECONAZOLE

(Spectazole® 1% cream in 15, 30 and 85 g tubes)

▨ INDICATIONS

- Candidiasis, cutaneous*
- Tinea*

▨ MECHANISM OF ACTION

It alters fungal cell membrane permeability by inhibiting 14-α-demethylase in ergosterol biosynthesis, which leads to cessation of cell growth.

▨ DOSAGE

CANDIDIASIS, CUTANEOUS: Apply bid.

TINEA: Apply qd.

▨ DRUG INTERACTIONS

None

■ SIDE EFFECTS

COMMON: erythema, pruritus, burning

RARE: rash

■ MONITORING

None

■ CONTRAINDICATIONS

Hypersensitivity to drug/class, pregnancy

■ PREGNANCY CLASS

C

EFALIZUMAB

(Raptiva® 125 mg vials SC injection)

■ INDICATIONS

Psoriasis, moderate to severe plaque-stage * (see pg. 392)

■ MECHANISM OF ACTION

Recombinant humanized monoclonal antibody that binds lymphocyte surface marker CD11a, which binds to intercellular adhesion molecule (ICAM) and therefore inhibits activation and trafficking of T cells.

■ DOSAGE

0.7 mg/kg SC injection for first dose, then 1 mg/kg SC injection 1 week after first dose and weekly thereafter

▓ DRUG INTERACTIONS

INCREASED RISK OF IMMUNOSUPPRESSION: immunosuppressants, leflunomide, tumor necrosis factor–blocking agents

▓ SIDE EFFECTS

COMMON: headache, infection, fever, chills, asthenia, flu-like symptoms, myalgias, back pain, nausea, diarrhea, pharyngitis, rhinitis, sinusitis, herpes simplex virus infection, rash

RARE: thrombocytopenia, leukocytosis, lymphocytosis, elevated liver function test results, elevated C-reactive protein, antibody formation, new form of psoriasis/flare, arthritis, interstitial pneumonitis, angioedema, malignancy, hypersensitivity reaction, laryngospasm

▓ MONITORING

BASELINE: platelets

MONTHLY FOR 3 MONTHS, THEN EVERY 3 MONTHS: platelets

▓ CONTRAINDICATIONS

Hypersensitivity to drug/class, thrombocytopenia, infection, malignancy, use of live vaccines, pregnancy

▓ PREGNANCY CLASS

C

EPOETIN ALPHA

(Procrit® 2,000, 3,000, 4,000, 10,000, 20,000, 40,000 U/mL in 1 mL single-use vials, 1,000 U/mL in 2 mL multi-use vials, 20,000, U/mL in 1 mL multi-use vials; Epogen® 2,000, 3,000, 4,000, 10,000, 40,000 U/mL in 1 mL single-use vials, 1,000 U/mL in 2 mL multi-use vials, 20,000 U/mL in 1 mL multi-use vials)

INDICATIONS

- Chemotherapy-induced anemia*
- Chronic renal failure–induced anemia*
- HIV-induced anemia*
- Preoperatively for transfusion reduction*

MECHANISM OF ACTION

It stimulates erythroid progenitor cell division and differentiation.

DOSAGE

CHEMOTHERAPY-INDUCED ANEMIA: 150 U/kg SC/IV 3 times a week for 8 weeks. If inadequate response, increase dose to 300 U/kg SC/IV 3 times a week.

CHRONIC RENAL FAILURE-INDUCED ANEMIA: 50–100 U/kg SC/IV 3 times a week, target dose of hematocrit 30–36. If hematocrit increases >4 in 2 weeks, decrease dose by 25 U/kg. If inadequate response after 8 weeks, increase dose by 50–100 U/kg q4–8 weeks.

HIV-INDUCED ANEMIA: 40,000 U SC every week or 100 U/kg SC/IV 3 times a week for 8 weeks. Increase dose by 50–100 U/kg q4–8 weeks to maximum of 300 U/kg 3 times a week.

PREOPERATIVELY FOR TRANSFUSION REDUCTION: 300 U/kg SC qd for 14 days (10 days prior surgery and 4 days after surgery), or 600 U/kg SC every week for 4 doses (given 21, 14, 7 days prior to surgery and the day of surgery). If hemoglobin 10–13, give with iron and daunorubicin-vincristine-prednisone prophylaxis.

DRUG INTERACTIONS

None

SIDE EFFECTS

COMMON: headache, arthralgia, tachycardia, nausea, diarrhea, fever, vomiting, dyspnea, edema, rash, dizziness, fatigue, asthenia, paresthesias, injection site reaction, vascular access thrombosis

RARE: hypertension, congestive heart failure, thromboembolism, vascular access thrombosis, myocardial infarction, stroke, seizures, dyspnea, edema, asthenia, paresthesias

▒ MONITORING

BASELINE: complete blood count. If chronic renal failure, renal function, electrolytes, phosphorus, and uric acid should be checked.

TWICE A WEEK FOR 2–6 WEEKS, THEN AT REGULAR INTERVALS: complete blood count. If chronic renal failure, renal function, electrolytes, phosphorus, and uric acid should be checked at regular intervals.

▒ CONTRAINDICATIONS

Hypersensitivity to drug/class, hypersensitivity to albumin, hypersensitivity to mammal-derived products, uncontrolled hypertension, iron deficiency, folate or vitamin B12 deficiency, congestive heart failure, coronary artery disease, seizures, sickle cell disease, hemolytic anemia, porphyria, hematologic disorders, Jehovah's witness, pregnancy

▒ PREGNANCY CLASS

C

ERYTHROMYCIN, TOPICAL

(ATS® 2% gel in 30, 60 g tubes; solution in 60 mL bottles; Erygel® 2% gel in 30, 60, 65 g tubes; Theramycin Z® 2% solution in 60 mL bottles; T-stat® 2% solution in 60 mL bottles and 2% pads in boxes of 60)

▒ INDICATIONS

- Acne vulgaris* (good gram positive coverage) (see pg. 347)
- Erythrasma (erythromycin$)
- Perioral dermatitis (erythromycin$)
- Rosacea (erythromycin$) (see pg. 395)
- Tufted folliculitis (erythromycin$)

MECHANISM OF ACTION

It binds to the bacterial 50S ribosomal subunit and interferes with protein synthesis (macrolide).

DOSAGE

Apply bid.

DRUG INTERACTIONS

DECREASED EFFICACY/ANTAGONISM OF ERYTHROMYCIN: topical clindamycin

INCREASED IRRITATION/DRYNESS: isotretinoin, topical tretinoin

SIDE EFFECTS

COMMON: burning, peeling, dryness, erythema, oily skin, pruritus, bacterial resistance (when erythromycin used alone)

RARE: contact dermatitis, sensitizer

MONITORING

None

CONTRAINDICATIONS

Hypersensitivity to drug/class

PREGNANCY CLASS

B

ETANERCEPT

(Enbrel® 25 mg SC vials, 50 mg/mL prefilled syringes)

▤ INDICATIONS

- Ankylosing spondylitis*
- Aphthous stomatitis+ (see pg. 352)
- Behçet's syndrome^ (see pg. 355)
- Cicatricial pemphigoid+ (see pg. 356)
- Histiocytosis X+
- Psoriasis*, chronic moderate to severe plaque stage (see pg. 392)
- Psoriatic arthritis*
- Rheumatoid arthritis*, juvenile*
- Scleroderma$ (see pg. 398)
- Wegener's syndrome^ (see pg. 404)

▤ MECHANISM OF ACTION

Recombinant human tumor necrosis factor alpha (TNF-α) receptor fusion protein consisting of two TNF-α receptor p75 extracellular domains and Fc region of immunoglobulin G1. It also inhibits soluble and membrane-bound TNF-α.

▤ DOSAGE

PSORIASIS: 50 mg SC twice a week for 3 months, then 50 mg SC four times a week.

PSORIATIC ARTHRITIS, RHEUMATOID ARTHRITIS, ANKYLOSING SPONDYLITIS: 50 mg SC four times a week.

▤ DRUG INTERACTIONS

INCREASED RISK OF SERIOUS INFECTIONS: immunosuppressants

▤ SIDE EFFECTS

COMMON: Upper respiratory infection, injection site reactions

RARE: reactivation tuberculosis, demyelinating disorders, aplastic anemia, development of positive antinuclear antibody (ANA), development of positive double stranded DNA (dsDNA), drug-induced lupus, malignancy, alopecia, cough, pancytopenia, congestive heart failure, sepsis/serious infections, myelitis, optic neuritis, pharyngitis, headache, rhinitis, abdominal pain, nausea, vomiting, rash

▥ MONITORING

None

▥ CONTRAINDICATIONS

Malignancy, sepsis/infection, congestive heart failure, tuberculosis, use of live vaccines, hypersensitivity to drug/class

▥ PREGNANCY CLASS

B

ETHAMBUTOL

(Myambutol® 100, 400 mg tabs)

▥ INDICATIONS

- *Mycobacterium avium-intracellulare*^
- *Mycobacterium bovis*$
- *Mycobacterium gordonae*+
- *Mycobacterium kansasii*^
- *Mycobacterium scrofulaceum*+
- *Mycobacterium tuberculosis**
- *Mycobacterium ulcerans*+
- *Mycobacterium xenopi*^

See Appendix III.

▥ MECHANISM OF ACTION

It diffuses into mycobacterial cells and inhibits production of metabolites, which impairs cellular metabolism and multiplication, and ends in death of the cell.

▥ DOSAGE

15–25 mg/kg PO qd

RENAL DOSING
    Creatinine clearance (CrCl) 50–90 mL/min: q24h
    CrCl 10–50 mL/min: q24–36h
    CrCl < 10 mL/min: q48h
    Hemodialysis: extra 200 mg PO after dialysis
    Continuous arteriovenous hemofiltration: q24h
    Chronic peritoneal dialysis: q48h.

DRUG INTERACTIONS

DECREASED EFFICACY OF ETHAMBUTOL: antacids

SIDE EFFECTS

COMMON: blurred vision, joint pain, anorexia, nausea, vomiting, dyspepsia, abdominal pain, fever, malaise, headache, dizziness, disorientation, hallucinations, rash, hyperuricemia, pruritus

RARE: anaphylaxis, thrombocytopenia, optic neuritis, peripheral neuropathy, arthralgia, hyperuricemia, loss red-green perception, central scotoma, blindness, confusion, hallucinations, vertigo, anorexia, peripheral neuritis, numbness extremities, eosinophilia, elevated liver function results, retrobulbar neuritis

MONITORING

BASELINE: eye exam

MONTHLY: eye exam if dose > 15 mg/kg/d

CONTRAINDICATIONS

Hypersensitivity to drug/class, optic neuritis, gout, eye disorders, impaired renal function, neurotoxic agents, children

PREGNANCY CLASS

B

EXTRACORPOREAL PHOTOCHEMOTHERAPY (PHOTOPHERESIS)

▨ INDICATIONS

- Atopic dermatitis[+] (see pg. 353)
- Chronic Lyme disease[+]
- Cutaneous T-cell lymphoma stage 2 and 3[^], erythrodermic[*] (see pg. 358)
- Epidermolysis bullosa acquisita[+] (see pg. 363)
- Graft-versus-host disease[$] (see pg. 365)
- Lichen planus, erosive[+] (see pg. 371)
- Lupus[$], systemic[$], discoid[+], subacute cutaneous[+] (see pg. 375)
- Lymphomatoid papulosis[+] (see pg. 377)
- Pemphigus vulgaris[+] (see pg. 385)
- Psoriasis[+] (see pg. 392)
- Psoriatic arthritis[$]
- Scleredema[+]
- Scleroderma[$] (see pg. 398)
- Scleromyxedema[+]
- Transplant rejection, cardiac[^], renal[+], lung[$], liver[+]
- Urticaria, solar[+] (see pg. 403)

▨ MECHANISM OF ACTION

The patient is given 8-methoxypsoralen (8-MOP) prior to photopheresis. The blood is passed through the machine, which separates the plasma and white blood cells from the red blood cells. The red blood cell fraction is returned to the patient, while the plasma/white blood cell fraction is treated with ultraviolet A (UVA) radiation (320–400 nm) and then returned to the patient. This occurs over 6 cycles. Like psoralen and UVA (PUVA), 8-MOP conjugates to DNA after photoactivation, which leads to inhibition of DNA synthesis and cell proliferation. It is also thought that the use of 8-MOP increases the quantity of antigenic peptides in circulation, which leads to an enhanced cytotoxic response.

DOSAGE

Twice a week to monthly. 8-MOP at 0.4 mg/kg plus 10 mg extra. Take within 1.5–3 h before treatment. Liquid 8-MOP can be injected into the photopharesis bag.

DRUG INTERACTIONS

INCREASED PHOTOSENSITIVITY: anthralin, coal tar, griseofulvin, phenothiazines, nalidixic acid, halogenated salicylanilides, sulfonamides, tetracyclines, thiazides, methylene blue, toluidine blue, rose bengal, methyl orange

SIDE EFFECTS

COMMON: nausea, vomiting, pruritus, erythema, edema, headache, hypotension, leg cramps, photosensitivity

RARE: dizziness, nervousness, insomnia, depression, rash, urticaria

MONITORING

BASELINE: eye exam, complete blood count, antinuclear antibodies, liver function, renal function

YEARLY: eye exam

EVERY 6 MONTHS: complete blood count, antinuclear antibodies, liver function, renal function

CONTRAINDICATIONS

Hypersensitivity to drug/class, hepatic disease, renal disease, cataracts, pregnancy

PREGNANCY CLASS

C

FAMCICLOVIR

(Famvir® 125, 250, 500 mg tabs)

▧ INDICATIONS

- Chronic hepatitis B^
- Herpes simplex prophylaxis after laser resurfacing^
- Herpes zoster*
- Herpes zoster ophthalmicus^
- Immunocompromised herpes simplex^
- Mononucleosis⁺
- Primary herpes simplex$
- Recurrent herpes simplex*
- Varicella

▧ MECHANISM OF ACTION

It is the oral prodrug of penciclovir with increased bioavailability, which requires phosphorylation by viral thymidine kinase to become activated. It inhibits viral DNA polymerase and thus DNA synthesis.

▧ DOSAGE

CHRONIC HEPATITIS B: 500 mg PO tid for 12 months

HERPES SIMPLEX PROPHYLAXIS AFTER LASER RESURFACING: 500 mg PO bid for 10 days

HERPES ZOSTER: 500 mg PO q8h for 7 days

HERPES ZOSTER OPHTHALMICUS: 500 mg PO tid for 7 days

IMMUNOCOMPROMISED RECURRENT OROLABIAL AND GENITAL HERPES: 500 mg PO bid for 7 days

MONONUCLEOSIS: 500 mg PO tid for 3 days

RECURRENT GENITAL HERPES: 125 mg PO q12h for 5 days

RECURRENT OROLABIAL OR GENITAL HERPES: 500 mg PO q12h for 7 days

SUPPRESSION OF RECURRENT GENITAL AND OROLABIAL HERPES: 250 mg
PO q12h

VARICELLA: 1000 mg PO tid for 7days

RENAL DOSING
Creatinine clearance (CrCl) 50–90 mL/min: 500 mg PO q8h
CrCl 10–50 mL/min: 500 mg PO q12h–q24h
CrCl < 10 mL/min: 250 mg PO q24h
Hemodialysis: 250 mg PO q24h after dialysis
Continuous ambulatory peritoneal dialysis: no data
Continuous arteriovenous hemofiltration: 500 mg PO q12h–q24h

DRUG INTERACTIONS

INCREASED LEVELS OF FAMCICLOVIR: probenecid, cimetidine, theophylline

SIDE EFFECTS

COMMON: headache, nausea, diarrhea, paresthesias, migraine, fatigue, vomiting, flatulence, abdominal pain, pruritus, rash, dysmenorrhea

RARE: none

MONITORING

None

CONTRAINDICATIONS

Hypersensitivity to drug/class or penciclovir

PREGNANCY CLASS

B

FEXOFENADINE

(Allegra® 30, 60, 180 mg tabs)

INDICATIONS

- Allergic rhinitis*
- Atopic dermatitis^ (see pg. 353)
- Urticaria, chronic* (see pg. 403)

MECHANISM OF ACTION

It is the active metabolite of terfenadine, which blocks H_1 histamine receptors. It has low sedative and anticholinergic effects.

DOSAGE

120–180 mg PO qd

RENAL DOSING: 60 mg PO qd

DRUG INTERACTIONS

DECREASED LEVELS OF FEXOFENADINE: antacids

INCREASED LEVELS OF FEXOFENADINE: ketoconazole, erythromycin

SIDE EFFECTS

COMMON: headache, dizziness, drowsiness

RARE: hypersensitivity reaction, back pain, upper respiratory infection, dyspepsia, fatigue, cough, fever, otitis, sinusitis

MONITORING

None

CONTRAINDICATIONS

Hypersensitivity to drug/class, impaired renal function, pregnancy

PREGNANCY CLASS

C

FILGRASTIM

(Neupogen® 300 µg/mL in 1 mL vials; 480 µg/1.6 ml in 1.6 mL vials; 300 µg/ 0.5 mL in 1 mL pre-filled syringes; 480 µg/0.8 mL in 1 mL pre-filled syringes)

INDICATIONS

- AIDS neutropenia*
- Post–bone marrow transfusion neutropenia*
- Postchemotherapy neutropenia*
- Progenitor mobilization*

MECHANISM OF ACTION

It is a human recombinant granulocyte colony–stimulating factor that stimulates granulocyte and macrophage proliferation and differentiation, and activates some end-cell functions.

DOSAGE

AIDS NEUTROPENIA: 1–10 µg/kg SC qd

POST–BONE MARROW TRANSFUSION NEUTROPENIA: Start at least 24 h after chemotherapy at 10 µg/kg IV qd infused over 4 h or 24 h.

POSTCHEMOTHERAPY NEUTROPENIA: Start at least 24 h after chemotherapy at 5 µg/kg SC/IV qd. May increase dose by 5 µg/kg per cycle. Continue for 2 weeks.

PROGENITOR MOBILIZATION: Start 4 days before first leukapheresis at 10 μg/kg SC qd and continue through last leukopheresis.

DRUG INTERACTIONS

INCREASED SENSITIVITY OF RAPIDLY DIVIDING MYELOID CELLS CYTO-TOXIC EFFECTS: cytotoxic chemotherapy

INCREASED RISK OF LEUKOCYTOSIS: lithium

SIDE EFFECTS

COMMON: bone pain, musculoskeletal pain, splenomegaly, injection site reaction, elevated alkaline phosphatase levels, elevated lactate dehydrogenase levels, hyperuricemia, nausea, abdominal pain, flank pain, headache, thrombocytopenia, anemia, hypotension, leukocytosis, alopecia, diarrhea, neutropenic fever, mucositis, dyspnea, cough, rash

RARE: splenic rupture, acute respiratory distress syndrome, anaphylaxis, thrombocytosis, myocardial infarction, arrhythmias, epistaxis, transfusion reactions, chest pain, sore throat, constipation, hemorrhagic complications, Sweet's-like rash

MONITORING

BASELINE AND TWICE A DAY: complete blood count with absolute neutrophil count. May discontinue if absolute neutrophil count > 1000 for 3 days and after expected nadir.

CONTRAINDICATIONS

Hypersensitivity to drug/class, hypersensitivity to *Escherichia coli* proteins, sickle cell disease, myelodysplasia, myeloid malignancy, pregnancy

PREGNANCY CLASS

C

FINASTERIDE

(Propecia® 1 mg)

▦ INDICATIONS

- Androgenic alopecia, female⁺, male* (see pg. 351)
- Hidradenitis suppurativa⁺
- Hirsutism^

▦ MECHANISM OF ACTION

Inhibitor of type II 5-α-reductase, which stimulates conversion of testosterone to dihydrotestosterone.

▦ DOSAGE

1 mg PO qd

▦ DRUG INTERACTIONS

None

▦ SIDE EFFECTS

COMMON: decreased libido, decreased ejaculate volume, impotence, erectile dysfunction, gynecomastia, myopathy

RARE: hypersensitivity reaction, teratogenicity (male fetus)

▦ MONITORING

BASELINE: prostate-specific antigen in men over 50 years of age

▦ CONTRAINDICATIONS

Hypersensitivity to drug, pregnancy, women and children, liver disease

▓ PREGNANCY CLASS

X

FLUCONAZOLE

(Diflucan® 50, 100, 150, 200 mg tabs; 10 mg/mL and 40 mg/mL suspension in 35 mL bottles; 200 mg/100 mL and 400 mg/200 mL solution for IV)

▓ INDICATIONS

- Blastomycosis^
- Candidiasis, bacteremia*
- Candidiasis, bladder*
- Candidiasis, cut^
- Candidiasis, endocarditis*
- Candidiasis, esophageal*
- Candidiasis, HIV stomatitis/esophagitis/vaginitis*
- Candidiasis, oropharyngeal*
- Candidiasis, peritonitis*
- Candidiasis, prophylaxis bone marrow transplant (BMT)*
- Candidiasis, thrush*
- Candidiasis, vaginal*
- Coccidioidomycosis, meningitis, pulmonary with HIV^
- Cryptococcosis, meningitis, HIV, non-HIV, non-meningitis*
- Onychomycosis^
- Sporotrichosis, cutaneous and lymphonodular$
- Tinea capitis^
- Tinea corporis, cruris, pedis^
- Tinea versicolor

See Appendix I.

▓ MECHANISM OF ACTION

It is a fungistatic agent that inhibits fungal cytochrome P450 sterol C14 alpha-demethylation.

▓ DOSAGE

ONYCHOMYCOSIS: 150–300 mg PO every week for 3–6 months for fingernails, 6–12 months for toenails

TINEA CAPITIS: 8 mg/kg PO every week for 8–12 weeks

TINEA CORPORIS, CRURIS, PEDIS: 150 mg PO every week for 2–4 weeks

TINEA VERSICOLOR: 400 mg PO once

See Appendix I.

RENAL DOSING FOR IV
   Creatinine clearance (CrCL) 50–90 mL/min: normal dose of 200–400 mg IV qd
   CrCl < 50 mL/min, continuous arteriovenous hemofiltration, chronic ambulatory peritoneal dialysis: 50% of normal dose
   Hemodialysis: extra 200 mg IV after dialysis

DRUG INTERACTIONS

INCREASED CENTRAL NERVOUS SYSTEM DEPRESSION: alfentanil, benzodiazepines, propoxyphene, buprenorphine, fentanyl

INCREASED LEVELS OF: amiodarone, almotriptan, aprepitant, aripiprazole, bosentan, budesonide, buspirone, ergotamine, carbamazepine, celecoxib, cilostazol, cyclopsorin, digoxin, eletriptan, statins, imatinib, levobupivacaine, metformin, sulfonylureas, methadone, mifepristone, modafinil, nefazodone, phenytoin, quetiapine, quinidine, repaglinide, sildenafil, sirolimus, tacrolimus, theophylline, tolterodine, vinca alkaloids, warfarin, ziprasidone, zonisamide

INCREASED LEVELS OF FLUCONAZOLE: amprenavir, protease inhibitors, paclitaxel

DECREASED LEVELS OF FLUCONAZOLE: barbiturates, rifampins

INCREASED RISK OF HYPOTENSION: bepridil, calcium channel blockers

INCREASED QT PROLONGATION: cisapride, pimozide

INCREASED ARRHYTHMIAS: disopyramide

INCREASED HYPERGLYCEMIA: pioglitazone

SIDE EFFECTS

COMMON: nausea, headache, rash, vomiting, abdominal pain, diarrhea, dyspepsia, aguesia, dizziness

Rare: hepatotoxicity, Stevens-Johnson syndrome, angioedema, seizures, leukopenia, agranulocytosis, toxic epidermal necrolysis, alopecia, neutropenia, thrombocytopenia, hypercholesterolemia, hypertriglyceridemia, hypokalemia

MONITORING

None

CONTRAINDICATIONS

Hypersensitivity to drug/class, impaired liver or renal function, pregnancy

PREGNANCY CLASS

C

FLUCYTOSINE

(Ancobon® 250, 500 mg caps)

INDICATIONS

- Candidiasis, endocarditis*
- Candidiasis, peritonitis*
- Cryptococcosis*

See Appendix I.

MECHANISM OF ACTION

The exact mechanism of action is unknown.

DOSAGE

See Appendix I.

▨ DRUG INTERACTIONS

INCREASED LEVELS OF: adefovir, tenofovir

INCREASED NEPHROTOXICITY: adefovir, aminoglycosides, amphotericin, cidofovir, zoledronic acid

INCREASED BONE MARROW SUPPRESSION: bone marrow suppressants, carboplatin, cisplatin, clozapine, cytotoxic chemotherapy, interferon alpha, interferon beta, zidovudine

INCREASED ACIDOSIS: metformin, sulfonylureas, rituximab

▨ SIDE EFFECTS

COMMON: chest pain, dyspnea, rash, pruritus, nausea, vomiting, abdominal pain, diarrhea, azotemia, anemia, ataxia, headache, paresthesias, confusion, hallucinations, fatigue, hypoglycemia, hypokalemia, vertigo

RARE: cardiac arrest, ventricular dysfunction, respiratory arrest, gastrointestinal bleed, ulcerative colitis, renal failure, agranulocytosis, aplastic anemia, thrombocytopenia, pruritus, photosensitivity, anorexia, dry mouth, gastrointestinal ulcer, jaundice, hyperbilirubinemia, crystalluria, leukopenia, thrombocytopenia, eosinophilia, hearing loss, peripheral neuropathy, sedation, seizures, psychosis, weakness, toxic epidermal necrolysis

▨ MONITORING

BASELINE AND WEEKLY: renal function, complete blood count

▨ CONTRAINDICATIONS

Hypersensitivity to drug/class, impaired renal and liver function, bone marrow suppression, pregnancy

▨ PREGNANCY CLASS

C

FLUOCINOLONE ACETONIDE 0.01%, HYDROQUINONE 4%, TRETINOIN 0.05%

(Tri-Luma® cream in 30 g tubes)

INDICATIONS

- Melasma*

MECHANISM OF ACTION

Hydroquinone inhibits tyrosinase, which prevents conversion of tyrosine to dopa. Tretinoin is a topical retinoid that modifies abnormal follicular keratinization to promote the detachment of cornified cells and to enhance the shedding of corneocytes from the follicle. It also increases the mitotic activity of follicular epithelia, which increases the turnover of corneocytes. It also modulates the proliferation and differentiation of epidermal cells by activation of retinoic acid receptors, which alters gene expression. Fluocinolone is a topical steroid that exerts anti-inflammatory and immunosuppressive effects. It inhibits nuclear factor kappa B (NFkB) to decrease production of interleukin-1, tumor necrosis factor alpha, adhesion molecules, and growth factors. It also inhibits AP-1, which is a heterodimeric transcription factor composed of c-jun, c-fos and activating transcription factor, to decrease cytokine production. It causes lymphocyte and eosinophil apoptosis. It inhibits phospholipase-A2, which leads to decreased production of cyclooxygenase, prostaglandins, leukotrienes, and hydroxyeicosatetraenoic acid inflammatory mediators.

DOSAGE

Apply qhs. Should use with sunscreen qd.

DRUG INTERACTIONS

Do not use concurrently with hydroquinone, retinoid, or topical steroids.

■ SIDE EFFECTS

COMMON: erythema, burning, dryness, desquamation, rash, rosacea, acne, perioral dermatitis, telangiectasias, pruritus, irritation, pigmentary alterations

RARE: atrophy, striae, exogenous ochronosis, contact dermatitis, paresthesias, suppression of hypothalamic-pituitary adrenal (HPA) axis

■ MONITORING

None. If suspected HPA axis suppression develops, check adrenocorticotropic hormone or cosyntropin, morning plasma cortisol, and urinary free cortisol

■ CONTRAINDICATIONS

Avoid sun exposure and photosensitizing medications; hypersensitivity to drug/class or sulfites, pregnancy

■ PREGNANCY CLASS

C

FLUOROQUINOLONES, FIRST GENERATION

Nalidixic acid (NegGram® 0.25, 0.5, 1 g tabs; 250 mg/5 mL suspension)

■ INDICATIONS

- *Enterobacter* sp.*
- *Escherichia coli**
- *Klebsiella* sp.*
- *Proteus* sp.*

See Appendix II.

■ MECHANISM OF ACTION

It is a bactericidal agent that inhibits DNA gyrase.

DOSAGE

1 g PO qid

DRUG INTERACTIONS

DECREASED EFFICACY OF FLUOROQUINOLONES: antacids, calcium, didanosine, iron, multivitamins, sucralfate

DECREASED EFFICACY OF: oral contraceptives, quinapril

INCREASED SEIZURE RISK: nonsteroidal anti-inflammatory drugs

INCREASED BLEEDING RISK: warfarin

SIDE EFFECTS

COMMON: drowsiness, weakness, headache, vertigo, visual disturbances, abdominal pain, nausea, vomiting, diarrhea, rash, pruritus, urticaria, angioedema, photosensitivity, fever, headache

RARE: intracranial hypertension, seizures, leukopenia, thrombocytopenia, pseudomembranous colitis, hemolytic anemia, Stevens-Johnson syndrome, metabolic acidosis, cholestatic jaundice

MONITORING

FREQUENTLY IF LONG-TERM USE: complete blood count, renal function, liver function

CONTRAINDICATIONS

Hypersensitivity to drug/class, seizures, impaired liver/renal/pulmonary function, cardiovascular disease, pregnancy

PREGNANCY CLASS

C

FLUOROQUINOLONES, SECOND GENERATION

Ciprofloxacin (Cipro® 100, 250, 500, 750 mg tabs; 250, 500 mg/5 mL suspension; IV), enoxacin (Penetrex® 200, 400 mg tabs), lomefloxacin (Maxaquin® 400 mg tabs), norfloxacin (Noroxin® 400 mg tabs), ofloxacin (Floxin® 200, 300, 400 mg tabs)

▣ INDICATIONS

- *Bacillus anthracis* (ciprofloxacin*)
- *Bacteroides fragilis* (ciprofloxacin*)
- *Chlamydia trachomatis* (ofloxacin*)
- *Citrobacter freundii* and *diversus* (ciprofloxacin*, lomefloxacin*, norfloxacin*, ofloxacin*)
- *Enterobacter cloacae* and *aerogenes**
- *Enterococcus faecalis* (ciprofloxacin*, norfloxacin*)
- *Escherichia coli**
- *Haemophilus influenzae* (ciprofloxacin*, lomefloxacin*, ofloxacin*)
- *Haemophilus parainfluenzae* (ciprofloxacin*)
- *Klebsiella pneumoniae**
- *Moraxella catarrhalis* (ciprofloxacin*, lomefloxacin*)
- *Morganella morganii* (ciprofloxacin*)
- *Neisseria gonorrhoeae**
- *Proteus mirabilis**
- *Proteus vulgaris* (norfloxacin*, enoxacin*)
- *Providencia stuartii* (ciprofloxacin*)
- *Pseudomonas aeruginosa**
- *Serratia marcescens* (ciprofloxacin*, norfloxacin*, ofloxacin*)
- *Staphylococcus aureus,* methicillin sensitive (ciprofloxacin*, norfloxacin*, ofloxacin*)
- *Staphylococcus epidermidis**
- *Staphylococcus saprophyticus* (enoxacin*, norfloxacin*)
- *Streptococcus agalactiae* (norfloxacin*)
- *Streptococcus pneumoniae* (ciprofloxacin*, ofloxacin*, lomefloxacin*)
- *Streptococcus pyogenes* (ciprofloxacin*, norfloxacin*, ofloxacin*)

See Appendix II.

Usually effective:

- *Aeromonas* sp.
- *Chlamydia* sp. (lomefloxacin, ofloxacin)

- *Citrobacter* sp.
- *Enterobacter* sp.
- *Klebsiella* sp. (not enoxacin)
- *Legionella* sp. (ofloxacin, ciprofloxacin)
- *Listeria monocytogenes* (lomefloxacin)
- *Moraxella catarrhalis* (ofloxacin)
- *Morganella* sp.
- *Mycoplasma pneumoniae* (ciprofloxacin, ofloxacin)
- *Neisseria meningitidis* (ciprofloxacin, ofloxacin)
- *Pasteurella multocida* (ofloxacin, ciprofloxacin)
- *Proteus vulgaris* (lomefloxacin, ofloxacin, ciprofloxacin)
- *Providencia* sp.
- *Salmonella* sp. (not lomefloxacin)
- *Serratia* sp.
- *Shigella* sp. (not lomefloxacin)
- *Staphylococcus aureus*, methicillin sensitive (lomefloxacin)
- *Yersinia enterocolitica*

Clinical trials lacking:

- *Acinetobacter* sp. (ciprofloxacin, ofloxacin)
- *Actinomyces* sp. (ofloxacin)
- *Clostridium,* not *difficile* (ofloxacin, ciprofloxacin)
- *Peptostreptococcus* sp. (ofloxacin, ciprofloxacin)
- *Prevotella melaninogenica* (ofloxacin)

MECHANISM OF ACTION

They are bactericidal agents, which inhibit DNA gyrase.

DOSAGE

CIPROFLOXACIN

250–750 mg PO q12h; 200–400 mg IV q12h
  Gonorrhea: 500 mg PO once

RENAL DOSING
  Creatinine clearance (CrCl) 10–50 mL/min: 50–75%
  CrCl < 10 mL/min: 50%
  Hemodialysis: 250 mg PO or 200 mg IV q12h
  Chronic ambulatory peritoneal dialysis (CAPD): 250 mg PO or 200 mg IV q8h
  Continuous arteriovenous hemofiltration (CAVH): 200 mg IV q12h

OFLOXACIN

400 mg PO/IV q12h
  Gonorrhea: 400 mg PO once

HEPATIC DOSING: 400 mg PO qd

RENAL DOSING
  CrCl 10–50 mL/min: 200–400 q12h
  CrCl < 10 mL/min and CAPD: 200 mg q24h
  Hemodialysis: 100–200 mg after dialysis
  CAVH: 300 mg qd

ENOXACIN

200–400 mg PO bid
  Gonorrhea: 400 mg PO once

RENAL DOSING
  CrCl < 30 mL/min: normal dose for first dose, then 50% q12h

HEPATIC DOSING: decrease dose if advanced cirrhosis

LOMEFLOXACIN

400 mg PO qd
  Gonorrhea: 400 mg PO once

RENAL DOSING
  CrCL 10–40 mL/min: 400 mg PO once, then 200 mg PO qd

NORFLOXACIN

400 mg PO bid
  Gonorrhea: 800 mg PO once

RENAL DOSING
  CrCl < 30 mL/min: 400 mg PO qd

▇ DRUG INTERACTIONS

DECREASED EFFICACY OF FLUOROQUINOLONES: antacids, calcium, didanosine, iron, multivitamins, sucralfate, bismuth, ranitidine, didanosine, quercetin, zinc

DECREASED EFFICACY OF: oral contraceptives, quinapril

INCREASED SEIZURE RISK: nonsteroidal anti-inflammatory drugs

INCREASED BLEEDING RISK: warfarin

INCREASED CAFFEINE LEVELS: caffeine (not lomefloxacin)

NEPHROTOXICITY: carbonic anhydrase inhibitors (not lomefloxacin), urinary alkalinizers (not lomefloxacin)

INCREASED LEVELS OF: clozapine (not lomefloxacin), cyclosporin (not lomefloxacin), olanzapine (not lomefloxacin), phenytoin (not lomefloxacin), riluzole (not lomefloxacin), theophylline (not lomefloxacin), tolterodine (only with norfloxacin)

INCREASED LEVELS OF FLUOROQUINOLONES: probenecid

INCREASED HYPOGLYCEMIA: metformin (not lomefloxacin), sulfonylureas (not lomefloxacin)

INCREASED TENDON RUPTURE: steroids

SIDE EFFECTS

COMMON: nausea, vomiting, diarrhea, abdominal pain, dyspepsia, dizziness, restlessness, vaginitis, insomnia, photosensitivity, pruritus, rash, anxiety, agitation, confusion, tendinitis, arthralgia, elevated liver function test results

RARE: seizures, hypersensitivity reactions, phototoxicity, pseudomembranous colitis, superinfection, increased intracranial pressure, psychosis, tendon rupture, arthropathy

MONITORING

FREQUENTLY IF LONG-TERM USE: complete blood count, renal function, liver function

CONTRAINDICATIONS

Hypersensitivity to drug/class, children, impaired renal or liver function, seizures, central nervous system disorder, theophylline (ciprofloxacin, enoxacin), dehydration, diabetes mellitus, sun exposure, pregnancy, lactating, glucose-6-phosphate dehydrogenase deficiency (norfloxacin), myasthenia gravis (norfloxacin)

PREGNANCY CLASS

C

FLUOROQUINOLONES, THIRD GENERATION

Levofloxacin (Levaquin® 250, 500 mg tabs), sparfloxacin (Zagam® 200 mg tabs)

INDICATIONS

- *Chlamydia pneumoniae**
- *Enterobacter cloacae**
- *Enterococcus faecalis* (levofloxacin*)
- *Escherichia coli* (levofloxacin*)
- *Haemophilus influenzae**
- *Haemophilus parainfluenzae* (levofloxacin*)
- *Klebsiella pneumoniae**
- *Legionella pneumophila* (levofloxacin*)
- *Moraxella catarrhalis**
- *Mycoplasma pneumoniae**
- *Proteus mirabilis* (levofloxacin*)
- *Pseudomonas aeruginosa* (levofloxacin*)
- *Staphylococcus aureus,* methicillin sensitive*
- *Staphylococcus saprophyticus* (levofloxacin*)
- *Streptococcus pneumoniae**
- *Streptococcus pyogenes* (levofloxacin*)

See Appendix II.

Usually effective (levofloxacin):

- *Aeromonas* sp.
- *Chlamydia* sp.
- *Citrobacter* sp.
- *Clostridium,* not *difficile*
- *Morganella* sp.
- *Neisseria gonorrhoeae*

- *Neisseria meningitidis*
- *Pasteurella multocida*
- *Peptostreptococcus* sp.
- *Prevotella melaninogenica*
- *Proteus vulgaris*
- *Providencia* sp.
- *Salmonella* sp.
- *Serratia* sp.
- *Shigella* sp.
- *Staphylococcus epidermidis*
- *Streptococcus milleri*
- *Streptococcus viridans*
- *Yersinia enterocolitica*

Clinical trials lacking (levofloxacin):

- *Acinetobacter* sp.
- *Stenotrophomonas maltophilia*

MECHANISM OF ACTION

They are bactericidal agents that inhibit bacterial DNA gyrase.

DOSAGE

LEVOFLOXACIN

250–500 mg PO/IV qd

RENAL DOSING
Creatinine clearance (CrCl) 10–50 mL/min and continuous arteriovenous hemo-filtration (CAVH): 500 mg once, then 250 mg q24–48h
CrCl < 10 mL/min and hemodialysis and chronic ambulatory peritoneal dialysis (CAPD): 500 mg once, then 250 mg q48h

SPARFLOXACIN

400 mg PO once, then 200 mg PO qd

RENAL DOSING
CrCl 10–50 mL/min: 50–75%
CrCl < 10 mL/min and hemodialysis: 50% q48h
CAPD and CAVH: no data

▥ DRUG INTERACTIONS

DECREASED EFFICACY OF FLUOROQUINOLONES: antacids, calcium, didanosine, iron, multivitamins, sucralfate

DECREASED EFFICACY OF: oral contraceptives, quinapril

INCREASED SEIZURE RISK: nonsteroidal anti-inflammatory drugs

INCREASED BLEEDING RISK: warfarin

NEPHROTOXICITY: carbonic anhydrase inhibitors

INCREASED LEVELS OF FLUOROQUINOLONES: probenecid

INCREASED HYPOGLYCEMIA: metformin, sulfonylureas

INCREASED TENDON RUPTURE: steroids

INCREASED QT INTERVAL: thiazides, amphotericin, class IA and III antiarrhythmics, beta-2 agonists, cidofovir, cisapride, cisplatin, dolasetron, droperidol, erythromycin, foscarnet, haloperidol, halothane, mefloquine, meperidine, phenothiazines, pimozide, promethazine, risperidone, ziprasidone, tricyclic antidepressants

▥ SIDE EFFECTS

COMMON: nausea, vomiting, diarrhea, abdominal pain, headache, dyspepsia, dizziness, restlessness, lightheadedness, vaginitis, insomnia, pruritus, rash, photosensitivity, anxiety, agitation, confusion, tendinitis, arthralgia, elevated liver function test results

RARE: anaphylaxis, hypersensitivity reactions, phototoxicity, pseudomembranous colitis, superinfection, increased intracranial pressure, seizures, psychosis, tendon rupture, arthropathy, QT prolongation, torsades de pointes

▥ MONITORING

FREQUENTLY IF LONG-TERM USE: complete blood count, renal function, liver function

▥ CONTRAINDICATIONS

Hypersensitivity to drug/class, pregnancy, lactating, children, prolonged QT, class IA and III antiarrhythmics, impaired renal function, seizures, central nervous system disorder, dehydration, diabetes mellitus, sun exposure, hypo-kalemia, bradycardia, cardiomyopathy, proarrhythmic conditions

PREGNANCY CLASS

C

FLUOROQUINOLONES, FOURTH GENERATION

Gatifloxacin (Tequin® 200, 400 mg tabs; IV), moxifloxacin (Avelox® 400 mg tabs), trovafloxacin (Trovan® 100, 200 mg tabs)

INDICATIONS

- *Bacteroides fragilis* (trovafloxacin*)
- *Chlamydia pneumoniae**
- *Enterococcus faecalis* (trovafloxacin*)
- *Escherichia coli* (trovafloxacin*, gatifloxacin*)
- *Gardnerella vaginalis* (trovafloxacin*)
- *Haemophilus influenzae**
- *Haemophilus parainfluenzae* (gatifloxacin*, moxifloxacin*)
- *Klebsiella pneumoniae**
- *Legionella pneumophila* (gatifloxacin*, trovafloxacin*)
- *Moraxella catarrhalis**
- *Mycoplasma pneumoniae**
- *Neisseria gonorrhoeae* (gatifloxacin*)
- *Peptostreptococcus* sp. (trovafloxacin*)
- *Prevotella* sp. (trovafloxacin*)
- *Proteus mirabilis* (trovafloxacin*, gatifloxacin*)
- *Pseudomonas aeruginosa* (trovafloxacin*)
- *Staphylococcus aureus,* methicillin sensitive*
- *Streptococcus agalactiae* (trovafloxacin*)
- *Streptococcus pneumoniae**
- *Streptococcus pyogenes* (moxifloxacin*)
- *Streptococcus viridans* (trovafloxacin*)

See Appendix II.

Usually effective:

- *Actinomyces* sp. (moxifloxacin, gatifloxacin)
- *Aeromonas* sp.
- *Bacteroides fragilis* (moxifloxacin)
- *Chlamydia* sp.
- *Citrobacter* sp.
- *Clostridium,* not *difficile*
- *Enterobacter* sp.
- *Enterococcus faecalis* (gatifloxacin, moxifloxacin)
- *Escherichia coli* (moxifloxacin)
- *Legionella* sp.
- *Listeria monocytogenes* (trovafloxacin)
- *Morganella* sp.
- *Neisseria gonorrhoeae* (trovafloxacin, gatifloxacin)
- *Neisseria meningitidis*
- *Pasteurella multocida*
- *Peptostreptococcus* sp. (moxifloxacin, gatifloxacin)
- *Prevotella melaninogenica*
- *Proteus mirabilis* (moxifloxacin)
- *Proteus vulgaris*
- *Providencia* sp.
- *Salmonella* sp.
- *Serratia* sp.
- *Shigella* sp.
- *Staphylococcus epidermidis*
- *Stenotrophomonas maltophilia* (trovafloxacin, moxifloxacin)
- *Streptococcus milleri*
- *Yersinia enterocolitica*

Clinical trials lacking:

- *Acinetobacter* sp.
- *Bacteroides fragilis* (gatifloxacin)
- *Clostridium difficile*
- *Enterococcus faecium*
- *Pseudomonas aeruginosa* (moxifloxacin, gatifloxacin)

MECHANISM OF ACTION

They are bactericidal agents that inhibit bacterial DNA gyrase.

▓ DOSAGE

GATIFLOXACIN

400 mg PO/IV qd

RENAL DOSING
Creatinine clearance (CrCl) < 50 mL/min, continuous arteriovenous hemofiltration, and chronic ambulatory peritoneal dialysis: 200 mg qd
Hemodialysis: 200 mg qd after dialysis

MOXIFLOXACIN

400 mg PO/IV qd

TROVAFLOXACIN

200 mg PO/IV qd

HEPATIC DOSING: Decrease dose 50%.

▓ DRUG INTERACTIONS

DECREASED EFFICACY OF FLUOROQUINOLONES: antacids, calcium, didanosine, iron, multivitamins, sucralfate, morphine (trovafloxacin)

DECREASED EFFICACY OF: oral contraceptives, quinapril

INCREASED SEIZURE RISK: nonsteroidal anti-inflammatory drugs

INCREASED BLEEDING RISK: warfarin

NEPHROTOXICITY: carbonic anhydrase inhibitors (not trovafloxacin)

INCREASED LEVELS OF FLUOROQUINOLONES: probenecid (gatifloxacin)

INCREASED HYPOGLYCEMIA (NOT TROVAFLOXACIN): metformin, sulfonylureas

INCREASED TENDON RUPTURE: steroids

INCREASED QT INTERVAL (NOT TROVAFLOXACIN): thiazides, amphotericin, class IA and III antiarrhythmics, beta-2 agonists, cidofovir, cisapride, cisplatin, dolasetron, droperidol, erythromycin, foscarnet, haloperidol, halothane, mefloquine, meperidine, phenothiazines, pimozide, promethazine, risperidone, ziprasidone, tricyclic antidepressants

SIDE EFFECTS

COMMON: nausea, vomiting, diarrhea, abdominal pain, headache, dyspepsia, dizziness, restlessness, lightheadedness, vaginitis, insomnia, pruritus, rash, photosensitivity, anxiety, agitation, confusion, tendinitis, arthralgia, elevated liver function test results

RARE: anaphylaxis, hypersensitivity reactions, phototoxicity, pseudomembranous colitis, superinfection, increased intracranial pressure, seizures, psychosis, tendon rupture, arthropathy, QT prolongation, torsades de pointes, hypoglycemia

MONITORING

FREQUENTLY IF LONG-TERM USE: complete blood count, renal function, liver function

CONTRAINDICATIONS

Hypersensitivity to drug/class, pregnancy, lactating, children, prolonged QT, class IA and III antiarrhythmics, impaired renal function, seizures, central nervous system disorder, dehydration, diabetes mellitus, sun exposure, hypokalemia, bradycardia, proarrhythmic conditions, hypokalemia, myocardial ischemia, impaired liver function (trovafloxacin)

PREGNANCY CLASS

C

FLUOROURACIL

(Efudex® 2, 5% solution in 10 mL bottles, 5% cream in 25 g tubes; Carac® 0.5% cream in 30 g tubes)

INDICATIONS

- Actinic keratoses* (see pg. 348)
- Basal cell carcinoma, superficial* (see pg. 354)
- Bowen's disease$

- Condylomata acuminata$ (see pg. 406)
- Keratoacanthoma$
- Squamous cell carcinoma$ (see pg. 400)

MECHANISM OF ACTION

It blocks the methylation reaction of deoxyuridylic acid to thymidylic acid, which inhibits DNA and RNA synthesis.

DOSAGE

Apply with nonmetal applicator and gloves, and wash hands afterward. Avoid sun exposure. Complete healing should occur 1–2 months after finishing treatment.

ACTINIC KERATOSES: Apply bid for 2–4 weeks.

BOWEN'S DISEASE, SQUAMOUS CELL CARCINOMA, KERATOACANTHOMA: Apply bid for 2–8 weeks.

SUPERFICIAL BASAL CELL CARCINOMAS: Apply bid for 3–6 weeks. Use 5% strength only.

DRUG INTERACTIONS

None

SIDE EFFECTS

COMMON: pruritus, dermatitis, burning, erythema, peeling, erosions

RARE: hyperpigmentation, photosensitivity, scarring, leukocytosis, insomnia, irritability, eosinophilia, thrombocytopenia, toxic granulation, alopecia, blistering, bullous pemphigoid, scaling, urticaria, conjunctival reaction, corneal reaction, lacrimation, nasal irritation, herpes simplex

MONITORING

None

▨ CONTRAINDICATIONS

Hypersensitivity to drug/class, pregnancy

▨ PREGNANCY CLASS

X

FOSCARNET

(Foscavir® 24 mg/mL, 250 and 500 mL vials)

▨ INDICATIONS

- Acyclovir-resistant herpes simplex virus*
- Cytomegalovirus retinitis in AIDS patients*

▨ MECHANISM OF ACTION

It is an organic analog of an inorganic pyrophosphate that inhibits replication of herpesvirus by inhibition of DNA polymerases. It does not require activation by thymidine kinase.

▨ DOSAGE

CYTOMEGALOVIRUS RETINITIS: 90 mg/kg IV q12h for 2–3 weeks for induction, then 90 mg/kg/d IV for maintenance

ACYCLOVIR-RESISTANT HERPES SIMPLEX VIRUS: 40 mg/kg IV q8–12 h for 2–3 weeks, 750–1000 mL saline solution IV prior to infusion

RENAL DOSING INDUCTION
Creatinine Clearance (CrCl) > 1.4 mL/min/kg: 60 mg/kg IV q8h
CrCl 1–1.4 mL/min/kg: 45 mg/kg IV q8h
CrCl 0.8–1 mL/min/kg: 50 mg/kg IV q12h
CrCl 0.6–0.8 mL/min/kg: 40 mg/kg IV q12h
CrCl 0.5–0.6 mL/min/kg: 60 mg/kg q24h
CrCl 0.4–0.5 mL/min/kg: 50 mg/kg IV q24h
CrCl < 0.4 mL/min/kg: Do not use.

RENAL DOSING MAINTENANCE
CrCl > 1.4 mL/min/kg: 120 mg/kg IV q24h
CrCl 1–1.4 mL/min/kg: 90 mg/kg IV q24h
CrCl 0.8–1 mL/min/kg: 65 mg/kg IV q24h
CrCl 0.6–0.8 mL/min/kg: 105 mg/kg IV q48h
CrCl 0.5–0.6 mL/min/kg: 80 mg/kg IV q48h
CrCl 0.4–0.5 mL/min/kg: 65 mg/kg IV q48h
CrCl < 0.4 mL/min/kg: Do not use.

DRUG INTERACTIONS

NEPHROTOXICITY: adefovir, aminoglycosides, cidofovir, nephrotoxic agents, tenofovir, zoledronic acid

INCREASED BORE MARROW SUPPRESSION: bone marrow suppressants, carboplatin, cisplatin, clozapine, cytotoxic chemotherapy, interferon alpha and beta, oxaliplatin, rituximab, zidovudine

INCREASED PERIPHERAL NEUROPATHY: didanosine

INCREASED SEIZURES: imipenem

INCREASED LACTIC ACIDOSIS: metformin/sulfonylureas, metformin

INCREASED LEVELS OF GANCICLOVIR: mycophenolate mofetil, probenecid

INCREASED HYPOKALEMIA: angiotensin receptor blockers/hydrochlorothiazide combinations, carbonic anhydrase inhibitors

INCREASED QT PROLONGATION: class III antiarrhythmics, bepridil, cisapride, dolasetron, droperidol, meperidine/promethazine, phenothiazides, pimozide, quinolones

SIDE EFFECTS

COMMON: fever, nausea, diarrhea, vomiting, headache, asthenia, hypocalcemia, hypophosphatemia, hypokalemia, local burning, elevated creatinine, hypo/hypermagnesemia

RARE: pancreatitis, renal failure, anemia, granulocytopenia, leukopenia, bone marrow suppression, thrombocytopenia, bronchospasms, seizures

MONITORING

BASELINE: creatinine, calcium, phosphorus, potassium, magnesium

2–3 TIMES A WEEK DURING INDUCTION: creatinine, calcium, phosphorus, potassium, magnesium

EVERY 1–2 WEEKS DURING MAINTENANCE: creatinine, calcium, phosphorus, potassium, magnesium
Discontinue if creatinine clearance < 0.4 mL/min/kg.

CONTRAINDICATIONS

Hypersensitivity to drug/class, pregnancy

PREGNANCY CLASS

C

GABAPENTIN

(Neurontin® 100, 300, 400, 800 mg cap; 600 mg tabs; 250 mg/5 mL in 40 mL bottle of solution)

INDICATIONS

- Neuropathic pain^
- Partial seizures*
- Postherpetic neuralgia^ (see pg. 389)
- Pruritus, brachoradial+

MECHANISM OF ACTION

It is structurally related to the neurotransmitter gamma-aminobutyric acid (GABA) but does not interact with its receptors, inhibit uptake/degradation, or convert into GABA. The exact mechanism is unknown.

▦ DOSAGE

Start at 300 mg PO qd day 1, then bid day 2, tid day 3. Stop at maximum dose of 3600 mg/d.

NEUROPATHIC PAIN: 300–1200 mg PO tid

PARTIAL SEIZURES: 300–1200 mg PO tid

POSTHERPETIC NEURALGIA, BRACHORADIAL PRURITUS: 300–600 mg PO tid

RENAL DOSING
Creatinine clearance (CrCl) 30–60: maximum 300 mg PO bid
CrCl 15–30: maximum 300 mg PO qd
CrCl < 15: maximum 300 mg PO qod

▦ DRUG INTERACTIONS

DECREASED BIOAVAILABILITY OF DRUG: antacids

INCREASED CENTRAL NERVOUS SYSTEM DEPRESSION: alcohol

▦ SIDE EFFECTS

COMMON: somnolence, dizziness, ataxia, fatigue, nystagmus, tremor, diplopia, rhinitis, blurred vision, nausea, vomiting, nervousness, dysarthria, weight gain, dyspepsia, rash, acne, back pain, edema, vasodilation, dry mouth, constipation, myalgia, amnesia, cough, pruritus, impotence, amblyopia, hypertension, hypotension, migraine

RARE: leukopenia, tachycardia, glossitis, hepatomegaly, hyper-/hypothyroid, arthralgia, arthritis, anxiety, paresthesias, increased/decreased reflexes, pneumonia, dyspnea, apnea, alopecia, eczema, increased sweating, seborrhea, herpes simplex, hematuria, dysuria, urinary retention/incontinence, vaginal bleeding

CHILDREN: viral infection, fever, hostility, emotional lability, bronchitis, hyperkinesia

▦ MONITORING

None

CONTRAINDICATIONS

Hypersensitivity to drug/class, renal impairment, pregnancy. Avoid abrupt withdrawal of drug.

PREGNANCY CLASS

C

GANCICLOVIR

(Cytovene® 250, 500 mg cap, 500 mg vials)

INDICATIONS

- Cytomegalovirus (CMV) colitis^
- CMV pneumonia^
- CMV retinitis*
- Herpes simiae$
- Herpes simplex virus keratitis^
- Prophylaxis against CMV in transplant and advanced HIV patients*

MECHANISM OF ACTION

It is a nucleoside analog of deoxyguanosine that inhibits viral DNA synthesis by inhibiting viral DNA polymerases and by incorporating into viral DNA, to result in chain termination.

DOSAGE

CMV RETINITIS

INDUCTION: 5 mg/kg IV q12h for 14–21 days

MAINTENANCE: 5 mg/kg IV qd or 1000 mg PO tid

PROPHYLAXIS

5 mg/kg IV q12h for 7–14 days, then 5 mg/kg IV qd; or 1000 mg PO tid

RENAL DOSING INDUCTION
Creatinine clearance (CrCl) 50–90 mL/min: 5 mg/kg IV q12h
CrCl 10–50 mL/min: 1.25–2.5 mg/kg IV q24h
CrCl < 10 mL/min: 1.25 mg/kg IV three times a week
Continuous ambulatory peritoneal dialysis: 1.25 mg/kg IV 3 times a week after dialysis
Hemodialysis: dose after dialysis

RENAL DOSING MAINTENANCE
Creatinine clearance (CrCl) 50–90 mL/min: 2.5–5 mg/kg IV q24h
CrCl 10–50 mL/min: 0.6–1.25 mg/kg IV q24h
CrCl < 10 mL/min: 0.625 mg/kg IV 3 times a week
Hemodialysis: 0.6 mg/kg IV after dialysis
Continuous ambulatory peritoneal dialysis: 0.625 mg/kg IV 3 times a week

▧ DRUG INTERACTIONS

NEPHROTOXICITY: adefovir, aminoglycosides, cidofovir, nephrotoxic agents, tenofovir

INCREASED BONE MARROW SUPPRESSION: bone marrow suppressants, carboplatin, cisplatin, clozapine, cytotoxic chemotherapy, interferon alpha and beta, oxaliplatin, rituximab, zidovudine

INCREASED PERIPHERAL NEUROPATHY: didanosine

INCREASED SEIZURES: imipenem

INCREASED LACTIC ACIDOSIS: metformin/sulfonylureas, metformin

INCREASED LEVELS OF GANCICLOVIR: mycophenolate mofetil, probenecid

▧ SIDE EFFECTS

COMMON: diarrhea, fever, leukopenia, anorexia, vomiting, anemia, sweating, chills, fever, pruritus, neuropathy, paresthesias, elevated liver transaminase levels, impaired fertility, elevated creatinine levels, infection, phlebitis

RARE: thrombocytopenia, neutropenia, pancytopenia, seizures, coma, sepsis, retinal detachment, nephrotoxicity, hypertension, pancreatitis, gastrointestinal perforation, impaired fertility, depression

▦ MONITORING

BASELINE, THEN PERIODICALLY: complete blood count, creatinine

▦ CONTRAINDICATIONS

Hypersensitivity to drug/class, bone marrow suppressants, renal dysfunction, pregnancy

▦ PREGNANCY CLASS

C

GENTAMICIN, TOPICAL

(Garamycin topical® 0.1% cream in 15 g tube, ointment in 15 g tube)

▦ INDICATIONS

- Acne, pustular with *pseudomonas sp.*[+]
- Bacterial skin infections[*] (some gram-positive, good gram-negative, including *Staphylococcus aureus* and *Pseudomonas spp.*)
- Cutaneous leishmaniasis[$] (with paromomycin)
- Hot tub folliculitis[+]
- Infected burn wounds[^]
- Infected ulcers[$]
- Tufted folliculitis[+]

MECHANISM OF ACTION

It is a bactericidal agent that binds to the bacterial 30S ribosomal subunit and inhibits protein (aminoglycoside) synthesis.

▦ DOSAGE

Apply tid to qid.

DRUG INTERACTIONS

None

SIDE EFFECTS

COMMON: irritation, erythema, photosensitivity, burning

RARE: none

MONITORING

None

CONTRAINDICATIONS

Hypersensitivity to drug/class, pregnancy

PREGNANCY CLASS

D

GRISEOFULVIN

(Griseofulvin V® 250, 500 mg microsized tabs; Grisactin® 250, 500 mg microsized tabs; Gris-PEG® 125, 250 mg ultramicrosized tabs)

INDICATIONS

- Onychomycosis*
- Tinea barbae*
- Tinea capitis*
- Tinea corporis*
- Tinea cruris*
- Tinea imbricata^
- Tinea pedis*

See Appendix I.

▓ MECHANISM OF ACTION

It is a fungistatic agent that deposits in the keratinocytes, which are gradually exfoliated and replaced by new, uninfected cells.

▓ DOSAGE

ONYCHOMYCOSIS: 750–1000 mg PO qd for 4 months for fingernails, 6 months for toenails (microsized); 250 mg PO qd for 4 months for fingernails, 6 months for toenails (ultramicrosized)

TINEA CAPITIS: 500 mg PO qd for 4–6 weeks (microsized), 375 mg PO qd for 4–6 weeks (ultramicrosized; should treat patient and household with selenium sulfide or ketoconazole shampoo qd for 6 weeks.)

TINEA BARBAE, CORPORIS, CRURIS: 500 mg PO qd for 2–4 weeks (microsized), 375 mg PO qd for 2–4 weeks (ultramicrosized)

TINEA IMBRICATA: 500 mg PO bid for 4 weeks

TINEA PEDIS: 500 mg PO qd for 4–8 weeks (microsized), 250 mg PO qd for 4–8 weeks (ultramicrosized)

▓ DRUG INTERACTIONS

DECREASED LEVELS OF: alfentanil, amiodarone, aprepitant, aripiprazole, bortezomib, bosentan, buprenorphine, benzodiazepines, carbamazepine, calcium channel blockers, clarithromycin, oral contraceptives, cyclosporin, delavirdine, disopyramide, efavirenz, erythromycins, fentanyl, geftinib, itraconazole, ketoconazole, levonorgestrel, paclitaxel, protease inhibitors, repaglinide, sirolimus, statins, tacrolimus, voriconazole, warfarin, zonisamide

DECREASED LEVELS OF GRISEOFULVIN: barbiturates

DISULFIRAM REACTION: ethanol

▓ SIDE EFFECTS

COMMON: rash, urticaria, nausea, headache, confusion, vomiting, candidiasis, photosensitivity, lupus-like reaction, estrogenic effects, paresthesias, dizziness, fatigue, insomnia, diarrhea, flatulence, increased thirst, proteinuria

RARE: granulocytopenia, hepatotoxicity, neutropenia, nephrotoxicity, erythema multiforme, angioedema, mental confusion

■ MONITORING

BASELINE: complete blood count, liver function

■ CONTRAINDICATIONS

Hypersensitivity to drug/class, porphyria, pregnancy, penicillin allergy, impaired liver function

■ PREGNANCY CLASS

C

HYDROQUINONE

(Claripel® 4% cream with sunscreen in 28 and 45 g tubes; Eldoquin forte® 4% cream in 30 g tubes; Eldopaque forte® 4% cream with sunscreen in 40 g tubes; Solaquin forte® 4% cream or gel with sunscreen in 30 g tubes; Lustra® 4% cream with glycolic acid in 28.4 and 56.8 g tubes; Lustra AF® 4% cream with glycolic acid and sunscreen in 28.4 and 56.8 g tubes; Melanex® 3% solution in 29 ml bottles, Triluma® cream in 30 g tubes)

■ INDICATIONS

- Ephelides*
- Melasma*
- Photodamage with salicylic acid peels^
- Post-laser resurfacing hyperpigmentation^
- Senile lentigines*

■ MECHANISM OF ACTION

Reversible depigmentation occurs via enzymatic oxidation of tyrosine to dopa by inhibiting tyrosinase and by suppression of other melanocytic metabolic processes.

■ DOSAGE

Apply qd to bid. Should be used with a sunscreen if the product does not already contain one.

■ DRUG INTERACTIONS

None

■ SIDE EFFECTS

COMMON: contact dermatitis, dryness, fissuring, erythema, burning, irritation

RARE: exogenous ochronosis, urticaria, anaphylaxis

■ MONITORING

None

■ CONTRAINDICATIONS

Hypersensitivity to drug/class or sulfites, pregnancy

■ PREGNANCY CLASS

C

HYDROXYCHLOROQUINE

(Plaquenil® 200 mg tabs)

■ INDICATIONS

- Angioedema with deficiency of C1 esterase inhibitor[+] (see pg. 351)
- Atopic dermatitis[+] (see pg. 353)
- Dermatomyositis[+] (see pg. 361)
- Erythema nodosum[+]
- Granuloma annulare[+]

- Idiopathic panniculitis[+]
- Lupus erythematosus, systemic and chronic discoid[*] (see pg. 375)
- Lupus panniculitis[+] (see pg. 375)
- Lymphocytoma cutis[+]
- Malaria prophylaxis[*]
- Malaria treatment[*]
- Oral lichen planus[$] (see pg. 371)
- Pemphigus[+] (see pg. 383–385)
- Polymorphous light eruption[*]
- Porphyria cutanea tarda[^] (see pg. 388)
- Psoriatic arthritis[$]
- Reticular erythematous mucinosis[+]
- Rheumatoid arthritis[*]
- Sarcoidosis, cutaneous[$] (see pg. 396)
- Scleroderma[+] (see pg. 398)
- Urticarial vasculitis[+] (see pg. 404)
- Weber-Christian panniculitis[+]

MECHANISM OF ACTION

The exact mechanism is unknown. It is thought to inhibit certain enzymes by interacting with DNA to exert its plasmodicidal action. It affects light filtration by altering prostaglandin synthesis, inhibiting superoxide production and binding to DNA. It inhibits antigen-antibody complex formation, decreases lymphocyte responsiveness, and decreases the ability of macrophages to express cell surface antigens, which leads to immunosuppression. It decreases lysosomal size and function and impairs chemotaxis to exert its anti-inflammatory action. It also inhibits platelet aggregation.

DOSAGE

Each 200 mg tab contains 155 mg hydroxychloroquine base. Avoid daily doses >6.5 mg/kg.

ANGIOEDEMA WITH DEFICIENCY OF C1 ESTERASE INHIBITOR, RHEUMATOID ARTHRITIS, DERMATOMYOSITIS, ERYTHEMA NODOSUM, RETICULAR ERYTHEMATOUS MUCINOSIS, PEMPHIGUS: 200 mg PO bid

ATOPIC DERMATITIS, ORAL LICHEN PLANUS, SCLERODERMA: 200–400 mg PO qd

CUTANEOUS SARCOIDOSIS: 2–3 mg/kg/d PO 4–12 weeks

DERMATOMYOSITIS: 2–5 mg/kg/d PO

GRANULOMA ANNULARE: 6 mg/kg/d PO

LUPUS ERYTHEMATOSUS: 400 mg PO qd to bid

LUPUS PANNICULITIS: 3.5 mg/kg/d PO

MALARIA PROPHYLAXIS: Start 2 weeks before and continue for 6–8 weeks after exposure, 400 mg PO every week.

MALARIA TREATMENT: Start 800 mg PO once, then 400 mg PO 6 h later, then 400 mg PO qd for 2 days.

PORPHYRIA CUTANEA TARDA: 200 mg PO twice a week

WEBER-CHRISTIAN PANNICULITIS: 4 mg/kg/d PO

DRUG INTERACTIONS

None

SIDE EFFECTS

COMMON: dizziness, ataxia, headache, abdominal pain, nausea, vomiting, diarrhea, pruritus, weight loss, hair bleaching, alopecia, pigmentary changes

RARE: agranulocytosis, thrombocytopenia, aplastic anemia, seizures, exfoliative dermatitis, visual changes, ototoxicity, urticaria, lichenoid and purpuric eruptions, erythema annulare centrifigum, diarrhea, abdominal cramps, corneal opacities, scotomas, irritability, nervousness, psychosis, nightmares, nystagmus, nerve deafness, extraocular muscle palsies, muscle weakness, absent or hypoactive deep tendon reflexes, disturbances of ocular accommodation, edema/atrophy/abnormal pigmentation of macula, optic disk pallor/atrophy, retinopathy (>6.5 mg/kg/d)

MONITORING

BASELINE: eye exam, complete blood count, glucose-6-phosphate dehydrogenase level, 24 h urine for porphyrin

EVERY 6 MONTHS: eye exam

MONTHLY FOR 3 MONTHS, THEN EVERY 4–6 MONTHS: complete blood count

CONTRAINDICATIONS

Hypersensitivity to drug/class, porphyria, retinal/visual field changes, psoriasis, pregnancy, concomitant use of chloroquine

PREGNANCY CLASS

C

HYDROXYUREA

(Hydrea® 500 mg caps)

INDICATIONS

- Hypereosinophilic syndrome[§] (see pg. 368)
- Melanoma* (see pg. 378)
- Ovarian carcinoma*
- Psoriasis[^] (see pg. 392)
- Pyoderma gangrenosum[+] (see pg. 394)
- Resistant chronic myelogenous leukemia (CML)*
- Sickle cell disease*
- Squamous cell carcinoma of head and neck with radiation* (see pg. 400)
- Sweet's syndrome[+] (see pg. 401)

MECHANISM OF ACTION

It inhibits DNA synthesis and repair and gene regulation by acting as a ribonucleotide reductase inhibitor.

DOSAGE

0.5–1.5 g/d PO in divided doses

DRUG INTERACTIONS

INCREASED RISK OF IMMUNOSUPPRESSION: alefacept, bone marrow suppressants/cytotoxic chemotherapy, clozapine, interferon alpha 2a/2b, interferon beta 1a/1b, rituximab, zidovudine

INCREASED RISK OF HEPATOTOXICITY: stavudine

INCREASED RISK OF INFECTION: tumor necrosis factor–blocking agents, live
vaccines

SIDE EFFECTS

COMMON: bone marrow suppression, stomatitis, anorexia, nausea, vomiting, diarrhea, constipation, rash, erythema, dysuria, headache, dizziness,
hallucinations, alopecia, dermatitis

RARE: seizures, leukopenia, leukemia, anemia, pulmonary fibrosis, dermatomyositis, hyperpigmentation, leg ulcers, lichen planus, vasculitis, radiation recall, fixed drug, photosensitivity, urticaria, acral erythema, erythema
multiforme, cutaneous carcinoma, elevated transaminase level, elevated
blood urea nitrogen/creatinine levels, loss of libido, arthralgia, epistaxis,
fever, diaphoresis, thrombocytopenia, leg ulcers

MONITORING

BASELINE: complete blood count, serum chemistry, urinalysis

WEEKLY FOR FIRST MONTH, THEN MONTHLY IF UNREMARKABLE: complete blood count

MONTHLY, THEN EVERY 3–6 MONTHS IF UNREMARKABLE: serum chemistry, urinalysis

CONTRAINDICATIONS

Hypersensitivity to drug/class, bone marrow depression, pregnancy, impaired renal function, use of myelosuppressive agents, lactation, impaired
hepatic function, cardiopulmonary disease, unstable/fulminant psoriasis,
psoriatic arthritis, ongoing infection, blood dyscrasias

PREGNANCY CLASS

D

HYDROXYZINE

(Atarax® 10, 25, 50, 100 mg tabs; 10 mg/5 mL liquid in 240 mL bottles)

▨ INDICATIONS

- Anxiety*
- Atopic dermatitis^(see pg. 353)
- Insomnia*
- Nausea/vomiting*
- Pruritus* (see pg. 391)
- Sedation*
- Urticaria, chronic^, cold^ (see pg. 403)

▨ MECHANISM OF ACTION

It is a first-generation peripheral and central H_1 histamine receptor blocker. Because it acts centrally, it causes sedation.

▨ DOSAGE

25–100 mg PO q6h

▨ DRUG INTERACTIONS

INCREASED CENTRAL NERVOUS SYSTEM DEPRESSION: opiates, propoxyphene, tramadol, antidepressants, antihistamines, barbiturates, benzodiazepines, central alpha-2 agonists, droperidol, dronabinol, ethanol, meperidine, meprobamate, metoclopramide, muscle relaxants, phenothiazines, promethazine

INCREASED ANTICHOLINERGIC ACTIVITY: anticholinergics, central alpha-2 agonists, cyclopentolate/phenylephrine, dexmedetomide, disopyramide

DECREASED EFFICACY OF HYDROXYZINE: cholinergics

▨ SIDE EFFECTS

COMMON: dry mouth, drowsiness, dizziness, ataxia, weakness, slurred speech, headache, agitation, bitter taste, nausea

RARE: wheezing, dyspnea, seizures, respiratory depression, tremor

▨ MONITORING

None

▨ CONTRAINDICATIONS

Hypersensitivity to drug/class, pregnancy, asthma

▨ PREGNANCY CLASS

C

IMIQUIMOD

(Aldara® 5% cream in boxes of twelve 250 mg packets)

▨ INDICATIONS

- Actinic keratoses* (see pg. 348)
- Basal cell carcinoma, superficial* (see pg. 354)
- Cutaneous T-cell lymphoma, stage IA+ (see pg. 358)
- Erythroplasia of Queyrat
- Extramammary Paget's disease+
- Foreign-body granuloma+
- Genital/perianal warts* (see pg. 406)
- Granuloma annulare+ (see pg. 365)
- Herpes simplex type II+
- Infantile hemangioma+
- Keloid$ (see pg. 371)
- Keratoacanthoma+
- Lentigo maligna, amelanotic+, melanotic+
- Lupus, discoid+ (see pg. 375)

- Melanoma with or without metastasis[+] (see pg. 378)
- Molluscum contagiosum (1% cream tid for 5 days a week^, 5% cream qd[$]) (see pg. 380)
- Porokeratosis of Mibelli[+]
- Squamous cell carcinoma[$], invasive[+] (see pg. 400)
- Verrucous carcinoma (with CO_2 laser)[+]

■ MECHANISM OF ACTION

It is an immunomodulator with antiviral and antitumor properties that induce tumor necrosis factor alpha, interferon gamma and alpha, interleukin 6-/-1/-8/-12, granulocyte-macrophage colony–stimulating factor, and granulocyte colony–stimulating factor.

■ DOSAGE

ACTINIC KERATOSIS: Apply twice a week for 16 weeks.

BASAL CELL CARCINOMA (SUPERFICIAL): Apply 5 times a week for 6 weeks.

MELANOMA METASTASIS: Apply qd to bid.

MOLLUSCUM CONTAGIOSUM: Apply 1% cream tid for 5 days a week or 5% cream qd.

POROKERATOSIS OF MIBELLI: Apply 5 times a week.

VERRUCOUS CARCINOMA, SQUAMOUS CELL CARCINOMA, CUTANEOUS T-CELL LYMPHOMA, MELANOMA WITH OR WITHOUT METASTASIS, FOREIGN-BODY GRANULOMA, GRANULOMA ANNULARE, KELOID: Apply qd.

WARTS, PAGET'S DISEASE, KERATOACANTHOMA, HEMANGIOMA, HERPES, ERYTHROPLASIA OF QUEYRAT, EXTRAMAMMARY, LENTIGO MALIGNA: Apply 3 times a week for 16 weeks.

Apply at bedtime, then wash off in 6–10 h. Do not use occlusion. Avoid sexual contact while cream is on the skin. Local reactions are common.

■ DRUG INTERACTIONS

None

▩ SIDE EFFECTS

COMMON: erythema, burning, hypopigmentation, irritation, pruritus, tenderness, stinging, rash, erosions, excoriations, flaking, edema

RARE: pain, fatigue, fever, flu-like symptoms, headache, diarrhea, myalgia

▩ MONITORING

None

▩ CONTRAINDICATIONS

Hypersensitivity to drug/class

▩ PREGNANCY CLASS

B

INFLIXIMAB

(Remicade® 100 mg vials)

▩ INDICATIONS

- Acrodermatitis continua of Hallopeau[+]
- Behçet's syndrome[$] (see pg. 355)
- Crohn's disease[*]
- Graft-versus-host disease[$] (see pg. 365)
- Hidradenitis suppurativa[$]
- Psoriasis[^] (see pg. 392)
- Psoriatic arthritis[^]
- Pyoderma gangrenosum[$] (see pg. 394)
- Rheumatoid arthritis[*]
- Sarcoidosis[$] (see pg. 396)
- Sneddon-Wilkinson disease[+]
- Toxic epidermal necrolysis[+] (see pg. 402)

MECHANISM OF ACTION

It is a chimeric monoclonal immunoglobulin G1(IgG1) antibody containing human constant region and mouse variable region that inhibits tumor necrosis factor alpha (TNFα) activity and triggers complement-mediated lysis of TNFα-expressing cells. It neutralizes soluble and blocks membrane receptor-bound TNFα.

DOSAGE

3–5 mg/kg/infusion IV, may increase to 10 mg/kg/infusion. Given once; given at weeks 0, 2, and 6 (then may be repeated every 4–8 weeks); or given monthly. Should be administered with methotrexate or other immuno-suppressants to decrease chance of antibody formation.*

DRUG INTERACTIONS

INCREASED RISK OF SERIOUS INFECTIONS: immunosuppressants

SIDE EFFECTS

COMMON: injection site reactions, headache, nausea, abdominal pain, fever, upper respiratory infection, fatigue, cough, urinary tract infection, myalgias, back pain, arthralgia, dizziness, rash

RARE: antibody formation/anaphylaxis/serum sickness, development of positive antinuclear antibody (ANA), development of positive double stranded DNA (dsDNA), drug-induced lupus, malignancy, sepsis/serious infection, tuberculosis reactivation, elevated liver function test results, chest pain, dyspnea, hyper-/hypotension, congestive heart failure, chest pain, bronchospasm

MONITORING

BASELINE: Purified protein derivative (PPD) and chest x-ray

■ CONTRAINDICATIONS

Malignancy, infection/tuberculosis/sepsis, congestive heart failure, antibody formation, hypersensitivity reaction to drug/class, demyelinating disorders, hypersensitivity to murine products, use of live vaccines

■ PREGNANCY CLASS

B

INTERFERON ALPHA 2A

(Roferon A® 3, 6, 9, 36 million unit single-use vials; 3, 6, 9 million unit pre-filled syringes; 9, 18 million unit multiuse vials)

■ INDICATIONS

- Acyclovir-resistant herpes simplex[+]
- Angiosarcoma of scalp[+]
- Atopic dermatitis[^] (see pg. 353)
- Basal cell carcinoma[$] (see pg. 354)
- Behçet's syndrome[^] (see pg. 355)
- Chronic hepatitis C[*]
- Cryoglobulinemia type 2[^]
- Cutaneous T-cell lymphoma[^] (see pg. 358)
- Eosinophilic cellulitis[+]
- Hairy cell leukemia[*]
- Hemangioma[$]
- Herpes zoster[^]
- Hypereosinophilic syndrome[+] (see pg. 368)
- Kaposi's sarcoma in AIDS[*], Mediterranean type[+] (see pg. 370)
- Keratoacanthoma[$]
- Langerhans cell histiocytosis[+]
- Lupus, discoid[$], subacute cutaneous[$] (see pg. 375)
- Necrobiotic xanthogranuloma[+]
- Philadelphia chromosome–positive chronic myelogenous leukemia[*]
- POEMS (Polyneuropathy, Organomegaly, Endocrinopathy, Monoclonal gammopathy, Skin lesions)[+]
- Recurrent genital herpes[$]
- Squamous cell carcinoma[$] (see pg. 400)
- Urticaria, chronic/mastocytosis[$] (mixed results) (see pg. 403)

▓ MECHANISM OF ACTION

It binds to specific membrane receptors, inducing a complex sequence of intracellular events. These include induction of certain enzymes, suppression of cellular proliferation, immunomodulating activities such as enhancement of phagocytic activities of macrophages and augmentation of specific cytotoxicity of lymphocytes for target cells, and inhibition of viral replication.

▓ DOSAGE

CHRONIC HEPATITIS C: 3 million units SC/IM 3 times a week for 12 months; or 6 million units SC/IM 3 times a week for 3 months, then 3 million units SC/IM for 9 months.

HAIRY CELL LEUKEMIA: 3 million units SC/IM 3 times a week (start 3 million units qd for 16–24 weeks. Maximum of 3 million units/dose)

KAPOSI'S SARCOMA IN AIDS: 3–6 million units SC/IM 3 times a week for 10–12 weeks

▓ DRUG INTERACTIONS

INCREASED BONE MARROW SUPPRESSION: angiotensin-converting enzyme inhibitors, zidovudine

INCREASED IMMUNOSUPPRESSION: alefacept, bone marrow suppressants, rituximab

INCREASED LEVELS OF: theophyllines

INCREASED RISK OF NEUROTOXICITY: vinca alkaloids

▓ SIDE EFFECTS

COMMON: flu-like symptoms, rash, anorexia, nausea, vomiting, diarrhea, arthralgia, throat irritation, dry mouth, dizziness, depression, headache, paresthesias, emotional lability, impaired thought, anxiety, injection site reactions, lymphadenopathy, cough, gingival bleeding, flatulence, epistaxis, rhinitis, sinusitis, diaphoresis, alopecia, menstrual irregularities, psoriasis, pruritus, eczema, conjunctivitis, seborrhea, dry skin

RARE: leukopenia, thrombocytopenia, anemia, seizures, anaphylaxis, hepatotoxicity, pulmonary toxicity, suicidal ideation, delirium, peripheral neuropathy, arrhythmias, cardiomyopathy, myocardial infarction, gastrointestinal bleed, hypertension, autoimmune disorders

█ MONITORING

BASELINE, THEN MONTHLY: complete blood count, clinical chemistry

PATIENTS WITH CARDIAC ABNORMALITIES: electrocardiogram before and periodically during treatment

PATIENTS WITH CHRONIC HEPATITIS C: liver function tests at baseline, after 2 weeks, then monthly

PATIENTS WITH NEUTROPHIL COUNTS < 1,500/MM^3, PLATELET COUNTS < 75,000/MM^3, HEMOGLOBIN < 10 G/DL, CREATININE > 1.5 MG/DL: baseline complete blood count, then monitored closely thereafter

PATIENTS WITH THYROID ABNORMALITIES: may be treated if thyroid-stimulating (TSH) can be maintained at normal levels with medications. TSH should be checked at baseline, then every 3 months.

█ CONTRAINDICATIONS

Hypersensitivity to drug, pregnancy, autoimmune hepatitis, myelosuppression, seizures, cardiac disease, liver disease, renal disease, depression, central nervous system disorder, diabetes, thyroid disorder, nephrotoxic agents, cardiotoxic agents, autoimmune disorders, use of live vaccines

█ PREGNANCY CLASS

C

INTERFERON ALPHA 2B

(Intron® 3, 5, 10, 18, 25, 50 million units single-use vials; 18, 25 million unit multidose vials; 3, 5, 10 million unit pens with 6 doses in each)

█ INDICATIONS

- Angiosarcoma[+]
- Atopic dermatitis[^] (see pg. 353)
- Basal cell carcinoma[^] (see pg. 354)

- Behçet's disease^ (see pg. 355)
- Chronic hepatitis B*
- Chronic hepatitis C*
- Condylomata acuminata* (see pg. 406)
- Cryoglobulinemia type 2^
- Cutaneous T-cell lymphoma$ (see pg. 358)
- Follicular non-Hodgkin's lymphoma*
- Genital herpes$
- Hairy cell leukemia*
- Hemangioma$
- Herpes zoster$
- Hypereosinophilic syndrome$ (see pg. 368)
- Kaposi's sarcoma in AIDS* (see pg. 370)
- Langerhans cell histiocytosis+
- Lupus, discoid$ (see pg. 375)
- Melanoma, adjuvant* (see pg. 378)
- Schnitzler's syndrome+
- Squamous cell carcinoma$ (see pg. 400)
- Urticaria, chronic/mastocytosis+ (mixed results) (see pg. 403)

MECHANISM OF ACTION

It binds to specific membrane receptors, inducing a complex sequence of intracellular events. These include induction of certain enzymes, suppression of cellular proliferation, immunomodulating activities such as enhancement of phagocytic activities of macrophages and augmentation of specific cytotoxicity of lymphocytes for target cells, and inhibition of viral replication.

DOSAGE

ADJUVANT FOR MELANOMA: 10 million units/m^2 SC/IM 3 times a week for 48 weeks

CHRONIC HEPATITIS B: 10 million units SC/IM 3 times a week for 16 weeks or 5 million units SC/IM qd for 16 weeks

CHRONIC HEPATITIS C: 3 million units SC/IM 3 times a week for 24–48 weeks or 3 million units SC/IM 3 times a week for 18–24 months (monotherapy)

CONDYLOMATA ACUMINATA: 1 million units intralesionally (IL)3 times a week for 3 weeks (maximum of 5 condyloma per treatment)

FOLLICULAR NON-HODGKIN'S LYMPHOMA: 5 million units SC/IM 3 times a week for 18 months

HAIRY CELL LEUKEMIA: 2 million units/m² SC/IM 3 times a week for 6 months

KAPOSI'S SARCOMA IN AIDS: 30 million units/m² SC/IM 3 times a week

DRUG INTERACTIONS

INCREASED BONE MARROW SUPPRESSION: angiotensin-converting enzyme inhibitors, zidovudine

INCREASED IMMUNOSUPPRESSION: alefacept, bone marrow suppressants, rituximab

INCREASED LEVELS OF: theophyllines

INCREASED RISK OF NEUROTOXICITY: vinca alkaloids

SIDE EFFECTS

COMMON: flu-like symptoms, rash, anorexia, nausea, vomiting, diarrhea, arthralgia, throat irritation, dry mouth, dizziness, depression, headache, paresthesias, emotional lability, impaired thought, anxiety, injection site reactions, lymphadenopathy, cough, gingival bleeding, flatulence, epistaxis, rhinitis, sinusitis, diaphoresis, alopecia, menstrual irregularities, psoriasis, pruritus, eczema, conjunctivitis, seborrhea, dry skin

RARE: leukopenia, thrombocytopenia, anemia, seizures, anaphylaxis, hepatotoxicity, pulmonary toxicity, suicidal ideation, delirium, peripheral neuropathy, arrhythmias, cardiomyopathy, myocardial infarction, gastrointestinal bleed, hypertension, autoimmune disorders

MONITORING

BASELINE, THEN MONTHLY THEREAFTER: complete blood count, electrolytes, liver function, thyroid-stimulating hormone, renal function

BASELINE, THEN AS NECESSARY: chest x-ray

PATIENTS WITH CARDIAC ABNORMALITIES: baseline electrocardiogram and periodically thereafter

PATIENTS WITH MELANOMA: complete blood count and liver function at baseline, weekly during induction, then monthly thereafter

PATIENTS WITH HEPATITIS B OR C: liver function, prothrombin time, albumin, and bilirubin at baseline, then close monitoring during therapy

▦ CONTRAINDICATIONS

Hypersensitivity to drug, pregnancy, autoimmune hepatitis, myelosuppression, seizures, cardiac disease, liver disease, renal disease, depression, central nervous system disorder, diabetes, thyroid disorder, nephrotoxic agents, cardiotoxic agents, autoimmune disorders, use of live vaccines

▦ PREGNANCY CLASS

C

INTERFERON GAMMA

(Actimmune® 100 μg [2 million unit] vials)

▦ INDICATIONS

- Atopic dermatitis^
- Basal cell carcinoma^ (see pg. 354)
- Bowenoid papulosis^
- Chronic granulomatous disease*
- Condylomata acuminata^ (see pg. 406)
- Keloids (with surgery)^ (see pg. 371)
- Localized sclerosis/morphea (decreases new lesions)^ (see pg. 381)
- Malignant osteopetrosis*
- Psoriasis^ (see pg. 392)
- Systemic sclerosis^ (see pg. 398)
- Visceral leishmaniasis^ (with pentivalent antimony)

▦ MECHANISM OF ACTION

It is produced by Th1 T lymphocytes and regulates the function of the immune system. It interacts with interleukins, suppresses immunoglobulin E levels, stimulates phagocyte function to increase superoxide production, and inhibits production of collagen.

DOSAGE

ATOPIC DERMATITIS: 50 μg/m^2 SC 3 times a week

BASAL CELL CARCINOMA: 0.05 mg IL 3 times a week for 3 weeks

BOWENOID PAPULOSIS: 4 million units SC 3 times a week for 13 weeks

CHRONIC GRANULOMATOUS DISEASE AND MALIGNANT OSTEOPETROSIS: 50 μg/m^2 SC 3 times a week if body surface area (BSA) > 0.5 m^2, or 1.5 μg/kg/dose SC 3 times a week if BSA ≤0.5 m^2

CONDYLOMATA ACUMINATA: 2 million units/m^2 SC 3 times a week for 6 weeks

KELOID WITH SURGERY: 0.1 mg IL once a week for 3 weeks

LOCALIZED SCLEROSIS/MORPHEA: 100 μg SC qd for 5 consecutive days for 2 weeks, then 100 μg SC once a week for 4 weeks

PSORIASIS: 100 μg SC qd for 2 weeks, then 3 times a week for 9 months

SYSTEMIC SCLEROSIS: 100 μcg SC 3 times a week for 1 month

VISCERAL LEISHMANIASIS WITH PENTAVALENT ANTIMONY: 25 μg/m^2 SC day 1, then 50 μg/m^2 SC day 2, then 100 μg SC days 3–30

DRUG INTERACTIONS

None

SIDE EFFECTS

COMMON: fever, headache, rash, chills, injection site reaction, fatigue, nausea, vomiting, diarrhea, myalgia, arthralgia

RARE: back pain, abdominal pain, depression, hypotension, syncope, tachyarrhythmia, heart block, heart failure, myocardial infarction, confusion, disorientation, gait disturbances, Parkinsonian attacks, seizures, hallucinations, transient ischemic attacks, hepatic insufficiency, renal insufficiency, pancreatitis, gastrointestinal bleeding, deep venous thrombosis, pulmonary embolism, tachypnea, bronchospasm, interstitial pneumonitis, hyponatremia, hyperglycemia, exacerbation of dermatomyositis

▓ MONITORING

BASELINE AND EVERY 3 MONTHS: complete blood count, urinalysis, renal and hepatic function

▓ CONTRAINDICATIONS

Hypersensitivity to drug/class or *Escherichia coli*–derived products, pregnancy

▓ PREGNANCY CLASS

C

INTRAVENOUS IMMUNOGLOBULIN

(BayGam® IV; Gamimune® 5, 10% IV; Gammagard® IV; Gammar-P® IV; Iveegam® IV; Sandoglobulin® IV; Panglobulin® IV; Polygam® IV; Venoglobulin-S® 5, 10% IV)

▓ INDICATIONS

- Atopic dermatitis[§] (see pg. 353)
- B-cell chronic lymphocytic leukemia[*]
- Bone marrow transplantation[*]
- Bullous pemphigoid[§] (see pg. 355)
- Dermatomyositis[^] (see pg. 361)
- Epidermolysis bullosa acquisita[+] (see pg. 363)
- Erythema multiforme[§] (see pg. 364)
- Graft-versus-host disease[*] (see pg. 365)
- Hepatitis A[*]
- Herpes gestationis[+] (see pg. 368)
- Hypereosinophilic syndrome[+] (see pg. 368)
- Idiopathic thrombocytopenic purpura[*]
- Kawasaki's disease[*]
- Leukocytoclastic vasculitis[+] (see pg. 404)
- Linear immunoglobulin A (IgA)[+] (see pg. 374)
- Livedoid vasculitis[+] (see pg. 404)
- Measles[*]

- Mixed connective tissue disease[+]
- Nephrogenic fibrosing dermopathy[+]
- Oral pemphigoid[^] (see pg. 356)
- Pediatric HIV[*]
- Pemphigus foliaceus[$] (see pg. 383)
- Pemphigus vulgaris[$] (see pg. 385)
- Polyarteritis nodosa, cutaneous[+] (see pg. 404)
- Primary humoral immunodeficiency[*]
- Psoriasis[+] (see pg. 392)
- Pyoderma gangrenosum[+] (see pg. 394)
- Rubella[*]
- Scleromyxedema[+]
- Stevens-Johnson syndrome, recurrent[+] (see pg. 400)
- Toxic epidermal necrolysis[$] (see pg. 402)
- Urticaria, delayed pressure[+], chronic[$] (see pg. 403)
- Varicella[*]

■ MECHANISM OF ACTION

It blocks Fc receptors, prevents complement-mediated damage, reduces circulating pathogens and antibodies, alters cytokines, has anti-idiotypic actions, increases immunoglobulin catabolism, acts as a colloid with a half-life of 17 days, and inhibits Fas-FasL interactions.

■ DOSAGE

DERMATOMYOSITIS, IMMUNOBULLOUS, VIRAL, PYODERMA GANGRENO-SUM, NEPHROGENIC FIBROSING DERMOPATHY, SCLEROMYXEDEMA, STEVENS-JOHNSON SYNDROME, URTICARIA (DELAYED PRESSURE): 2 g/kg/month IV, divided into either 2 doses of 1 g/kg/d or 5 doses of 0.4 g/kg/d

LINEAR IGA: 0.4 g/kg/d IV for 5 days with salazosulphapyridine 3 g PO qd

ERYTHEMA MULTIFORME: 750 mg IM once a month

TOXIC EPIDERMAL NECROLYSIS: 1 g/kg/d for 4 days

■ DRUG INTERACTIONS

May interfere with live vaccines, such as measles-mumps-rubella, yellow fever, and varicella. Use should be deferred until 6 months after treatment complete.

▦ SIDE EFFECTS

COMMON: headache, flushing, chills, myalgia, wheezing, tachycardia, back pain, nausea

RARE: hypotension, neutropenia, serum sickness, disseminated intravascular coagulation, aseptic meningitis, eczema, alopecia, oliguria/anuria, acute renal failure, acute tubular necrosis, proximal tubular nephropathy, osmotic nephrosis, thrombosis.

▦ MONITORING

BASELINE: liver function, renal function, complete blood count, IgA, HIV, hepatitis A/B/C, rheumatoid factor, cryoglobulins

BEFORE EACH SUBSEQUENT INFUSION: liver function, renal function, complete blood count

ANNUALLY: HIV, hepatitis A/B/C

▦ CONTRAINDICATIONS

Hypersensitivity to drug/class or anti-IgA, IgA deficiency, sensitivity to thimerosal, renal dysfunction, pregnancy. Can decrease efficacy of measles-mumps-rubella, varicella, and yellow fever vaccines.

▦ PREGNANCY CLASS

C

ISONIAZID

(Nydrazid®100, 300 mg tabs; 50 mg/5 mL suspension in 473 mL bottles; IV), isoniazid and rifampin (Rifamate® 150/300 g tabs), isoniazid, rifampin, and pyrazinamide (Rifater® 50/120/300 mg tabs)

▦ INDICATIONS

- *Mycobacterium bovis*$
- *Mycobacterium haemophilum*+

- *Mycobacterium kansasii^*
- *Mycobacterium scrofulaceum+*
- *Mycobacterium tuberculosis**

See Appendix III.

▩ MECHANISM OF ACTION

It is a bactericidal agent which inhibits lipid and nucleic acid synthesis in my-cobacterial organisms.

▩ DOSAGE

TUBERCULOSIS PROPHYLAXIS IN HIGH RISK, PURIFIED PROTEIN DERIVA-TIVE (PPD) POSITIVE: 5 mg/kg PO qd, maximum of 300 mg qd, for 9 months (prophylaxis) or 12 months (PPD positive). Give with vitamin B6 25–50 mg PO qd to prevent peripheral neuropathy.

RENAL DOSING
Creatinine clearance < 10 mL/min: decrease dose by 50%
Continuous ambulatory peritoneal dialysis: 50% of normal dose q24h
Hemodialysis and peritoneal dialysis: dose after dialysis

▩ DRUG INTERACTIONS

HEPATOTOXICITY: acetaminophen, ethanol, pyrazinamide, rifampin, ri-fabutin, ethionamide

CENTRAL NERVOUS SYSTEM DEPRESSION: cycloserine, alfentanil, fentanyl, meperidine

RESPIRATORY DEPRESSION: alfentanil, fentanyl

DECREASED EFFICACY OF ISONIAZID: antacids, prednisone

DECREASED EFFICACY OF: enflurane, oral hypoglycemics, insulin, isoflu-rane, sevoflurane, ketoconazole, itraconazole

INCREASED LEVELS OF: aripiprazole, bosentan, buprenorphine, benzodi-azepines, gefitinib, paclitaxel, phenytoin, riluzole, voriconazole, warfarin, carbamazepine, ethosuximide, ketoconazole, primidone, propranolol

THEOPHYLLINE TOXICITY: theophylline

INCREASED SEIZURES: valproic acid

DECREASED LEVELS OF: verapamil

WORSENED PARKINSON'S DISEASE: levodopa

PELLAGRA: niacin

INCREASED PERIPHERAL NEUROPATHY: didanosine, stavudine, zalcitabine

INCREASED ATAXIA: disulfiram

INCREASED LEVELS OF ISONIAZID: aspirin, procainamide

HYPOGLYCEMIA: chlorpropamide

SIDE EFFECTS

COMMON: nausea, vomiting, epigastric discomfort, diarrhea, dizziness, rash, acne, elevated liver function test results, euphoria, agitation, tinnitus, paresthesias

RARE: agranulocytosis, aplastic anemia, thrombocytopenia, hepatotoxicity, optic neuritis, peripheral neuropathy, seizures, leukopenia

MONITORING

BASELINE: liver function tests, opthalmologic and neurologic testing

MONTHLY: liver function tests

CONTRAINDICATIONS

Hypersensitivity to drug/class, liver disease, impaired liver function, impaired renal function, alcohol use, caution if >35 years of age, peripheral neuropathy, pregnancy, IV drug abuse, HIV positive

PREGNANCY CLASS

C

ISOTRETINOIN

(Accutane® 10, 20, 40 mg caps; Sotret® 10, 20, 30 and 40 mg tabs)

▮ INDICATIONS

- Acne, nodulocystic in patients on hemodialysis^, nodulocystic* (see pg. 347)
- Atrophoderma vermiculatum[+]
- Cancer (cutaneous), chemoprevention[$]
- Condylomata acuminata[$] (see pg. 406)
- Cutis verticis gyrata[+]
- Darier's disease[$] (see pg. 359)
- Diffuse dermal angiomatosis of the breast[+]
- Dissecting cellulitis[+]
- Epidermolysis bullosa simplex[+] (see pg. 363)
- Epidermolytic hyperkeratosis[$]
- Erosive oral lichen planus[$] (see pg. 371)
- Extranodal Rosai-Dorfman disease[+]
- Fordyce spots[+]
- Fox-Fordyce disease[+]
- Gram-negative folliculitis[$]
- Granuloma annulare[+] (see pg. 365)
- Granulomatous rosacea[+] (see pg. 395)
- Grover's disease[+] (see pg. 366)
- Hidradenitis suppurativa[$]
- HIV-associated eosinophilic folliculitis[$]
- Human papillomavirus–induced ulcers[+]
- Hyperimmunoglobulin (Ig) E syndrome[+]
- IgA pemphigus[+] (see pg. 384)
- Keratoacanthoma[+]
- Keratodermas[$]
- Lamellar ichthyosis[$] (see pg. 369)
- Langerhans cell histiocytosis[+]
- Lichen planus[+] (see pg. 371)
- Lupus, discoid[+], hypertrophic[+], subacute cutaneous[$] (see pg. 375)
- Lupus miliaris disseminatus faciei[+]
- Nipple hyperkeratosis[+]
- Papular mucinosis[+]

- Perforating folliculitis[+]
- Persistent facial edema of acne[+]
- Pityriasis rubra pilaris[$] (see pg. 387)
- Psoriasis[^] (with psoralen–ultraviolet A) (see pg. 392)
- Pyoderma faciale[+]
- Rosacea, papulopustular[^] (see pg. 395)
- Sarcoidosis, cutaneous[+] (see pg. 396)
- Scleromyxedema[+]
- Sebaceous hyperplasia[+]
- Ulerythema ophryogenes[+]

MECHANISM OF ACTION

It activates retinoid acid receptor on keratinocytes to induce cellular differentiation and to exert antiproliferative and anti-inflammatory effects. It also inhibits sebaceous gland differentiation and proliferation to decrease amount of sebum secreted and thus decrease *Propionibacterium acnes* colonization. It also down-regulates cutaneous androgen receptors.

DOSAGE

Start 0.5 mg/kg/d for first month, then increase to 1 mg/kg/d to maximum of 2 mg/kg/d if needed. For acne, give for 20 weeks; may need to repeat course after 2–3 months. Defects in keratinization may require treatment with doses up to 4 mg/kg/d for long period of time.

DRUG INTERACTIONS

INCREASED DRY SKIN: topical benzoyl peroxide and topical tretinoin

HYPERVITAMINOSIS A: vitamin A, acitretin

PSEUDOTUMOR CEREBRI: tetracycline, doxycycline, minocycline

INCREASED LEVELS OF: cyclosporin, isotretinoin

DECREASED LEVELS OF: rifampin, rifabutin, phenobarbital, carbamazepine

DECREASED EFFICACY OF ISOTRETINOIN: progestin-only contraceptives

INCREASED RISK OF BONE LOSS: systemic steroids, phenytoin

■ SIDE EFFECTS

COMMON: chelitis, dry skin, skin fragility, pruritus, epistaxis, dry mucous membranes, conjunctivitis, photosensitivity, arthralgia/myalgia, hypertriglyceridemia, desquamation of palms and soles, hair thinning/loss, nail changes, elevated liver enzyme levels, contact lens intolerance, decreased night vision, visual disturbances, depression, tinnitus, back pain, photosensitivity, pyogenic granulomas, paronychia, onycholysis, photophobia, headache, nausea, diarrhea, abdominal pain

RARE: pseudotumor cerebri, osteopenia/osteoporosis, hepatotoxicity, anaphylaxis, allergic vasculitis, major birth defects, violent behavior/aggression, psychosis, suicidal ideation, hearing impairment, cataracts/corneal opacities, premature epiphyseal closure, neutropenia, rhabdomyolysis, agranulocytosis, inflammatory bowel disease, pancreatitis, vascular thrombosis, stroke, seizures

■ MONITORING

BASELINE: Two forms of birth control must be started 1 month before commencing isotretinoin and for 1 month after completion. Serum and urine pregnancy test, complete blood count, liver function tests, fasting lipid profile, renal function tests, urinalysis. Consider x-rays of wrists, ankles, and spine if long-term use is needed. Consider eye exam if history of cataracts or retinopathy.

MONTHLY FOR FIRST 3–6 MONTHS, THEN EVERY 3 MONTHS: complete blood count, liver function tests, fasting lipid profile, renal function tests

MONTHLY DURING TREATMENT: serum and urine pregnancy test

YEARLY: x-rays and eye exam if necessary

■ CONTRAINDICATIONS

Hypersensitivity to drug/class, hypersensitivity to parabens, pregnancy, lactating, prolonged ultraviolet light exposure, depression/suicidal ideation, osteoporosis/osteomalacia, inflammatory bowel disease flare, seizure disorder, hyperlipidemia, pancreatitis, diabetes, hyperuricemia/gout, anorexia, vasculitis

▨ PREGNANCY CLASS

X

ITRACONAZOLE

(Sporanox® 100 mg caps; 10 mg/mL solution in 25 mL ampules and 50 ml bags; 10 mg/mL suspension in 150 mL bottles)

▨ INDICATIONS

- Aspergillosis, pulmonary and extrapulmonary*
- Blastomycosis, pulmonary and extrapulmonary*
- Candidiasis, stomatitis/esophagitis/vaginitis HIV^
- Candidiasis, thrush^
- Candidiasis, vaginitis^
- Chromomycosis$
- Coccidioidomycosis, pulmonary HIV^
- Cryptococcosis, not meningeal non-HIV^
- Histoplasmosis, HIV pulmonary and disseminated (not meningeal)*
- Histoplasmosis, pulmonary and disseminated (not meningeal)*
- Majocchi's granuloma$
- Onychomycosis*
- Paracoccidioidomycosis^
- Penicilliosis$
- Phaeohyphomycosis+
- Pityrosporum folliculitis^
- Pseudoallescheria boydii+
- Seborrheic dermatitis$
- Sporotrichosis, cutaneous and lymphocutaneous$
- Tinea capitis, corporis, cruris, pedis^
- Tinea imbricata^
- Tinea versicolor^

See Appendix I.

▨ MECHANISM OF ACTION

It inhibits fungal cytochrome P450–dependent ergosterol synthesis.

▓ DOSAGE

MAJOCCHI'S GRANULOMA: 200 mg PO bid for 7 days, then off for 14 days (repeat 3 times total)

SEBORRHEIC DERMATITIS: 200 mg PO qd for first week of month, then first 2 days of every month for 11 months

TINEA IMBRICATA: 100 mg PO qd for 4 weeks

See Appendix I.

RENAL DOSING
Creatinine clearance (CrCl) 10–90 mL/min: 100% of normal dose of 100–200 mg IV q12h
CrCl < 10 mL/min: 50% of normal dose
Hemodialysis, continuous ambulatory peritoneal dialysis, continuous arterio-venous hemofiltration: 100 mg IV q12–24h

▓ DRUG INTERACTIONS

INCREASED CENTRAL NERVOUS SYSTEM DEPRESSION: alfentanil, benzodiazepines, propoxyphene, buprenorphine, fentanyl

INCREASED LEVELS OF: amiodarone, almotriptan, aprepitant, aripiprazole, bosentan, budesonide, buspirone, ergotamine, carbamazepine, celecoxib, cilostazol, cyclosporin, digoxin, eletriptan, statins, imatinib, levobupivacaine, metformin, sulfonylureas, methadone, mifepristone, modafinil, nefazodone, phenytoin, quetiapine, quinidine, repaglinide, sildenafil, sirolimus, tacrolimus, theophylline, tolterodine, vinca alkaloids, warfarin, ziprasidone, zonisamide

INCREASED LEVELS OF ITRACONAZOLE: amprenavir, protease inhibitors, paclitaxel

DECREASED LEVELS OF ITRACONAZOLE: barbiturates, rifampins, didanosine, griseofulvin, H_2 blockers, proton pump inhibitors

INCREASED RISK OF HYPOTENSION: bepridil, calcium channel blockers

INCREASED QT PROLONGATION: cisapride, pimozide

INCREASED ARRHYTHMIAS: disopyramide

INCREASED HYPERGLYCEMIA: pioglitazone

▓ SIDE EFFECTS

COMMON: nausea, vomiting, diarrhea, hypokalemia, elevated transaminase and bilirubin levels, injection site reaction, rash, vasculitis, abdominal pain, elevated creatinine levels, headache, fever, hypertension, hypertriglyceridemia

RARE: hepatotoxicity, hepatic failure, congestive heart failure, pulmonary edema, anaphylaxis, peripheral neuropathy, Stevens-Johnson syndrome, toxic epidermal necrolysis, malaise, anorexia, pruritus, dizziness, decreased libido, somnolence, vertigo, impotence, albuminuria, depression, constipation, dyspepsia, stomatitis, sinusitis, pain, fatigue, alopecia, neutropenia

▓ MONITORING

BASELINE: complete blood count, liver function

EVERY 6 WEEKS: liver function

▓ CONTRAINDICATIONS

Hypersensitivity to drug/class, congestive heart failure, left ventricular dysfunction, CrCl < 30 mL/min, cardiovascular disease, pulmonary disease, impaired liver and renal function, pregnancy

▓ PREGNANCY CLASS

C

IVERMECTIN

(Stromectol® 3 and 6 mg tabs)

▓ INDICATIONS

- Body cavity filariasis (*Mansonella ozzardi*)^
- Cutaneous larva migrans (*Ancylostoma braziliense*)^
- Demodex[+]
- Gnathostomiasis[$]
- Head lice (*Pediculus humanus,* not nits)[+]

- Intestinal helminths (*Trichuris trichiura* and *Ascaris lumbricoides*)^
- Lymphatic filariasis (microfilariae of *Wuchereria bancrofti, Brugia malayi* and *timori*)^
- Mite dermatitis (*Cheyletiella blakei*)+
- Onchocerciasis (microfilariae of *Onchocerca volvulus,* not adult forms)*
- Scabies (*Sarcoptes scabiei*)^
- Strongyloidiasis (intestinal stages of *Strongyloides stercoralis*)*

MECHANISM OF ACTION

It is a member of the avermectin class of antiparasitics, which bind selectively and with high affinity to glutamate-gated chloride ion channels in invertebrate nerve and muscle cells. This causes an increase in nerve and muscle cell membrane permeability, leading to hyperpolarization of the nerve or muscle, which results in paralysis and death.

DOSAGE

BODY CAVITY FILARIASIS: 200 µg/kg PO once with water

CUTANEOUS LARVA MIGRANS: 200 µg/kg PO once with water

DEMODEX: 200 µg/kg PO once with water and weekly with permethrin

GNATHOSTOMIASIS: 200 µg/kg PO once with water

HEAD LICE: 200 µg/kg PO once with water

INTESTINAL HELMINTHS: 200 µg/kg PO once with water and albendazole 400 mg PO once

LYMPHATIC FILARIASIS: 100–440 µg/kd PO once with water

MITE DERMATITIS: 200 µg/kg PO once with water

ONCHOCERCIASIS: 150 µg/kg PO once with water, may need to repeat treatment

SCABIES: 200 µg/kg PO once with water, may need to repeat one week later

STRONGYLOIDIASIS: 200 µg/kg PO once with water

DRUG INTERACTIONS

None

SIDE EFFECTS

COMMON: cutaneous and/or systemic reactions of varying severity (Mazzotti reaction) and ophthalmologic reactions in patients with onchocerciasis due to allergic and inflammatory responses to the death of microfilariae. The Mazzotti reaction consists of pruritus, rash, fever, edema, lymphadenopathy, dizziness, chest pain, abdominal distension, tachycardia, limbitis, and abnormal eye sensation.

RARE: hypotension, elevated liver function test results, leukopenia, anemia, asthenia/fatigue, abdominal pain, anorexia, constipation, diarrhea, nausea, vomiting, somnolence, vertigo, tremor, urticaria, dizziness, rash

MONITORING

None

CONTRAINDICATIONS

Hypersensitivity to drug/class, hyper-reactive onchodermatitis (sowda), pregnancy

PREGNANCY CLASS

C

KETOCONAZOLE

(Nizoral® 200 mg tabs; 2% cream in 15, 30, 60 g tubes; 2% shampoo)

INDICATIONS

- Blastomycosis*
- Candidiasis, bladder*

- Candidiasis, mucocutaneous*
- Candidiasis, thrush*
- Chromomycosis*
- Coccidioidomycosis*
- Histoplasmosis*
- Onychomycosis^
- Paracoccidioidomycosis*
- Pityrosporum folliculitis^
- Reiter's syndrome$
- Seborrheic dermatitis (oral and topical)^ (see pg. 399)
- Tinea capitis^
- Tinea corporis, cruris, pedis (oral and topical)*
- Tinea versicolor (oral and topical)*

See Appendix I.

MECHANISM OF ACTION

It inhibits cell membrane ergosterol synthesis.

DOSAGE

PITYROSPORUM FOLLICULITIS: 200 mg PO qd for 4 weeks

SEBORRHEIC DERMATITIS: Apply topically bid for 4 weeks; 200 mg PO qd for 4 weeks.

TINEA CAPITIS: 3.3–6.6 mg/kg/d

TINEA PEDIS: Apply topically bid for 6 weeks; 200 mg PO qd for 4 weeks.

TINEA VERSICOLOR, CORPORIS, CRURIS: Apply topically bid for 2 weeks; 200 mg PO qd for 4 weeks (except Tinea versicolor, 400 mg PO once).

See Appendix I.

DRUG INTERACTIONS (ORAL)

INCREASED CENTRAL NERVOUS SYSTEM DEPRESSION: alfentanil, benzodiazepines, propoxyphene, buprenorphine, fentanyl

INCREASED LEVELS OF: amiodarone, almotriptan, aprepitant, aripiprazole, bosentan, budesonide, buspirone, ergotamine, carbamazepine, celecoxib, cilostazol, cyclosporin, delavirdine, digoxin, eletriptan, statins, imatinib, levobupivacaine, metformin, sulfonylureas, methadone, mifepristone, modafinil, nefazodone, phenytoin, quetiapine, quinidine, repaglinide, sildenafil, sirolimus, tacrolimus, theophylline, tolterodine, vinca alkaloids, warfarin, ziprasidone, zonisamide

INCREASED LEVELS OF KETOCONAZOLE: amprenavir, protease inhibitors, paclitaxel

DECREASED LEVELS OF KETOCONAZOLE: barbiturates, rifampins, didanosine, griseofulvin, H2 blockers, proton pump inhibitors

INCREASED RISK OF HYPOTENSION: bepridil, calcium channel blockers

INCREASED QT PROLONGATION: cisapride, pimozide

INCREASED ARRHYTHMIAS: disopyramide

INCREASED HYPERGLYCEMIA: pioglitazone

SIDE EFFECTS

TOPICAL

COMMON: rash, pruritus, irritation, burning

RARE: systemic absorption

ORAL

COMMON: nausea, dizziness, abdominal pain, diarrhea, headache, pruritus, lethargy, nervousness, somnolence, rash, elevated transaminases, gynecomastia

RARE: adrenal insufficiency, thrombocytopenia, hepatic failure, hepatotoxicity, anaphylaxis, leukopenia, hemolytic anemia, fever, chills, photophobia, alopecia, impotence, increased intracranial pressure, paresthesias, hypertriglyceridemia, suicidal, depression, prolonged QT interval

MONITORING (ORAL)

BASELINE: complete blood count, liver function

EVERY 6 WEEKS: liver function

▓ CONTRAINDICATIONS

TOPICAL: hypersensitivity to drug/class, pregnancy

ORAL: hypersensitivity to drug/class, achlorhydria, fungal meningitis, impaired liver function, pregnancy

▓ PREGNANCY CLASS

C

LIDOCAINE, TOPICAL

(Xylocaine® 2% jelly in 30 mL tubes, 2.5% ointment [over the counter], 5% ointment in 35 g tubes; LMX® 4% and 5% cream in 5, 30 g tubes [over the counter]; EMLA® 2.5% cream in 5, 30 g tubes, lidocaine 2.5% and prilocaine 2.5%)

▓ INDICATIONS

- Notalgia paresthetica⁺
- Post-burn pruritus$
- Postherpetic neuralgia^ (see pg. 389)
- Post-trichloroacetic acid (TCA) peel pain^
- Prior to IV insertion^
- Prior to wound débridement^
- Temporary relief of pain from minor cuts, abrasions, minor burns, sunburns, insect bites, irritation*

▓ MECHANISM OF ACTION

Topical application leads to the accumulation of the drug in the vicinity of pain receptors and nerve endings. It stabilizes neuronal membranes by inhibiting the ionic fluxes required for the initiation and conduction of impulses, thereby affecting local anesthetic action.

▓ DOSAGE

Apply thin layer q4h.

DRUG INTERACTIONS

SYNERGISM WITH: class I antiarrhythmics

SIDE EFFECTS

Related to amount and duration of use.

COMMON: erythema, edema, abnormal sensation in treated area, irritation

RARE: seizures, respiratory depression, cardiac arrest, malignant hyperthermia, anaphylaxis, anxiety, dizziness, nausea, vomiting, tissue necrosis, hypotension, blurred vision, numbness, tremors

MONITORING

None

CONTRAINDICATIONS

Hypersensitivity to drug/class, methemoglobinemia, glucose-6-phosphate dehydrogenase deficiency, impaired liver function

PREGNANCY CLASS

B

LINDANE

(Lindane® 1% lotion and shampoo in 60 and 480 mL bottles)

INDICATIONS

- Demodex folliculitis[+]
- Furuncular myiasis[+]
- Mite dermatitis (*Cheyletiella yasguri*)[+]
- Pediculosis capitis (*Pediculus humanus*)[^]
- Scabies (*Sarcoptes scabiei*)* (see pg. 397)

▨ MECHANISM OF ACTION

It exerts its antiparasiticidal action by being directly absorbed into parasites and ova.

▨ DOSAGE

PEDICULOSIS CAPITIS: Apply 15–30 mL shampoo to clean dry hair, wait 4 min, add water and lather, rinse immediately. Remove nits with comb or tweezer. Do not retreat.

SCABIES: Apply thin layer from head to toes (maximum 30 mL), bathe after 8–12 hours, do not retreat.

▨ DRUG INTERACTIONS

None

▨ SIDE EFFECTS

COMMON: dizziness, dermatitis, alopecia, headache, pain, paresthesias, pruritus, urticaria

RARE: neurotoxicity, seizures, death

▨ MONITORING

None

▨ CONTRAINDICATIONS

Hypersensitivity to drug, seizure disorder, inflamed or raw skin, Norwegian scabies, premature infants and pediatric use, adult use within past 3 months, central nervous system tumor, HIV, head injury, pregnancy, alcohol abuse, use as first-line therapy, concomitant use of oils/ointments/creams

▨ PREGNANCY CLASS

C

LINEZOLID

(Zyvox® 600 mg tabs; 100 mg/5 mL suspension; IV)

▓ INDICATIONS

- *Enterococcus faecium,* vancomycin resistant*
- *Staphylococcus aureus,* methicillin resistant*
- *Staphylococcus aureus,* methicillin sensitive*
- *Streptococcus agalactiae**
- *Streptococcus pneumoniae**
- *Streptococcus pyogenes**

See Appendix II.

Usually effective:

- *Clostridium,* not *difficile*
- *Enterococcus faecalis*
- *Enterococcus faecium*
- *Listeria monocytogenes*
- *Mycobacterium avium*
- *Peptostreptococcus* sp.
- *Staphylococcus epidermidis*

Clinical trials lacking:

- *Bacteroides fragilis*
- *Clostridium difficile*
- *Haemophilus influenzae*
- *Legionella* sp.
- *Moraxella catarrhalis*
- *Mycoplasma pneumoniae*

▓ MECHANISM OF ACTION

It is a bactericidal and bacteriostatic agent that binds to the 50S ribosomal subunit to inhibit protein synthesis.

▓ DOSAGE

400–600 mg IV/PO q12h

RENAL DOSING: No data for continuous arteriovenous hemofiltration or chronic ambulatory peritoneal dialysis. Dose after hemodialysis

DRUG INTERACTIONS

SEROTONIN SYNDROME: tramadol, dextromethorphan, buspirone, meperidine, nefazodone, sibutramine, serotonin reuptake inhibitors, trazodone, tricyclic antidepressants, venlafaxine

SEIZURES: tramadol, carbamazepine, cyclobenzaprine, maprotiline, mertazapine

INCREASED LEVELS OF: almotriptan, bupropion, rizatriptan, sumatriptan, zolmitriptan

HYPERTENSION: alpha-2 agonists, decongestants, carbidopa/levodopa, pseudoephedrine, catechol-O-methyltransferase inhibitors, epinephrine, monoamine oxidase inhibitors, metoclopramide, modafinil, reserpine, stimulants, sympathomimetics

CARDIOVASCULAR: beta-2 agonists

HYPOTENSION: phenothiazines

SIDE EFFECTS

COMMON: diarrhea, headache, nausea, vomiting, hypertension, tongue discoloration, pruritus, vaginal candidiasis, rash, abdominal pain

RARE: thrombocytopenia, pseudomembranous colitis, leukopenia, pancytopenia, anemia, neuropathy

MONITORING

FREQUENTLY IF LONG-TERM USE: complete blood count

CONTRAINDICATIONS

Hypersensitivity to drug/class, uncontrolled hypertension, pheochromocytoma, carcinoid syndrome, uncontrolled thyroid disease, monoamine oxidase inhibitors, thrombocytopenia, phenylketonuria, severe liver disease, myelosuppression, pregnancy

PREGNANCY CLASS

C

LORATADINE

(Claritin® 10 mg tabs, 5 mg/5 mL liquid in 150 mL bottles; Claritin Reditabs®
10 mg tabs that dissolve in mouth)

INDICATIONS

- Allergic rhinitis*
- Atopic dermatitis^ (see pg. 353)
- Pruritus, mosquito bites^ (see pg. 391)
- Urticaria, chronic* (see pg. 403)

MECHANISM OF ACTION

It is a long-acting H_1 histamine receptor blocker with minimal sedation and
anticholinergic effects.

DOSAGE

10 mg PO qd

RENAL DOSING
Creatinine clearance < 30 mL/min: 10 mg PO qod

HEPATIC DOSING: 10 mg PO qod

DRUG INTERACTIONS

None

SIDE EFFECTS

COMMON: headache, somnolence, fatigue, dry mouth, nervousness, abdominal pain, bronchospasm, hyperkinesia, conjunctivitis, dysphonia,
malaise, upper respiratory infection

RARE: hepatitis, hypersensitivity reaction, altered lacrimation, altered salivation, flushing, impotence, increased sweating, thirst, edema, asthenia, back pain, blurred vision, chest pain, earache, eye pain, fever, leg cramps, rigors, tinnitus, weight gain, hypertension, hypotension, palpitations, syncope, tachycardia, blepharospasm, migraine, paresthesia, vertigo, altered taste, anorexia, constipation, diarrhea, dyspepsia, flatulence, gastritis, increased appetite, stomatitis, arthralgia, myalgia, agitation, amnesia, decreased libido, depression, insomnia, irritability, breast pain, dysmenorrhea, vaginitis, menorrhagia, bronchitis, cough, dyspnea, epistaxis, hemoptysis, laryngitis, sinusitis, dermatitis, dry skin, purpura, pruritus, rash, urticaria, urinary incontinence/retention, urinary discoloration.

■ MONITORING

None

■ CONTRAINDICATIONS

Hypersensitivity to drug/class, impaired liver or renal function

■ PREGNANCY CLASS

B

MACROLIDES

Azithromycin (Zithromax® 250, 500, 600 mg tabs; 200 mg/5 mL suspension; IV; Z Pak® six 250 mg tabs; Tri Pak® three 500 mg tabs), clarithromycin (Biaxin® 250, 500 mg tabs; Biaxin SR® 500 mg extended release tabs), erythromycin base (E-Mycin® 250, 333 mg tabs; Ery-Tab® 250, 333, 500 mg tabs; Eryc® 250 mg tabs), erythromycin estolate (Ilosone® 125, 250, 500 mg tabs; 100, 125, 250 mg/5 mL suspension), erythromycin ethyl succinate (EES® 400 mg tabs; 200, 400 mg/5 mL suspension; EryPed® 200 mg chewable tabs; 200, 400 mg/5 mL suspension), erythromycin lactobionate (Erythrocin IV® IV), erythromycin stearate (Erythrocin® 250, 500 mg tabs)

▥ INDICATIONS

- Acne (azithromycin$) (see pg. 347)
- *Bordetella pertussis* (erythromycin*)
- *Chlamydia pneumoniae* (clarithromycin*)
- *Chlamydia trachomatis* (not clarithromycin*)
- *Corynebacterium diphtheriae* (erythromycin*)
- *Corynebacterium minutissimum* (erythromycin*)
- *Entamoeba histolytica* (erythromycin*)
- *Haemophilus influenzae**
- *Haemophilus parainfluenzae* (clarithromycin*)
- *Helicobacter pylori* (clarithromycin*)
- *Legionella pneumoniae* (erythromycin*)
- *Listeria monocytogenes* (erythromycin*)
- *Moraxella catarrhalis* (not clarithromycin)*
- *Mycobacterium abscessus* (clarithromycin$)
- *Mycobacterium avium-intracellulare* (azithromycin,* clarithromycin*)
- *Mycobacterium chelonae* (clarithromycin$)
- *Mycobacterium haemophilum* (clarithromycin*)
- *Mycobacterium marinum* (clarithromycin$)
- *Mycobacterium scrofulaceum* (clarithromycin⁺)
- *Mycoplasma pneumoniae* (erythromycin,* clarithromycin*)
- *Neisseria gonorrhoeae* (erythromycin*)
- *Staphylococcus aureus,* methicillin sensitive*
- *Streptococcus agalactiae* (azithromycin*)
- *Streptococcus pneumoniae**
- *Streptococcus pyogenes**
- *Ureaplasma urealyticum* (erythromycin*)

See Appendix II.

Usually effective:

- *Actinomyces* sp.
- *Chlamydia* sp.
- *Clostridium,* not *difficile* (azithromycin, clarithromycin)
- *Haemophilus ducreyi* (azithromycin, erythromycin)
- *Legionella* sp. (azithromycin, clarithromycin)
- *Listeria monocytogenes* (azithromycin, clarithromycin)
- *Moraxella catarrhalis* (clarithromycin)
- *Mycoplasma pneumoniae* (azithromycin)
- *Neisseria meningitidis* (azithroymcin, erythromycin)
- *Peptostreptococcus* sp. (azithromycin)
- *Prevotella melaninogenica* (azithromycin, clarithromycin)

Clinical trials lacking:

- *Clostridium,* not *difficile* (erythromycin)
- *Neisseria gonorrhoeae* (azithromycin, clarithromycin)
- *Peptostreptococcus* sp. (erythromycin, clarithromycin)
- *Rickettsia* sp. (erythromycin)
- *Salmonella* sp. (azithromycin)
- *Shigella* sp. (azithromycin)

MECHANISM OF ACTION

They bind to the 50S ribosomal subunit to interfere with bacterial protein synthesis.

DOSAGE

AZITHROMYCIN

500 mg PO qd for 1 day, then 250 mg PO qd for 4 more days

ACNE: 250 mg PO 3 times a week

CLARITHROMYCIN

250–500 mg PO bid or 1000 mg PO qd (extended-release tabs)

RENAL DOSING
Creatinine clearance (CrCl) 10–50 mL/min: 75% of normal dose
CrCL < 10 mL/min: 50–75% of normal dose
Hemodialysis: dose after dialysis

ERYTHROMYCIN

BASE: 333 mg PO tid or 250–500 mg PO q6h

ESTOLATE: 250–500 mg PO q6–12h, maximum of 2 g/d

ETHYL SUCCINATE: 400 mg PO q6d, maximum of 4 g/d

LACTOBIONATE: 15–50 mg/kg IV qd divided q6h

STEARATE: 250–500 mg PO q6–12h

RENAL DOSING
CrCl < 10 mL/min: 50–75% of normal dose

DRUG INTERACTIONS (APPLY TO ERYTHROMYCIN AND CLARITHROMYCIN UNLESS OTHERWISE INDICATED)

DECREASED EFFICACY OF MACROLIDES: antacids (azithromycin)

INCREASED LEVELS OF: digoxin (all), warfarin (all), almotriptan, amiodarone, benzodiazepines, aprepitant, aripiprazole, calcium channel blockers, bortezomib, bosentan, budesonide, buprenorphine, buspirone, carbamazepine, cilostazol, clozapine, cyclosporin, delavirdine, elatriptan, gefitinib, imatinib, levobupivacaine, methadone, mifepristone, modafinil, paclitaxel, phenytoin, protease inhibitors, quetiapine, repaglinide, sildenafil, sirolimus, tacrolimus, theophylline, tolterodine, valproic acid, vinca alkaloids, ziprasidone, zonisamide

DECREASED EFFICACY OF: oral contraceptives (all), fosfomycin (erythromycin)

INCREASED CENTRAL NERVOUS SYSTEM AND RESPIRATORY DEPRESSION: alfentanil, fentanyl

INCREASED ERGOT TOXICITY: ergotamine, ergot alkaloids

INCREASED QT PROLONGATION: cisapride, disopyramide, dofetilide, pimozide, quinidine, droperidol (erythromycin), halothane (erythromycin), mefloquine (erythromycin), quinolones (erythromycin), ziprasidone

DECREASED LEVELS OF MACROLIDES: efavirenz, griseofulvin, rifabutin, rifapentine

HYPERKALEMIA: eplerenone

RHABDOMYOLYSIS: statins

SIDE EFFECTS (APPLY TO ALL THREE UNLESS OTHERWISE INDICATED)

COMMON: diarrhea, nausea, vomiting, abdominal pain and cramping, vaginitis, dyspepsia, dizziness, rash, anorexia, pruritus, ageusia (clarithromycin), headache, stomatitis (erythromycin), melena (erythromycin), elevated liver function test results (erythromycin), jaundice (erythromycin), eosinophilia (erythromycin)

RARE: angioedema, anaphylaxis, cholestatic jaundice, Stevens-Johnson syndrome, toxic epidermal necrolysis, pseudomembranous colitis, hepatotoxicity (clarithromycin), QT prolongation (clarithromycin), ventricular arrhythmias (clarithromycin, erythromycin), pancreatitis (clarithromycin), thrombophlebitis (erythromycin), bradycardia (erythromycin), hypotension (erythromycin), ototoxicity (erythromycin IV), glossitis, stomatitis, confusion, vertigo, urticaria, sweating, jaundice, psychosis, change in taste or smell, elevated liver function test results, arrhythmias, hypoglycemia, anemia, elevated renal function test results

▧ MONITORING

None

▧ CONTRAINDICATIONS

Hypersensitivity to drug/class, impaired liver function, astemizole or terfenadine use (azithromycin, erythromycin), impaired liver function (clarithromycin), pregnancy (clarithromycin), myasthenia gravis (erythromycin)

▧ PREGNANCY CLASS

B (azithromycin, erythromycin); C (clarithromycin)

MAGIC MOUTHWASH

▧ INDICATIONS

- Aphthous stomatitis[+] (see pg. 352)
- Autoimmune bullous disease[+] (see pg. 355, 382–385)
- Candidal infection[+]
- Medication-induced ulcers[+]
- Radiation-induced ulcers[^]
- Stomatitis from chemotherapy[^]

▧ MECHANISM OF ACTION

This combination helps to relieve the pain, inflammation, irritation, and any candidal infection associated with the various causes of stomatitis.

DOSAGE

COMPOUNDS: nystatin suspension 60 mL; diphenhydramine suspension
    30 mL; triamcinolone suspension 40 mg/mL, 5 mL; viscous lidocaine 2%
    40 mL; Maalox® 200 mL.
    Swish (for 5–10 min) and swallow 5–10 mL PO qid.

DRUG INTERACTIONS

None

SIDE EFFECTS

COMMON: burning, tingling, pruritus, bad tasting, dermatitis

RARE: methemoglobinemia (lidocaine)

MONITORING

None

CONTRAINDICATIONS

Hypersensitivity to drugs/classes, methemoglobinemia (lidocaine), pregnancy

PREGNANCY CLASS

C

MEBENDAZOLE

(Vermox® 100 mg chewable tabs)

INDICATIONS

- Capillariasis (*Capillaria philippinensis*)^
- Filariasis, body cavity (*Mansonella perstans*$, *Loa loa*$)

- Hookworm (*Ancylostoma duodenale, Necator americanus*)*
- Pinworm (*Enterobius vermicularis*)*
- Roundworm (*Ascaris lumbricoides**, *Angiostrongylus cantonensis* and *costaricensis* [in vitro])
- Toxocariasis/visceral larva migrans (*Toxocara canis* and *catis*,^ *Ancylostoma*,^ *Gnathostoma spinigerum*+, *Spirometra mansonoides*+)
- Trichinosis (*Trichinella spiralis*^)
- Whipworm (*Trichuris trichiura*)*

MECHANISM OF ACTION

It inhibits microtubule formation and glucose uptake.

DOSAGE

CAPILLARIASIS: 200 mg PO bid for 20 days

FILARIASIS: 100 mg PO bid for 30 days

HOOKWORM: 100 mg PO bid for 3–5 days

PINWORM: 100 mg PO once

ROUNDWORM: 100 mg PO bid for 5 days (except *A. costaricensis*, 200–400 mg PO tid for 10 days)

SPIROMETRA: 40 mg/kg/d for 6 months

TOXOCARIASIS/VISCERAL LARVA MIGRANS: 100–300 mg PO bid for 5 days

TRICHINOSIS: 200–400 mg PO tid for 3 days

WHIPWORM: 100 mg PO bid for 3–5 days

DRUG INTERACTIONS

DECREASED EFFICACY OF MEBENDAZOLE: cimetidine

SIDE EFFECTS

COMMON: abdominal pain, diarrhea, nausea, vomiting, rash, pruritus

RARE: angioedema, seizures, neutropenia, agranulocytosis, hepatitis, angioedema, elevated liver function tests, alopecia, fever, dizziness, headache

▓ MONITORING

None

▓ CONTRAINDICATIONS

Hypersensitivity to drug/class, children <2 years of age, prolonged use, pregnancy

▓ PREGNANCY CLASS

C

MECHLORETHAMINE (NITROGEN MUSTARD), TOPICAL

(Mustargen® 10 mg in each vial)

▓ INDICATIONS

- Acrodermatitis of Hallopeau⁺
- Alopecia areata$ (see pg. 349)
- Cutaneous chronic granulocytic leukemia⁺
- Cutaneous Hodgkin's disease⁺
- Cutaneous T-cell lymphoma (with electron beam^, monotherapy$) (see pg. 358)
- Multicentric reticulohistiocytosis⁺
- Psoriasis (with ultraviolet B^, monotherapy$) (see pg. 392)
- Pyoderma gangrenosum⁺ (see pg. 394)

▓ MECHANISM OF ACTION

It is an alkylating agent that inhibits DNA replication.

DOSAGE

TOPICAL AQUEOUS SOLUTION: 10 mg in 60 mL of tap water applied qd. May use up to 40 mg in 60 mL with a 4–6 month rest period between treatment courses.

TOPICAL OINTMENT: 10 mg in 10 mL of 95% absolute alcohol, then mix with 100 g of Aquaphor® or white petrolatum and apply qd. May use up to 40 mg in 100 g. 4–6 month rest periods between treatment courses.

DRUG INTERACTIONS

None

SIDE EFFECTS

COMMON: urticaria, contact or irritant dermatitis, erythema, pruritus, burning/stinging

RARE: anaphylaxis, squamous and basal cell carcinoma, Stevens-Johnson syndrome, eruptive epidermoid cysts, bullous pemphigoid

MONITORING

None

CONTRAINDICATIONS

Hypersensitivity to drug/class, pregnancy

PREGNANCY CLASS

D

MELPHALAN

(Alkeran® 2 mg tabs; IV)

▓ INDICATIONS

- Amyloidosis^ (see pg. 350)
- Cryoglobulinemia⁺
- Metastatic melanoma^ (see pg. 378)
- Multiple myeloma*
- Necrobiotic xanthogranuloma⁺
- Ovarian cancer*
- Pyoderma gangrenosum⁺ (see pg. 394)
- Scleromyxedema§

▓ MECHANISM OF ACTION

It is a derivative of nitrogen mustard, which alkylates and cross-links DNA to inhibit DNA synthesis.

▓ DOSAGE

AMYLOIDOSIS: 70–200 mg/m^2 IV per infusion

CRYOGLOBULINEMIA: 0.25 mg/kg/d for 4 days, every 4 weeks

METASTATIC MELANOMA: 10–13 mg/L limb perfusion for 60 min

MULTIPLE MYELOMA: 6 mg PO qd or 16 mg/m^2 IV every 2 weeks for 4 doses, then monthly thereafter

NECROBIOTIC XANTHOGRANULOMA: 0.15 mg/kg/d IV for 5 days, given monthly

PYODERMA GANGRENOSUM: 2 mg PO qod

SCLEROMYXEDEMA: 9–18 mg PO qd for 4–7 days, every 4–6 weeks

■ DRUG INTERACTIONS

INCREASED IMMUNOSUPPRESSION: alefacept

INCREASED MYELOSUPPRESSION: bone marrow suppressants, rituximab, ibritumomab tiuxetan, zidovudine

ANTAGONISTIC EFFECTS WITH: colony-stimulating factors

INADEQUATE RESPONSE OF: toxoids

■ SIDE EFFECTS

COMMON: stomatitis, nausea, vomiting, diarrhea, alopecia, sterility, myelo-suppression

RARE: anaphylaxis, bone marrow failure, hemolytic anemia, oral ulcers, hepatotoxicity, pulmonary fibrosis, interstitial pneumonitis, vasculitis

■ MONITORING

BASELINE AND MONTHLY: complete blood count

■ CONTRAINDICATIONS

Hypersensitivity to drug/class, pregnancy, hypersensitivity to chlorambucil, impaired renal function, leukopenia, thrombocytopenia, anemia, chronic lymphocytic leukemia, use of live vaccines

■ PREGNANCY CLASS

D

METHOTREXATE

(Rheumatrex® 2.5 mg tabs, 25 mg/mL in 2 and 10 mL vials, 25 mg/mL in 2, 4, 8, 10 mL preservative-free vials; Trexall® 2.5, 5, 7.5, 15 mg tabs)

INDICATIONS

- Atopic dermatitis§ (see pg. 353)
- Behçet's disease$^+$ (see pg. 355)
- Bullous pemphigoid§ (see pg. 355)
- Cutaneous T-cell lymphoma§ (see pg. 358)
- Dermatitis herpetiformis$^+$ (see pg. 360)
- Dermatomyositis$^\wedge$ (see pg. 361)
- IgA pemphigus$^+$ (see pg. 384)
- Keloids$^+$ (see pg. 371)
- Keratoacanthomas§
- Leukocytoclastic vasculitis$^+$ (see pg. 404)
- Lupus, discoid$^+$, subacute cutaneous§, systemic$^\wedge$ (see pg. 375)
- Lymphomatoid papulosis§, topical$^+$ (see pg. 377)
- Morphea§ (see pg. 381)
- Pemphigus foliaceus$^+$ (see pg. 383)
- Pemphigus vulgaris§ (see pg. 385)
- Pityriasis lichenoides et varioliformis acuta§ (see pg. 386)
- Pityriasis rubra pilaris§ (see pg. 387)
- Polyarteritis nodosa, cutaneous$^+$ (see pg. 404)
- Prevention of antibody formation to infliximab$^\wedge$
- Psoriasis* (see pg. 392)
- Psoriatic arthritis$^\wedge$
- Pyoderma gangrenosum$^+$ (see pg. 394)
- Reiter's disease$^+$ (see pg. 395)
- Rheumatoid arthritis*
- Sarcoidosis$^\wedge$ (see pg. 396)
- Scleroderma$^\wedge$ (see pg. 398)
- Sezary's syndrome* (see pg. 358)

MECHANISM OF ACTION

It competitively and irreversibly inhibits dihydrofolate reductase, preventing the conversion of dihydrofolate to tetrahydrofolate and thus inhibiting DNA synthesis. It also competitively and reversibly inhibits thymidylate synthetase. Lymphocyte proliferation is also blocked.

DOSAGE

ATOPIC DERMATITIS: 7.5–12 mg PO weekly

BEHÇET'S DISEASE, LYMPHOMATOID PAPULOSIS, PEMPHIGUS: 2.5–15 mg PO weekly

BULLOUS PEMPHIGOID, DERMATOMYOSITIS: 2.5–30 mg PO weekly

CUTANEOUS T-CELL LYMPHOMA: 5–75 mg PO weekly

LEUKOCYTOCLASTIC VASCULITIS: 15 mg IM weekly

PSORIASIS, PITYRIASIS RUBRA PILARIS, CUTANEOUS LUPUS: 10–30 mg PO/IM/SC weekly

PSORIATIC ARTHRITIS: 2.5–15 mg PO weekly

REITER'S DISEASE: 20–30 mg PO weekly

RHEUMATOID ARTHRITIS, PITYRIASIS LICHENOIDES ET VARIOLIFORMIS ACUTA (PLEVA): 7.5–30 mg PO/IM/SC weekly

SEZARY'S SYNDROME: 2.5–80 mg PO/IM weekly

SYSTEMIC LUPUS, SCLERODERMA, MORPHEA: 15–20 mg PO weekly

LYMPHOMATOID PAPULOSIS: 0.83 mg topical per lesion qd

RENAL DOSING
Creatinine clearance (CrCl) 60–80 mL/min: decrease by 25%
CrCl 50–60 mL/min: decrease by 33%
CrCl 10–50 mL/min: decrease by 50–70%
CrCl < 10 mL/min: avoid use

May divide into 3 doses q12h once a week. Give folic acid 1 mg PO qd or leucovorin 5 mg PO weekly (begin 24 h after dosing methotrexate). May start at 5–10 mg weekly, increasing by 2.5–5 mg weekly. May taper down with same frequency.

▓ DRUG INTERACTIONS

INCREASED LEVELS OF METHOTREXATE: cyclooxygenase-2 inhibitors, nonsteroidal anti-inflammatory drugs, sulfonamides, salicylates, probenecid, penicillins, trimethoprim, dipyridamole, chloramphenicol, phenothiazines, phenytoin, tetracycline

INCREASED RISK OF HEPATOTOXICITY: acitretin, leflunomide, alcohol

INCREASED RISK OF BLOOD DYSCRASIAS: lamotrigine

INCREASED HEMATOLOGIC TOXICITY: trimethoprim, sulfonamides, leflunomide, dapsone

SIDE EFFECTS

COMMON: nausea, vomiting, stomatitis, malaise, fatigue, fever, chills, dizziness, diarrhea, rash, pruritus, alopecia, photosensitivity

RARE: thrombocytopenia, leukopenia, anemia, aplastic anemia, hepatotoxicity, nephrotoxicity, immunosuppression, infection, leukoencephalopathy, seizures, neurotoxicity, arachnoiditis and subacute myelopathy with intrathecal injection, pulmonary fibrosis, pneumonitis, Stevens-Johnson syndrome, exfoliative dermatitis, erythema multiforme, toxic epidermal necrolysis, radiation recall reaction

MONITORING

BASELINE: complete blood count, liver function, renal function, hepatitis A/B/C, HIV, liver biopsy if high-risk patient

WEEKLY FOR 2–4 WEEKS, GRADUALLY DECREASING TO EVERY 3 MONTHS, 5–6 DAYS AFTER DOSE ESCALATION: complete blood count, liver function

TWICE YEARLY: renal function

LIVER BIOPSY
After first 3–6 months: baseline liver biopsy (in long-term use only)
After every 1.5–2 g total dose if low risk, 1 g if high risk: liver biopsy
After every 6 months if grade IIIA on liver biopsy: liver biopsy

Liver biopsy grades:

- I: normal, mild fatty infiltration, mild portal inflammation
- II: moderate to severe fatty infiltration, moderate to severe portal inflammation
- IIA: mild fibrosis
- IIIB: moderate to severe fibrosis
- IV: cirrhosis

Discontinue if grade IIIB or IV. Discontinue if liver function test results are twice the upper limits of normal, white blood cells < 3500 cells/mm^3, or platelet count < 100,000 cells/mm^3. May restart after rest period of 2–3 weeks.

CONTRAINDICATIONS

Hypersensitivity to drug/class, pregnancy, lactation, alcohol abuse, liver dysfunction, infection, pleural/peritoneal effusion, immunodeficiency, impaired renal function, bone marrow depletion, peptic ulcer disease, infection, concomitant radiotherapy, immunodeficiency, blood dyscrasias

▓ PREGNANCY CLASS

X

METHOXSALEN

(8MOP® 10 mg tabs, Oxsoralen-Ultra® 10 mg caps, Oxsoralen® 1% lotion in 1 oz bottles, UVADEX® 20 µg/mL in 10 mL vials)

▓ INDICATIONS

ORAL
- Cutaneous T-cell lymphoma with ultraviolet (UV) A and photopheresis* (see pg. 358)
- Psoriasis with UVA* , pustular with UVA$ (see pg. 392)
- Vitiligo* with UVA (see pg. 405)

TOPICAL
- Cutaneous T-cell lymphoma with bexarotene 300 mg/m² PO qd⁺ (see pg. 358)
- Dyshidrotic eczema^
- Palmoplantar pustulosis$
- Psoriasis^, with narrow-band UVB^ (see pg. 392)
- Vitiligo* (see pg. 405)

▓ MECHANISM OF ACTION

It binds and cross-links to DNA to prevent DNA synthesis. Upon photoactivation with UVA or photopheresis, it also inhibits lymphocyte function, decreases Langerhans cell numbers, influences adhesion molecule expression, decreases antigen-presenting cell function, decreases cell proliferation, and increases cytotoxic function.

■ DOSAGE

PHOTOPHERESIS: 0.4 mg/kg PO plus 10 mg extra, 1.5–3 h before UVA treatment. 10 mL vial of UVADEX® can be added to photopheresis bag during first cycle.

ORAL PSORALEN UVA (PUVA): <30 kg, 10 mg; 30–50 kg, 20 mg; 51–65 kg, 30 mg; 66–80 kg, 40 mg; 81–90 kg, 50 mg; 91–115 kg, 60 mg; >115 kg, 70 mg PO 1.5–3 h before treatment

TOPICAL PUVA: applied in physician's office once a week to daily, then treated with UVA

■ DRUG INTERACTIONS

INCREASED PHOTOSENSITIVITY: anthralin, coal tar, griseofulvin, phenothiazines, nalidixic acid, halogenated salicylanilides, sulfonamides, tetracyclines, thiazides, methylene blue, toluidine blue, rose bengal, methyl orange

■ SIDE EFFECTS

ORAL

COMMON: nausea, vomiting, pruritus, erythema, rash, headache, urticaria, leg cramps, photosensitivity

RARE: herpes simplex, skin cancers

TOPICAL

COMMON: sunburn, skin thickening

RARE: skin cancers, hypotension, edema, dizziness, nervousness, insomnia, depression

■ MONITORING FOR ORAL USE

BASELINE: eye exam, complete blood count, anti-nuclear antibodies, liver function, renal function

EVERY 6 MONTHS: complete blood count, anti-nuclear antibodies, liver function, renal function

▨ CONTRAINDICATIONS

ORAL: hypersensitivity to drug/class, children <12 years old, hepatic disease, renal disease, cataracts, photosensitivity, invasive squamous cell carcinoma, melanoma, aphakia, basal cell carcinoma, prior arsenic or radiation exposure, cardiac disease, porphyria, lupus, xeroderma pigmentosum, pregnancy

TOPICAL: hypersensitivity to drug/class, melanoma, invasive skin cancers, porphyria, lupus, xeroderma pigmentosum, children <12 years old, pregnancy

▨ PREGNANCY CLASS

C

METRONIDAZOLE

(Flagyl® 250, 375, 500 mg tabs, 500 mg powder for IV; Flagyl ER® 750 mg tabs)

▨ INDICATIONS

- Amebiasis, intestinal*
- Amebic abscess (*Entamoeba histolytica*)*
- Bacterial vaginosis (*Gardnerella vaginalis*,^ *Bacteroides fragilis*,* *Peptococcus**)
- *Bacteroides fragilis, distasonis, oavtus, thetaiotaomicron,* and *vulgatus**
- *Clostridium difficile* and others*
- Dracunculosis (*Dracunculus medinensis*)^
- *Eubacterium* sp.*
- *Fusobacterium* sp.*
- Giardiasis (*Giardia lamblia*)^
- *Peptococcus niger* and others*
- *Peptostreptococcus* sp.*
- *Porphyromonas gingivalis*^
- *Prevotella melaninogenica*^
- Protozoa, intestinal (*Balantidium coli*,^ *Blastocystis hominis*^)
- Trichomoniasis (*Trichomonas vaginalis*)*

See Appendix II.

▦ MECHANISM OF ACTION

It disrupts DNA and inhibits nucleic acid synthesis.

▦ DOSAGE

AMEBIASIS, INTESTINAL: 750 mg PO tid for 5–10 days with iodoquinol 650 mg PO tid for 20 days or paromycin 500 mg PO tid for 7 days

AMEBIC ABSCESS: 500–750 mg PO tid for 5–10 days

BACTERIAL INFECTIONS: 500 mg PO q6–8 h for 7–14 days or 15 mg/kg IV once, then 7.5 mg/kg IV q6h, maximum 1 g/d

BACTERIAL VAGINOSIS: 500 mg PO bid for 7 days, or vaginal cream qhs for 5 days

CLOSTRIDIUM DIFFICILE **COLITIS:** 500 mg PO tid for 7–14 days

DRACUNCULOSIS: 250 mg PO tid for 10 days

GIARDIASIS: 250 mg PO tid for 5–7 days

PROTOZOA, INTESTINAL: 750 mg PO tid for 5 days (*B. coli*), for 10 days (*B. hominis*)

TRICHOMONIASIS: 2 g PO once or 500 mg PO bid for 7 days

RENAL DOSING
   Creatinine clearance < 10 mL/min and chronic peritoneal dialysis: 50% of 7.5 mg/kg IV q6h
   Hemodialysis: dose after dialysis

▦ DRUG INTERACTIONS

INCREASED RISK OF PROPYLENE GLYCOL TOXICITY: amprenavir

INCREASED LEVELS OF: bosentan, cyclosporin, lithium, phenytoin, sildenafil, tacrolimus, voriconazole, warfarin

INCREASED ERGOT TOXICITY: ergotamine, ergot alkaloids

DECREASED EFFICACY OF METRONIDAZOLE: oral contraceptives

INCREASED PERIPHERAL NEUROPATHY: didanosine, stavudine, zalcitabine

PSYCHOSIS: disulfiram

DISULFIRAM-LIKE REACTION: ethanol, lopinavir/ritonavir, ritonavir

▩ SIDE EFFECTS

COMMON: nausea, vomiting, dyspepsia, diarrhea, metallic taste, dry mouth, rash, pruritus, headache, dizziness, syncope, ataxia, confusion, thrombo-phlebitis, fever, vertigo, paresthesias, furry tongue, red-brown urine

RARE: seizures, neutropenia, peripheral neuropathy, constipation, flattened T waves on electrocardiogram, flushing, dry mouth, nasal congestion, decreased libido

▩ MONITORING

None

▩ CONTRAINDICATIONS

Hypersensitivity to drug/class, first-trimester use, blood dyscrasias, impaired liver function, central nervous system disorder, ethanol

▩ PREGNANCY CLASS

B

METRONIDAZOLE, TOPICAL

(MetroCream® 0.75% cream in 45 g tubes, MetroGel® 0.75% gel in 45 g tubes, MetroLotion® 0.75% lotion in 59 mL bottles, MetroGel vaginal® 0.75% vaginal gel in 70 g tubes, Noritate® 1% cream in 30 g tubes)

▩ INDICATIONS

- Acne vulgaris^ (see pg. 347)
- Childhood granulomatous perioral dermatitis+

- Demodex folliculitis^
- Malodorous wounds^
- Perioral dermatitis^
- Rosacea (see pg. 395)
- Seborrheic dermatitis^ (see pg. 399)
- Skin ulcers$

MECHANISM OF ACTION

It inhibits nucleic acid and DNA synthesis.

DOSAGE

Apply bid.

DRUG INTERACTIONS

None

SIDE EFFECTS

COMMON: burning, stinging, erythema, dryness, pruritus

RARE: metallic taste, numbness of extremities, nausea, contact dermatitis

MONITORING

None

CONTRAINDICATIONS

Hypersensitivity to drug/class, blood dyscrasias

PREGNANCY CLASS

B

MICONAZOLE

(Zeasorb® AF 2% lotion/powder in 56 g bottles; Zeasorb® AF 2% powder in 70 g bottles; Monistat® 2% cream [over the counter]; Monistat 1® 6.5% vaginal cream and 1200 mg vaginal suppository [over the counter]; Monistat 3® 4% vaginal cream and 200 mg vaginal suppository [over the counter]; Monistat 7® 2% vaginal cream and 100 mg vaginal suppository [over the counter]; Micatin® 2% cream, powder, spray [over the counter])

■ INDICATIONS

- Candidiasis, cutaneous (cream)*
- Candidiasis, vaginal (vaginal cream, vaginal suppository)*
- Tinea (cream)*

See Appendix I

■ MECHANISM OF ACTION

It alters fungal cell membrane permeability by inhibiting 14-α-demethylase in ergosterol biosynthesis, which leads to cessation of cell growth.

■ DOSAGE

CANDIDIASIS, CUTANEOUS: Apply cream bid for 2–4 weeks.

CANDIDIASIS, VAGINAL: Insert vaginal suppository or vaginal cream qhs for 1–7 days.

TINEA: Apply cream bid for 2–4 weeks.

■ DRUG INTERACTIONS

None

■ SIDE EFFECTS

CREAM

COMMON: irritation, burning, stinging, pruritus, erythema

RARE: maceration, contact dermatitis

VAGINAL SUPPOSITORY AND VAGINAL CREAM

COMMON: burning, pruritus, soreness, swelling

RARE: pain, cramps, abdominal pain

MONITORING

None

CONTRAINDICATIONS

Hypersensitivity to drug/class, pregnancy

PREGNANCY CLASS

C

MINOXIDIL

(Rogaine® 2, 5% solution [over the counter])

INDICATIONS

- Alopecia areata (see pg. 349)^
- Androgenic alopecia, 5% for men,* 2% for women, 5% for women^
  (see pg. 351)
- Chemotherapy-induced alopecia^

MECHANISM OF ACTION

The exact mechanism of action is unknown. However, it is thought to increase cutaneous blood flow.

DOSAGE

Apply bid.

■ DRUG INTERACTIONS

None

■ SIDE EFFECTS

COMMON: hypertrichosis, dryness, irritation, edema, contact dermatitis, pruritus

RARE: cardiac irregularities (especially in children using > 2 mL/qd of 5% solution).

■ MONITORING

None

■ CONTRAINDICATIONS

Hypersensitivity to drug/class, pregnancy

■ PREGNANCY CLASS

C

MUPIROCIN

(Bactroban® 2% ointment in 15 and 30 g tubes, cream in 15 and 30 g tubes, Bactroban nasal® 2% ointment in 1 g single-use tubes)

■ INDICATIONS

- Bacterial skin infections caused by methicillin-resistant *Staphylococcus aureus* (MRSA), *Staphylococcus aureus*, *Streptococcus pyogenes*, or beta-hemolytic *Streptococcus**
- Impetigo, caused by MRSA, *Staphylococcus aureus*, *Streptococcus pyogenes*, or beta-hemolytic *Streptococcus**
- MRSA nasal colonization* (nasal ointment)
- Wound healing^ (see pg. 407)

■ MECHANISM OF ACTION

It selectively binds to bacterial isoleucyl transfer-RNA synthetase to inhibit bacterial protein synthesis.

■ DOSAGE

SKIN INFECTIONS: Apply tid.

MRSA NASAL COLONIZATION: Apply bid for first week of every month to the inside of each nostril.

■ DRUG INTERACTIONS

None

■ SIDE EFFECTS

COMMON: burning, pruritus, erythema, dryness, tenderness, headache (nasal), rhinitis (nasal), cough (nasal), pharyngitis (nasal), taste change (nasal)

RARE: superinfection, respiratory disorders (nasal), contact dermatitis

■ MONITORING

None

■ CONTRAINDICATIONS

Hypersensitivity to drug/class, large open wounds, ophthalmic use

■ PREGNANCY CLASS

B

MYCOPHENOLATE MOFETIL

(CellCept® 250 mg caps, 500 mg tabs, 200 mg/mL suspension in 225 mL bottles, 500 mg in 20 mL vials)

■ INDICATIONS

- Atopic dermatitis$ (see pg. 353)
- Bowel-associated arthritis dermatitis syndrome+
- Bullous pemphigoid+ (see pg. 355)
- Churg-Strauss syndrome+ (see pg. 404)
- Cicatricial pemphigoid$ (see pg. 356)
- Dyshidrotic eczema+
- Epidermolysis bullosa acquisita+ (see pg. 363)
- Erythema nodosum+
- Graft-versus-host disease, chronic+ (see pg. 365)
- Lichen planus+, oral+ (see pg. 371)
- Linear IgA+ with dapone 25 mg PO qd (see pg. 374)
- Lupus, discoid+, subacute cutaneous+ (see pg. 375)
- Metastatic Crohn's disease+
- Paraneoplastic pemphigus+ (see pg. 382)
- Pemphigus foliaceus$ (see pg. 383)
- Pemphigus vulgaris$ (see pg. 385)
- Psoriasis$ (see pg. 392)
- Pyoderma gangrenosum+ (see pg. 394)
- Recurrent erythema multiforme/Stevens-Johnson syndrome+ (see pg. 364, 400)
- Renal/cardiac/hepatic allograft rejection*
- Sarcoidosis, cutaneous+ (see pg. 396)
- Urticarial vasculitis+ (see pg. 404)
- Weber-Christian disease+

■ MECHANISM OF ACTION

Mycophenolate mofetil (MMF) inhibits de novo purine synthesis by competitively blocking inosine monophosphate dehydrogenase (converts inosine-5-phosphate and xanthine-5-phosphate to guanosine-5-phosphate). T and B cells that lack the purine salvage pathway cannot proliferate, thus leading to decreased levels of immunoglobulins and delayed hypersensitivity.

■ DOSAGE

Bowel-Associated Arthritis Dermatitis Syndrome: 1 g PO qd

Lichen Planus, Erythema Nodosum, Sarcoidosis, Discoid Lupus: 1.5 g PO bid

Linear IgA: 155 mg/m^2 PO qd with dapsone 25 mg PO qd

Metastatic Crohn's Disease: 500 mg PO bid

All Others: 1 g PO bid

■ DRUG INTERACTIONS

Increased Levels of MMF: acyclovir, ganciclovir, probenecid

Decreased Levels of MMF: antacids, cholestyramine, iron salts

Increased Risk of Immunosuppression: alefacept

Increased Risk of Bone Marrow Suppression: azathioprine

Decreased Levels of: levonorgestrel

Increased Risk of Nephrotoxicity: nonsteroidal anti-inflammatory drugs (NSAIDS)

Increased Risk of Gastrointestinal Bleed: NSAIDS

Increased Risk of Infection: tumor necrosis factor blocking agents

■ SIDE EFFECTS

Common: nausea, vomiting, diarrhea, abdominal pain, anorexia, dysuria, urinary urgency and increased frequency, sterile pyuria, herpes zoster, infections, weakness, fatigue, headaches, tinnitus, insomnia, gastrointestinal bleed/perforation/ulceration, hypertension, edema, elevated liver function test results, oral candidiasis, flatulence

Rare: squamous cell carcinomas, psychosis, thrombocytopenia, leukopenia, neutropenia, immunosuppression, sepsis, lymphoma/lymphoproliferative disorders/malignancies, hypotension with rapid IV infusion, dyspnea, cough, hypercholesterolemia, hypokalemia, tremor, acne, hypophospha-temia, hyperglycemia, increased blood urea nitrogen/creatinine, increased lactate dehydrogenase levels, bilirubinemia, hypervolemia, hyperuricemia, hypomagnesemia, acidosis, weight gain, hypocalcemia, hypoproteinemia, constipation, cholangitis, hepatitis, cholestatic jaundice, chest pain, ane-mia, ecchymosis, oliguria, bradycardia, pericardial effusion, heart failure, pharyngitis, rhinitis, sinusitis, asthma, atelectasis, rash, pruritus, sweating, hypertonia, dizziness, agitation, confusion, nervousness, depression, pares-thesias, anxiety, leg cramps, myalgia, amblyopia

MONITORING

BASELINE: complete blood count, serum chemistry, liver function

WEEKLY FOR FIRST MONTH: complete blood count

TWICE A MONTH FOR SECOND AND THIRD MONTHS: complete blood count

MONTHLY: complete blood count (after fourth month), liver function

CONTRAINDICATIONS

Hypersensitivity to drug/class, pregnancy, lactation, peptic ulcer disease, he-patic or renal disease, azathioprine use, cholestyramine use, IV use if allergic to polysorbate 80, avoid live vaccines, hereditary deficiency of hypoxanthine-guanine phosphoribosyl-transferase, phenylketonuria

PREGNANCY CLASS

C

NAFTIFINE

(Naftin® 1% cream in 30 g tubes, 1% gel in 40 and 60 g tubes)

INDICATIONS

- Candidiasis, cutaneous*
- Tinea*

See Appendix I.

MECHANISM OF ACTION

It is fungistatic and fungicidal. It inhibits squalene epoxidase for ergosterol biosynthesis.

DOSAGE

Apply qd.

DRUG INTERACTIONS

None

SIDE EFFECTS

COMMON: burning, pruritus, erythema

RARE: contact dermatitis, dryness, tingling, burning, irritation

MONITORING

None

CONTRAINDICATIONS

Hypersensitivity to drug/class

PREGNANCY CLASS

B

NALOXONE

(Narcan® 10 mL multidose vial with 0.4 mg/mL or 1 mg/mL, 1 mL ampule with 0.4 mg/mL, 2 mL ampule with 0.02 mg/mL or 1 mg/mL)

▧ INDICATIONS

- Increased blood pressure in septic shock*
- Opiate overdose*
- Opiate reversal post-surgery*
- Pruritus of cholestasis^ (see pg. 391)

▧ MECHANISM OF ACTION

It antagonizes opioids by competing for the same receptor sites.

▧ DOSAGE

OPIATE OVERDOSE: 0.4–2 mg SC/IV q2–3min for up to 10 min

OPIATE REVERSAL POST-SURGERY: 0.1–0.2 mg IV q2–3min as needed

PRURITUS OF CHOLESTASIS: 0.2 µg/kg/min IV for 4 days

▧ DRUG INTERACTIONS

MAY PRECIPITATE WITHDRAWAL: acetaminophen/opiates, acetaminophen/propoxyphene, acetaminophen/tramadol, aspirin/opiates, chlorpheniramine/hydrocodone, decongestants/opiates, meperidine/promethazine, opiates, promethazine/codeine, propoxyphene, tramadol

▧ SIDE EFFECTS

COMMON: tachycardia, hyper-/hypotension, nausea, vomiting, tremor, withdrawal symptoms, diaphoresis, pulmonary edema, irritability

RARE: ventricular fibrillation, cardiac arrest, seizures

MONITORING

None

CONTRAINDICATIONS

Hypersensitivity to drug, cardiovascular disease, opiate addiction, impaired liver function, impaired renal function, cardiotoxic drugs

PREGNANCY CLASS

B

NALTREXONE

(ReVia® 50 mg tabs)

INDICATIONS

- Alcohol dependence*
- Opiate addiction*
- Pruritus of cholestasis^, uremic^ (see pg. 391)

MECHANISM OF ACTION

It is an opioid antagonist that reversibly and competitively binds to opioid receptors to block the effects of opioids.

DOSAGE

50 mg PO qd

DRUG INTERACTIONS

MAY PRECIPITATE WITHDRAWAL: acetaminophen/opiates, acetaminophen/propoxyphene, acetaminophen/tramadol, aspirin/opiates, chlorpheniramine/hydrocodone, decongestants/opiates, meperidine/promethazine, opiates, promethazine/codeine, propoxyphene, tramadol

SIDE EFFECTS

COMMON: opiate withdrawal, insomnia, nausea, vomiting, anxiety, headache, abdominal pain, muscle aches, rash, dizziness, fatigue, somnolence, anorexia, constipation, liver dysfunction, chills, acne, cold sores, alopecia, pruritus

RARE: suicidal ideation

MONITORING

BASELINE: liver function tests and urine screen for opiates (if abuse suspected)

CONTRAINDICATIONS

Hypersensitivity to drug, opiate use, opiate dependence, opiate withdrawal, liver failure, acute hepatitis, failed naloxone challenge, failed naltrexone challenge, impaired liver function, pregnancy

PREGNANCY CLASS

C

NYSTATIN

(Mycostatin® 200,000 U lozenges, 100,000 U/mL suspension, 100,000 U/g cream in 30 g tubes, powder in 15 g bottles; Nystop® powder 100,000 U/g in 15 g bottles; Nilstat® 100,000 U/mL suspension; Nystatin® 100,000 U vaginal suppository)

■ INDICATIONS

- Candidiasis, cutaneous (topical)*
- Candidiasis, oral (lozenges, suspension)*
- Candidiasis, vaginal (suppositories)*

See Appendix I.

■ MECHANISM OF ACTION

It is fungistatic and fungicidal. It binds to fungal cell membranes and then causes a change in permeability, allowing leakage of intracellular components.

■ DOSAGE

CANDIDIASIS, CUTANEOUS: Apply topically bid to tid for 1–2 weeks.

CANDIDIASIS, ORAL: 1–2 lozenges 4–5 times a day for 14 days

CANDIDIASIS, ORAL: 4–6 mL PO qid for 1–2 weeks

CANDIDIASIS, VAGINAL: Insert 1 vaginal suppository qhs for 2 weeks.

■ DRUG INTERACTIONS

None

■ SIDE EFFECTS

LOZENGES, SUSPENSION, SUPPOSITORIES

COMMON: irritation, nausea, sensitization

RARE: diarrhea, gastrointestinal distress, vomiting, rash, urticaria, Stevens-Johnson syndrome, abdominal pain

TOPICAL

COMMON: rash, irritation, pruritus

RARE: eczema, pain, allergic reaction

MONITORING

None

CONTRAINDICATIONS

Hypersensitivity to drug/class, pregnancy (oral)

PREGNANCY CLASS

C (oral), A (suppositories), B (others)

OXICONAZOLE

(Oxistat® 1% cream in 15, 30 and 60 g tubes, 1% lotion in 30 mL bottles)

INDICATIONS

- Candidiasis, cutaneous*
- Tinea*

See Appendix I.

MECHANISM OF ACTION

It alters fungal cell membrane permeability by inhibiting 14-α-demethylase in ergosterol biosynthesis, which leads to cessation of cell growth.

DOSAGE

CANDIDIASIS, CUTANEOUS: Apply bid.

TINEA: Apply qd.

DRUG INTERACTIONS

None

■ SIDE EFFECTS

Common: pruritus, burning, erythema

Rare: irritation, maceration, fissuring

■ MONITORING

None

■ CONTRAINDICATIONS

Hypersensitivity to drug/class, pregnancy

■ PREGNANCY CLASS

C

PENCICLOVIR

(Denavir® 1% cream in 1.5 g tubes)

■ INDICATIONS

- Genital herpes
- Recurrent herpes labialis

■ MECHANISM OF ACTION

It is activated by viral thymidine kinase and then inhibits viral DNA polymerase and DNA synthesis.

■ DOSAGE

Apply q2h for 4 days.

▓ DRUG INTERACTIONS

None

▓ SIDE EFFECTS

COMMON: headache, taste changes, erythema, pruritus, hypesthesia/anesthesia, pain, rash

RARE: none

▓ MONITORING

None

▓ CONTRAINDICATIONS

Hypersensitivity to drug/class

▓ PREGNANCY CLASS

B

PENICILLAMINE

(Cuprimine® 125, 250 mg caps)

▓ INDICATIONS

- Cystinuria*
- Heavy metal poisoning*
- Menkes' kinky-hair syndrome+
- Rheumatoid arthritis*
- Scleroderma^ (see pg. 398)
- Wilson's disease*

MECHANISM OF ACTION

It chelates copper and decreases T-cell activity, which leads to decreased IgM rheumatoid factor levels.

DOSAGE

CYSTINURIA: 250–1000 mg PO qid

MENKES' KINKY-HAIR SYNDROME: 250 mg PO weekly or 150 mg PO q2d

RHEUMATOID ARTHRITIS: 250 mg PO bid to tid

SCLERODERMA: 125 mg PO qod

WILSON'S DISEASE: 250–500 mg PO tid to qid

DRUG INTERACTIONS

INCREASED NEPHROTOXICITY: adefovir, aminoglycosides, cidofovir, nephrotoxic agents, zoledronic acid, tenofovir

DECREASED EFFICACY OF PENCICLOVIR: antacids, iron salts, multivitamins with minerals, sucralfate

INCREASED LACTIC ACIDOSIS: metformin

INCREASED LEVELS OF PENCICLOVIR: probenecid

SIDE EFFECTS

COMMON: pruritus, rash, nausea, vomiting, dyspepsia, proteinuria, taste change, glossitis, stomatitis, hirsutism, diarrhea

RARE: thrombocytopenia, aplastic anemia, agranulocytosis, pancreatitis, exfoliative dermatitis, pemphigus, pemphigoid, myasthenia gravis, lupus-like syndrome, elastosis perforans serpiginosa, peptic ulcer, leukopenia, hematuria, tinnitus, dystonia, lichen planus, alopecia, dermatomyositis, anetoderma, Goodpasture's syndrome, toxic epidermal necrolysis, vasculitis, asthma, epidermolysis bullosa acquisita, pseudoxanthoma elasticum

■ MONITORING

BASELINE: urinalysis, complete blood count

EVERY 2 WEEKS FOR FIRST 6 MONTHS, MONTHLY THEREAFTER: urinalysis, complete blood count

■ CONTRAINDICATIONS

Hypersensitivity to drug/class, pregnancy, gold salt use, immunosuppressant use, antimalarial use, penicillin allergy, impaired renal function, history of anemia due to penicillamine, pregnancy

■ PREGNANCY CLASS

D

PENICILLINS, FIRST GENERATION

Benzathine penicillin (Bicillin LA® IM), procaine penicillin (Wycillin® IM), procaine and benzathine penicillin (Bicillin CR® IM), penicillin G aqueous (IV, IM), penicillin VK (Pen-Vee K® 250, 500 mg tabs, 125 and 250 mg/5 mL suspension; Veetids® 250, 500 mg tabs)

■ INDICATIONS

- *Actinomyces aerogenes* and *faecalis* (penicillin G*)
- *Bacillus anthracis* (penicillin G*)
- *Clostridium difficile* (penicillin G*)
- *Corynebacterium diphtheriae* (penicillin G*)
- Erysipeloid (penicillin G*)
- *Escherichia coli* (penicillin G*)
- *Fusobacterium fusifomisnas* (penicillin G*, penicillin VK*)
- *Listeria monocytogenes* (penicillin G*)
- *Neisseria gonorrhoeae* (penicillin G*)
- *Neisseria meningitidis* (penicillin G*)
- *Pasteurella multocida* (penicillin G*)
- *Proteus mirabilis* (penicillin G*)
- *Salmonella* sp. (penicillin G*)
- *Shigella* sp. (penicillin G*)

- *Spirillum minus* (penicillin G*)
- *Staphylococcus aureus* (penicillin G*)
- *Staphylococcus epidermidis* (penicillin VK*)
- *Streptobacillus moniliformis* (penicillin G*)
- *Streptococcus pneumoniae**
- *Streptococcus*, group A, C, G*
- *Treponema pallidum* (penicillin G*, benzathine penicillin*)

See Appendix II.

Usually effective:

- *Actinomyces* sp. (penicillin G)
- *Clostridium*, not *difficile*
- *Enterococcus faecalis*
- *Haemophilus ducreyi* (penicillin G)
- *Pasteurella multocida* (penicillin VK)
- *Peptostreptococcus* sp.
- *Prevotella melaninogenica* (penicillin G)
- *Streptococcus milleri*

Clinical trials lacking:

- *Actinomyces* sp. (penicillin VK)
- *Bacteroides fragilis* (penicillin VK)
- *Enterococcus faecium*
- *Streptococcus viridans*

▧ MECHANISM OF ACTION

They are bactericidal agents that inhibit bacterial cell wall synthesis.

▧ DOSAGE

BENZATHINE PENICILLIN

BACTERIAL INFECTION: 1.2 million units IM once
Syphilis: 2.4 million units IM once for primary and secondary, 2.4 million units IM weekly 3 times for tertiary

PROCAINE PENICILLIN

BACTERIAL INFECTION: 0.6–1.2 million units IM qd

GONORRHEA: 4.8 million units IM once, after 1 g of probenecid

PENICILLIN G AQUEOUS

BACTERIAL INFECTIONS, NEUROSYPHILIS: 4 million units IM/IV q4h

RENAL DOSING
Creatinine clearance (CrCl) 10–50 mL/min and continuous arteriovenous hemofiltration: 75%
CrCl < 10 mL/min and chronic ambulatory peritoneal dialysis: 20–50%
Hemodialysis: dose after dialysis

PENICILLIN VK

BACTERIAL INFECTION: 250–500 mg PO q6–8h

RENAL DOSING
CrCl < 10 mL/min: normal dose q8h

HEPATIC DOSING: Decrease dose.

▨ DRUG INTERACTIONS

INCREASED EFFICACY OF PENICILLIN: aminoglycosides

INCREASED LEVELS OF PENICILLIN: probenecid

INCREASED LEVELS OF: methotrexate

DECREASED EFFICACY OF: oral contraceptives, aminoglycosides, chloramphenicol

DECREASED EFFICACY OF PENICILLIN: tetracycline

▨ SIDE EFFECTS

COMMON: nausea, vomiting, diarrhea, rash, urticaria, fever, injection site pain (aqueous penicillin, benzathine penicillin)

RARE: thrombocytopenia, anaphylaxis, seizures, hemolytic anemia, interstitial nephritis, pseudomembranous colitis, myocardial depression (procaine penicillin), confusion (procaine penicillin, benzathine penicillin), hallucinations (procaine penicillin), lethargy (procaine penicillin, benzathine penicillin), dizziness (procaine penicillin, benzathine penicillin), Jarisch-Herxheimer reaction (procaine penicillin, benzathine penicillin), thrombophlebitis (aqueous penicillin), Stevens-Johnson syndrome (aqueous penicillin, benzathine penicillin)

MONITORING

None

CONTRAINDICATIONS

Hypersensitivity to drug/class, cephalosporin allergy, seizures, phenylketonuria, impaired renal function, neonates (procaine penicillin), live typhoid vaccine

PREGNANCY CLASS

B

PENICILLINS, SECOND GENERATION

Dicloxacillin (Dynapen® 250, 500 mg caps; 62.5 mg/5 mL suspension), methicillin (Celbenin® IV, Staphcillin® IV, Metin® IV), nafcillin (Nallpen® IM/IV), oxacillin (Bactocill® 250, 500 mg caps; 250 mg/5 mL suspension; IM/IV)

INDICATIONS

- *Staphylococcus aureus,* methicillin sensitive*
- *Staphylococcus epidermidis**
- *Streptococcus pyogenes* (dicloxacillin*)

See Appendix II.

Usually effective:

- *Peptostreptococcus* sp.
- *Streptococcus milleri*
- *Streptococcus pneumoniae*

Clinical trials lacking:

- *Streptococcus viridans*

MECHANISM OF ACTION

They are bactericidal agents that inhibit bacterial cell wall synthesis.

DOSAGE

DICLOXACILLIN

125–250 mg PO q6h

METHACILLIN

RENAL DOSING
  Glomerular filtration rate (GFR) 90–50 mL/min: normal dose q4–6h
  GFR 10–50 mL/min: normal dose q6–8h
  GFR < 10 mL/min: normal dose q8–12h

NAFCILLIN

0.5–2 g IV/IM q4–6h

RENAL AND HEPATIC DOSING: Reduce dose by 33–50%.

OXACILLIN

1–2 g IV/IM q4–6h, 0.5–1 g PO q4–6h

DRUG INTERACTIONS

INCREASED EFFICACY OF PENICILLINS: aminoglycosides

INCREASED LEVELS OF PENICILLINS: probenecid

INCREASED LEVELS OF: methotrexate

DECREASED EFFICACY OF: oral contraceptives, warfarin (nafcillin, dicloxacillin), nifedipine (nafcillin), cyclosporin (nafcillin)

DECREASED LEVEL OF: cyclosporin (nafcillin), gifitinib (nafcillin), tacrolimus (nafcillin)

SIDE EFFECTS

COMMON: epigastric pain, diarrhea, nausea, vomiting, dizziness, fatigue, eosinophilia, elevated liver function test results, rash, urticaria, interstitial nephritis (oxacillin)

RARE: seizures (dicloxacillin, nafcillin), thrombocytopenia, agranulocytosis, leukopenia, pseudomembranous colitis, anaphylaxis, anemia, thrombophlebitis (oxacillin)

MONITORING

Frequently. If long-term use: complete blood count, renal and liver function.

CONTRAINDICATIONS

Hypersensitivity to drug/class, cephalosporin allergy, acute lymphocytic leukemia (dicloxacillin), Epstein-Barr virus (dicloxacillin), cytomegalovirus (dicloxacillin), impaired renal function, neonates, impaired liver function (nafcillin), live typhoid vaccine

PREGNANCY CLASS

B

PENICILLINS, THIRD GENERATION

Amoxicillin (Amoxil® 250, 500, 875 mg tabs; 125, 200, 250, 400 mg chewable tabs; Trimox® 250, 500 mg tabs; 125, 250 mg/5 mL suspension), amoxicillin clavulanate (Augmentin® 250, 500, 875 mg tabs; 125, 200, 250, 400 mg/5 mL suspension), ampicillin (Principen® 250, 500 mg caps; 125, 250 mg/5 mL susp, IM/IV; Omnipen® 250, 500 mg caps; 125, 250 mg/5 mL; IM/IV), ampicillin sulbactam (Unasyn® IM/IV)

▓ INDICATIONS (FOR BETA-LACTAMASE STRAINS)

- *Acinetobacter calcoaceticus* (ampicillin/sulbactam*)
- *Bacteroides fragilis* (ampicillin/sulbactam*)
- *Enterobacter* sp. (amoxicillin/clavulanate,* ampicillin/sulbactam*)
- *Enterococcus faecalis* (amoxicillin,* ampicillin*)
- *Escherichia coli* (amoxicillin,* amoxicillin/clavulanate,* ampicillin/sulbactam*)
- *Haemophilus influenzae* (amoxicillin,* amoxicillin/clavulanate,* ampicillin*)
- *Haemophilus vaginalis* (ampicillin*)
- *Helicobacter pylori* (amoxicillin*)
- *Klebsiella pneumoniae* (amoxicillin/clavulanate,* ampicillin/sulbactam*)
- *Moraxella catarrhalis* (amoxicillin/clavulanate*)
- *Neisseria gonorrhoeae* (amoxicillin,* ampicillin*)
- *Proteus mirabilis* (amoxicillin,* ampicillin/sulbactam,* ampicillin*)
- *Salmonella* sp. (ampicillin*)
- *Shigella* sp. (ampicillin*)
- *Staphylococcus aureus,* methicillin sensitive*
- *Streptococcus,* alpha- and beta-hemolytic (amoxicillin,* ampicillin*)
- *Streptococcus pneumoniae* (amoxicillin,* ampicillin,* amoxicillin/clavulanate*)

See Appendix II.

Usually effective:

- *Actinomyces* sp.
- *Aeromonas* sp. (amoxicillin/clavulanate, ampicillin/sulbactam)
- *Bacteroides fragilis* (amoxicillin/clavulanate)
- *Clostridium difficile* (ampicillin/sulbactam)
- *Clostridium,* not *difficile*
- *Enterococcus faecalis* (amoxicillin/clavulanate, ampicillin/sulbactam)
- *Enterococcus faecium*
- *Haemophilus ducreyi* (amoxicillin/clavulanate, ampicillin/sulbactam)
- *Haemophilus influenzae* (ampicillin/sulbactam)
- *Listeria monocytogenes* (ampicillin, amoxicillin, ampicillin/sulbactam)
- *Moraxella catarrhalis* (ampicillin/sulbactam)
- *Morganella* sp. (ampicillin/sulbactam)
- *Neisseria gonorrhoeae* (amoxicillin/clavulanate, ampicillin/sulbactam)
- *Neisseria meningitidis*
- *Pasteurella multocida*
- *Peptostreptococcus* sp.
- *Prevotella melaninogenica*
- *Proteus mirabilis* (amoxicillin/clavulanate)
- *Proteus vulgaris* (amoxicillin/clavulanate, ampicillin/sulbactam)
- *Providencia* sp. (amoxicillin/clavulanate, ampicillin/sulbactam)

- *Salmonella* sp. (amoxicillin/clavulanate, ampicillin/sulbactam)
- *Shigella* sp. (amoxicillin/clavulanate, ampicillin/sulbactam)
- *Staphylococcus epidermidis* (amoxicillin/clavulanate, ampicillin/sulbactam)
- *Streptococcus milleri*

Clinical trials lacking:

- *Escherichia coli* (ampicillin)
- *Morganella* sp. (amoxicillin/clavulanate)
- *Salmonella* sp. (amoxicillin)
- *Shigella* sp. (amoxicillin)
- *Staphylococcus epidermidis* (amoxicillin, ampicillin)
- *Streptococcus viridans*
- *Yersinia enterocolitica* (amoxicillin/clavulanate, ampicillin/sulbactam)

MECHANISM OF ACTION

They are bactericidal agents that inhibit bacterial cell wall synthesis.

DOSAGE

AMOXICILLIN

BACTERIAL INFECTIONS: 250–500 mg PO q8h

GONORRHEA: 3 g PO once

RENAL DOSING
Creatinine clearance (CrCl) 10–30 mL/min: q12h
CrCl < 10 mL/min: q24h

AMOXICILLIN/CLAVULANATE

500–875 mg PO q12h

RENAL DOSING
CrCl 10–30 mL/min: 250–500 mg PO q12h
CrCl < 10 mL/min: 250–500 mg PO q24h

AMPICILLIN

BACTERIAL INFECTION: 250–500 mg PO q6h or 0.5–2 g IV/IM q6h

MENINGITIS: 1–2 g IV q3–4h

RENAL DOSING
   CrCl 50–90 mL/min: q6h
   CrCl 10–50 mL/min: q6–12h
   CrCl < 10 mL/min: q12–16h
   Hemodialysis: dose after hemodialysis
   Peritoneal dialysis: 250 mg PO q12h
   Continuous hemofiltration: 250–2000 mg PO q6–12h

AMPICILLIN/SULBACTAM

1.5–3 g IV/IM q6h

RENAL DOSING
   CrCl 15–30 mL/min: q12h
   CrCl 5–15 mL/min: q24h

▒ DRUG INTERACTIONS

INCREASED EFFICACY OF PENICILLINS: aminoglycosides

INCREASED LEVELS OF PENICILLINS: probenecid

INCREASED LEVELS OF: methotrexate, mefloquine (ampicillin)

DECREASED EFFICACY OF: oral contraceptives, raloxifene (ampicillin)

INCREASED RISK OF RASH: allopurinol

DECREASED BIOAVAILABILITY OF PENICILLINS: chloroquine (ampicillin)

▒ SIDE EFFECTS

COMMON: nausea, vomiting, diarrhea, rash, urticaria, elevated liver function test results, eosinophilia, abdominal pain, headache, candidiasis, confusion (ampicillin), dizziness (ampicillin), injection site pain (ampicillin/sulbactam), thrombophlebitis (ampicillin/sulbactam), elevated blood urea nitrogen/creatinine

RARE: thrombocytopenia, agranulocytosis, anaphylaxis, pseudomembranous colitis, Stevens-Johnson syndrome, toxic epidermal necrolysis, leukopenia, anemia, seizures, hepatotoxicity, interstitial nephritis

▓ MONITORING

None

▓ CONTRAINDICATIONS

Hypersensitivity to drug/class, cephalosporin allergy, Epstein-Barr virus, cytomegalovirus, acute lymphocytic leukemia, impaired renal function, phenylketonuria (amoxicillin), pseudomembranous colitis, children (ampicillin/sulbactam), impaired liver function (amoxicillin/clavulanate), cholestatic jaundice (amoxicillin/clavulanate)

▓ PREGNANCY CLASS

B

PENICILLINS, FOURTH GENERATION

Mezlocillin (Mezlin® IM/IV), piperacillin (Pipracil® IM/IV), piperacillin/tazobactam (Zosyn® IV), ticarcillin (Ticar® IM/IV), ticarcillin/clavulanate (Timentin® IV)

▓ INDICATIONS

- *Acinetobacter* sp. (piperacillin*)
- *Bacteroides fragilis,* * *ovatus* (piperacillin/tazobactam*), *thetaiotoamicron* (piperacillin/tazobactam*), and *vulgatus* (piperacillin/tazobactam*)
- *Citrobacter* sp. (ticarcillin/clavulanate,* ticarcillin*)
- *Clostridium difficile* (piperacillin*)
- *Enterobacter cloacae* (piperacillin,* ticarcillin/clavulanate,* ticarcillin,* mezlocillin*)
- *Enterococcus faecalis* (piperacillin*)
- *Escherichia coli**
- *Haemophilus influenzae**
- *Klebsiella pneumoniae* (piperacillin,* ticarcillin/clavulanate,* ticarcillin,* mezlocillin*)
- *Morganella morganii* (mezlocillin*)
- *Neisseria gonorrhoeae* (piperacillin,* mexlocillin*)
- *Peptococcus* sp. (mezlocillin*)
- *Peptostreptococcus* sp. (mezlocillin*)

- *Prevotella melaninogenica* (ticarcillin/clavulanate,* ticarcillin*)
- *Proteus mirabilis* (piperacillin,* mezlocillin*)
- *Proteus vulgaris* (mezlocillin*)
- *Providencia rettgeri* (mezlocillin*)
- *Pseudomonas aeruginosa**
- *Serratia marcescens* (ticarcillin/clavulanate, piperacillin,* mezlocillin,* ticarcillin*)
- *Staphylococcus aureus,* methicillin sensitive (ticarcillin/clavulanate,* ticarcillin,* piperacillin/tazobactam*)
- *Staphylococcus epidermidis* (ticarcillin*)
- *Streptococcus faecium* (mezlocillin*)
- *Streptococcus pneumoniae* (piperacillin*)
- *Streptococcus pyogenes* (piperacillin*)

See Appendix II.

Usually effective:

- *Acinetobacter* sp. (ticarcillin/clavulanate, piperacillin/tazobactam)
- *Actinomyces* sp. (piperacillin)
- *Aeromonas* sp.
- *Citrobacter* sp. (not ticarcillin/clavulanate)
- *Clostridium difficile* (mezlocillin)
- *Clostridium,* not *difficile*
- *Enterobacter* sp.
- *Enterococcus faecalis* (piperacillin/tazobactam)
- *Klebsiella* sp. (piperacillin)
- *Listeria monocytogenes* (ticarcillin, mezlocillin, piperacillin)
- *Moraxella catarrhalis* (piperacillin/tazobactam, ticarcillin/clavulanate)
- *Morganella* sp.
- *Neisseria gonorrhoeae* (not piperacillin)
- *Neisseria meningitidis*
- *Pasteurella multocida* (not piperacillin/tazobactam)
- *Peptostreptococcus* sp.
- *Prevotella melaninogenica* (not ticarcillin/clavulanate)
- *Proteus mirabilis* (not piperacillin)
- *Proteus vulgaris*
- *Providencia* sp.
- *Salmonella* sp. (not piperacillin/tazobactam)
- *Serratia sp.* (not piperacillin)
- *Shigella* sp. (piperacillin, mezlocillin, ticarcillin)
- *Staphylococcus epidermidis* (piperacillin/tazobactam)
- *Streptococcus milleri*
- *Yersinia enterocolitica* (piperacillin, mezlocillin, ticarcillin/clavulanate)

Clinical trials lacking:

- *Enterococcus faecalis* (ticarcillin, ticarcillin/clavulanate)
- *Enterococcus faecium* (not mezlocillin)
- *Moraxella catarrhalis* (piperacillin)
- *Staphylococcus epidermidis* (ticarcillin/clavulanate)
- *Stenotrophomonas maltophilia* (not ticarcillin)
- *Streptococcus viridans*
- *Yersinia enterocolitica* (ticarcillin)

MECHANISM OF ACTION

They are bactericidal agents that inhibit bacterial cell wall synthesis.

DOSAGE

MEZLOCILLIN

3–4 g IV/IM q4–6h

RENAL DOSING
  Creatinine clearance (CrCl) 10–50 mL/min: 3 g q6–8h
  CrCl < 10 mL/min: 2 g q8h
  Hemodialysis: 3–4 g after dialysis, then q12h
  Peritoneal dialysis: 3 g q12h

HEPATIC DOSING: Decrease dose by 50%.

PIPERACILLIN

3–4 g IV/IM q4–6h

RENAL DOSING
  CrCl 10–50 mL/min and continuous arteriovenous hemofiltration (CAVH): q6–8h
  CrCl < 10 mL/min and chronic ambulatory peritoneal dialysis (CAPD): q8h
  Hemodialysis: dose after dialysis

PIPERACILLIN/TAZOBACTAM

3.375 g IV q6h

RENAL DOSING
  CrCl 10–50 mL/min: 2.25 g IV q6h
  CrCl < 10 mL/min and CAPD: 2.25 g IV q8h
  Hemodialysis: 2.25 g IV q8h plus 0.75 g IV after dialysis

TICARCILLIN

3–4 g IV q4–6h

RENAL DOSING
   CrCl 30–60 mL/min: 1–2 g IV q4h
   CrCl 10–30 mL/min and CAVH: 1–2 g IV q8h
   CrCl < 10 mL/min and CAPD: 1–2 g IV q12h
   Hemodialysis: extra 2 g after dialysis
   Peritoneal dialysis: 3 g q12h

TICARCILLIN/CLAVULANATE

3.1 g IV q4–6h

RENAL DOSING
   CrCl 10–50 mL/min: 2 g IV q4–8h
   CrCl < 10 mL/min: 2 g IV q12h
   Hemodialysis: extra 3.1 g IV after dialysis
   CAPD: 3.1 g IV q12h

DRUG INTERACTIONS

INCREASED EFFICACY OF PENICILLINS: aminoglycosides

INCREASED LEVELS OF PENICILLINS: probenecid

INCREASED LEVELS OF: methotrexate, cyclosporin (ticarcillin)

DECREASED EFFICACY OF: oral contraceptives

INCREASED RISK OF BLEEDING: heparin, warfarin, thrombin inhibitors

PROLONGED NEUROMUSCULAR BLOCKADE: non-depolarizing neuromuscular blockers (piperacillin, piperacillin/tazobactam)

SIDE EFFECTS

COMMON: rash, pain at injection site, phlebitis, nausea, vomiting, diarrhea, eosinophilia, fever, pruritus, urticaria, hypokalemia (except mezlocillin), hyperbilirubinemia (piperacillin, piperacillin/tazobactam), elevated liver function test results (except mezlocillin)

Rare: seizures, neutropenia, thrombocytopenia, hemolytic anemia, leukopenia, pseudomembranous colitis, anaphylaxis, Stevens-Johnson syndrome (except mezlocillin), interstitial nephritis, prolonged bleeding time, hypernatremia (ticarcillin/clavulanate)

▓ MONITORING

Frequently If Long-Term Use: complete blood count, liver function, renal function, sodium, potassium

▓ CONTRAINDICATIONS

Hypersensitivity to drug/class, cephalosporin allergy, bleeding tendencies, hypokalemia, uremia, children (except mezlocillin), seizures, nephrotoxic agents, sodium restriction (except mezlocillin), hypokalemia (mezlocillin)

▓ PREGNANCY CLASS

B

PENTOXIFYLLINE

(Trental® 400 mg tabs)

▓ INDICATIONS

- Actinic granuloma[+]
- Aphthous stomatitis[$] (see pg. 352)
- Arterial ulcers[$]
- Behçet's disease[+] (see pg. 355)
- Calciphylaxis[+]
- Claudication[*]
- Cutaneous polyarteritis nodosa[+]
- Diabetic ulcers[$]
- Erythema nodosum leprosum[$]
- Granuloma annulare[+] (see pg. 365)
- Kasabach-Merritt syndrome[+]
- Kimura's disease with oral ulcers[+]
- Leischmaniasis[+]

- Leukocytoclastic vasculitis[+] (see pg. 404)
- Livedoid vasculitis[+], with enoxaparin 1 mg/kg SC q12h[+] (see pg. 404)
- Necrobiosis lipoidica diabeticorum[+] (see pg. 381)
- Polyarteritis nodosa, cutaneous[+] (see pg. 404)
- Radiation-induced fibrosis[^]
- Raynaud's phenomenon[+]
- Rheumatoid arthritis[$]
- Sarcoidosis[$] (see pg. 396)
- Schamberg's disease[+]
- Scleroderma[$] (see pg. 398)
- Sickle cell disease, crisis[^], leg ulcers[+]
- Toxic epidermal necrolysis[+] (see pg. 402)
- Urticarial vasculitis[+] (see pg. 404)
- Venous ulcers[^]

MECHANISM OF ACTION

It lowers blood viscosity and improves erythrocyte flexibility. It also increases leukocyte deformability and inhibits neutrophil adhesion and activation. It improves tissue oxygenation. It also inhibits tumor necrosis factor alpha synthesis.

DOSAGE

CLAUDICATION: 400–800 mg PO tid

DRUG INTERACTIONS

INCREASED LEVELS OF: theophylline

SIDE EFFECTS

COMMON: dyspepsia, nausea, vomiting, dizziness, headache, diarrhea, flushing, pruritus, rash, urticaria

RARE: arrhythmias, agitation, drowsiness, angina, hypotension, anorexia, cholecystitis, dry mouth, anxiety, confusion, depression, nasal congestion, epistaxis, laryngitis, brittle fingernails, angioedema, conjunctivitis, scotoma, excess salivation, sore throat, bad/metallic taste, leukopenia, malaise, insomnia, blurred vision

░ MONITORING

PERIODICALLY: blood pressure monitoring

░ CONTRAINDICATIONS

Hypersensitivity to drug/class, methylxanthine intolerance, recent cerebral bleed, recent retinal hemorrhage, concurrent use of anticoagulants or platelet aggregation inhibitors, pregnancy

░ PREGNANCY CLASS

C

PERMETHRIN

(Elimite® 5% cream in 60 g tube; Nix® 1% cream [over the counter]; Acticin® 5% cream in 60 g tube)

░ INDICATIONS

- Demodex+
- Eosinophilic folliculitis+
- Pediculosis (*Pediculus capitis* and *pubis*)^
- Rosacea, populopustular^ (see pg. 395)
- Scabies (*Sarcoptes scabiei*)* (see pg. 397)

░ MECHANISM OF ACTION

It disrupts parasitic nerve cell membrane sodium channel currents, which results in delayed repolarization and paralysis.

░ DOSAGE

EOSINOPHILIC FOLLICULITIS, DEMODEX, ROSACEA: Apply bid.

PEDICULOSIS: Wash hair, apply cream for 10 min, then rinse and comb. Retreat in 7–10 days.

Sᴄᴀʙɪᴇѕ: Massage into skin from head to toes. Bathe in 8–14 h to remove cream. If mites are found in 14 days, repeat treatment. Pruritus is not an indication to retreat.

DRUG INTERACTIONS

None

SIDE EFFECTS

Cᴏᴍᴍᴏɴ: burning, pruritus, erythema, numbness, tingling

Rᴀʀᴇ: none

MONITORING

None

CONTRAINDICATIONS

Hypersensitivity to drug/class

PREGNANCY CLASS

B

PIMECROLIMUS

(Elidel® 1% cream in 15, 30, 100 g tubes)

INDICATIONS

- Atopic dermatitis* (see pg. 353)
- Contact dermatitis$ (see pg. 357)
- Lichen planus, oral+ (see pg. 371)
- Lupus, cutaneous+ (see pg. 375)
- Psoriasis^ (see pg. 392)
- Seborrheic dermatitis+ (see pg. 399)

MECHANISM OF ACTION

Like cyclosporin, it has the structure of a macrolide antibiotic. It inhibits the activation of helper T cells by binding to intercellular protein, FKBP2, which inhibits calcineurin. This ultimately inhibits the dephosphorylation and translocation of the nuclear factor of activated T cells (NFAT), a nuclear component of gene transcription aids in the formation of lymphokines (e.g., interleukin-2 and interferon gamma). It also inhibits the production of interleukin-8.

DOSAGE

Apply qd to bid.

DRUG INTERACTIONS

None

SIDE EFFECTS

COMMON: skin burning, headache, erythema, pruritus

RARE: lymphadenopathy, herpes simplex/zoster infection, nasopharyngitis, influenza, cough, pharyngitis, pyrexia, hypersensitivity reaction, papilloma

MONITORING

None

CONTRAINDICATIONS

Hypersensitivity to drug/class, local infection, herpes simplex/zoster infection, sun exposure, pregnancy

PREGNANCY CLASS

C

PIMOZIDE

(Orap® 1, 2 mg tabs)

▓ INDICATIONS

- Bromhidrosis[+]
- Delusions of parasitosis[^] (see pg. 362)
- Tourette's syndrome[*]
- Trigeminal neuralgia[^]

▓ MECHANISM OF ACTION

It selectively antagonizes dopamine D_2 receptors.

▓ DOSAGE

BROMHIDROSIS, DELUSIONS OF PARASITOSIS: Start at 1 mg PO qd and increase by 1 mg q4–7d to maximum of 10 mg PO qd. Usually 4–6 mg PO qd is sufficient. Maintain symptom free for 1 month, then decrease dose by 1 mg PO qd every 1–2 weeks to minimum effective dosage.

TOURETTE'S SYNDROME: Start at 1–2 mg PO qd to maximum of 10 mg PO qd.

▓ DRUG INTERACTIONS

INCREASED QT PROLONGATION: angiotensin receptor blockers, angiotensin-converting enzyme inhibitors, amphotericin, antiarrhythmics class Ia/III, aprepitant, azoles, beta-2 agonists, beta blocker/thiazide combinations, budesonide, carbonic anhydrase inhibitors, cidofovir, cisapride, cisplatin, clarithromycin, systemic steroids, cyclosporin, diltiazem, loop diuretics, potassium-sparing diuretics, dolasetron, erythromycin, foscarnet, grapefruit, halothane, imatinib, mefloquine, meperidine, nefazodone, phenothiazines, promethazine, protease inhibitors, quinolones, quinupristin/dalfopristin, risperidone, sertraline, tricyclic antidepressants, verapamil, ziprasidone

INCREASED EFFECTS OF: anticholinergics

ALTERED PIMOZIDE LEVELS: efavirenz

DECREASED EFFECTS OF: epinephrine

SIDE EFFECTS

COMMON: tremors, rigidity, akinesia, nausea, vomiting, dyspepsia, rash, urticaria, increased salivation, diarrhea, constipation, sedation, lethargy

RARE: neuroleptic malignant syndrome, seizures, arrhythmias, dystonic reactions, akathesia, hypotension, palpitations, tachycardia, amenorrhea, extrapyramidal symptoms, tardive dyskinesia, hyperpyrexia, increased appetite and thirst, muscle cramps and tightness, depression, nervousness, change in taste, photophobia, visual disturbances, impotence

MONITORING

BASELINE: electrocardiogram (QT should be < 0.47 s)

WHEN DOSE REACHES 4–6 MG PO QD: electrocardiogram

CONTRAINDICATIONS

Hypersensitivity to drug/class, arrhythmia, central nervous system depression, coma, pregnancy

PREGNANCY CLASS

C

PODOFILOX

(Condylox® 0.5% gel in 3.5 g tubes with applicators, 0.5% solution in 3.5 mL bottles)

INDICATIONS

- Condylomata acuminata* (see pg. 406)
- Molluscum contagiosum^ (see pg. 380)

▨ MECHANISM OF ACTION

It is an antimitotic agent that arrests cells in metaphase by binding reversibly to tubulin.

▨ DOSAGE

Apply bid for 3 days, repeat weekly for 4 weeks. Do not use more than 0.5 g qd of gel or 0.5 mL qd of solution. Do not apply to surfaces >10 cm^2.

▨ DRUG INTERACTIONS

None

▨ SIDE EFFECTS

COMMON: inflammation, burning, erythema, erosions, pruritus, pain, bleeding, edema, tingling, tenderness, bullae

RARE: scarring

▨ MONITORING

None

▨ CONTRAINDICATIONS

Hypersensitivity to drug, use on mucosa, pregnancy

▨ PREGNANCY CLASS

C

PODOPHYLLIN

(Podocon-25® 25% liquid in 15 mL bottles)

■ INDICATIONS

- Condylomata acuminata* (see pg. 406)

■ MECHANISM OF ACTION

It is an antimitotic agent that arrests cells in metaphase by binding reversibly to tubulin.

■ DOSAGE

Must be applied by physician only. Not for at home use.
Apply sparingly to condyloma only and allow to dry. For the first application, the area should be cleansed with alcohol or soap and water after 30–40 min. Treatments thereafter should be cleansed in 1–4 h.

■ DRUG INTERACTIONS

None.

■ SIDE EFFECTS

COMMON: inflammation, burning, tingling, erosions, pruritus, pain, bleeding, tenderness, rash

RARE: paresthesia, polyneuritis, paralytic ileus, pyrexia, leukopenia, thrombocytopenia, coma, death

■ MONITORING

None

CONTRAINDICATIONS

Hypersensitivity to drug/class, diabetics, patients on steroids or with poor circulation, pregnancy, bleeding or inflamed warts

PREGNANCY CLASS

C

PRAZIQUANTEL

(Biltricide® 600 mg tabs)

INDICATIONS

- Intestinal fluke (*Heterophyes heterophyes*[+], *Metagonimus yokogawai*[^])
- Liver fluke (*Clonorchis sinensis, Opisthorchis viverrini*)[*]
- Lung fluke (*Paragonimus westermani*[^])
- Neuro cysticercosis (*Taenia solium*[^])
- Schistosomiasis (*Schistosoma haematobium, intercalatum, japonicum, mansoni,* and *mekongi*)[*]
- Tapeworm (*Diphyllobothrium latum,*[$] *Dipylidium caninum*[+], *Taenia saginata*[^]*, Taenia solium* and *Hymenolepsis diminuta*[+] and *nana*[$])

MECHANISM OF ACTION

It increases cell membrane permeability of worm.

DOSAGE

NEURO CYSTICERCOSIS: 50 mg/kg PO qd divided in 3 doses for 30 days

SCHISTOSOMIASIS: 20 mg/kg PO q4–6h for 1 day

LIVER AND INTESTINAL FLUKE: 25 mg/kg PO q4–6h for 1 day

LUNG FLUKE: 25 mg/kg PO q4–6h for 2 days

TAPEWORM: 5–25 mg/kg PO once

DRUG INTERACTIONS

INCREASED LEVELS OF: albendazole

SIDE EFFECTS

COMMON: malaise, headache, dizziness, abdominal pain, nausea, fever, bitter taste, drowsiness, anorexia, sweating

RARE: urticaria, elevated liver enzyme levels

MONITORING

None

CONTRAINDICATIONS

Hypersensitivity to drug/class, ocular schistosomiasis, ocular cysticercosis, children <4 years of age, impaired liver function

PREGNANCY CLASS

B

PYRANTEL

(Antiminth® 50 mg/mL suspension, Pin X® 50 mg/mL suspension)

INDICATIONS

- Hookworm (*Necator americanus,*^ *Ancylostoma duodenale*^)
- Pinworm (*Enterobius vermicularis**)
- Roundworm (*Ascaris lumbricoides,*^ *Trichostrongylus orientalis*^)
- Whipworm (*Trichuris trichiura*^)

▨ MECHANISM OF ACTION

It is a depolarizing neuromuscular blocking agent that causes worm paralysis and death.

▨ DOSAGE

HOOKWORM: 11 mg/kg PO qd for 3 days

PINWORM: 11 mg/kg PO once, repeat every 2 weeks twice

ROUNDWORM: 11 mg/kg PO qd once

WHIPWORM: 11 mg/kg PO qd once
    Maximum 1 g/d

▨ DRUG INTERACTIONS

None

▨ SIDE EFFECTS

COMMON: anorexia, nausea, vomiting, abdominal cramps, diarrhea, dizziness, drowsiness, insomnia, headache, rash, elevated liver function test results, tenesmus, weakness

RARE: none

▨ MONITORING

None

▨ CONTRAINDICATIONS

Hypersensitivity to drug/class, pregnancy, impaired liver function, malnutrition

▨ PREGNANCY CLASS

C

PYRETHRIN

(Rid® 0.33% lice-killing shampoo or mousse, egg and nit comb-out gel [over the counter]; Barc® 0.18, 0.3% lotion [over the counter])

▓ INDICATIONS

- Head and pubic lice*

▓ MECHANISM OF ACTION

It disables sodium transport mechanism of arthropods, which is responsible for polarization of cell membranes. This leads to paralysis.

▓ DOSAGE

Use on day 1 and day 10. Massage into clean, dry hair. Leave on for 10 min, then lather and rinse. Comb hair to remove eggs and remaining nits.

▓ DRUG INTERACTIONS

None

▓ SIDE EFFECTS

COMMON: burning, pruritus, erythema, tingling

RARE: none

▓ MONITORING

None

▓ CONTRAINDICATIONS

Hypersensitivity to drug/class

▓ PREGNANCY CLASS

B

QUINACRINE

(Mepacrine® 100 mg tabs)

▓ INDICATIONS

- Atopic dermatitis due to giardiasis$ (see pg. 353)
- Giardiasis*
- Lupus, discoid^, panniculitis+, subacute cutaneous+, systemic^ (see pg. 375)
- Malaria*
- Pemphigus vulgaris$ (see pg. 385)
- Reticular erythematous mucinosis$
- Rheumatoid arthritis^
- Sarcoidosis+ (see pg. 396)

▓ MECHANISM OF ACTION

The exact mechanism is unknown. It is thought to inhibit certain enzymes by interacting with DNA to exert its plasmodicidal action. It affects light filtration by altering prostaglandin synthesis and inhibiting superoxide production and binding to DNA. It inhibits antigen-antibody complex formation, decreases lymphocyte responsiveness, and decreases the ability of macrophages to express cell-surface antigens, leading to immunosuppression. It decreases lysosomal size and function and impairs chemotaxis, thus exerting its anti-inflammatory action. It also inhibits platelet aggregation.

▓ DOSAGE

100–300 mg PO qd

▓ DRUG INTERACTIONS

None

▓ SIDE EFFECTS

COMMON: nausea, vomiting, diarrhea, yellow pigmentation (especially shins, face, palate, nails), pruritus, eczematous dermatitis, urticaria, lichen planus–like dermatitis

RARE: restlessness, excitement, confusion, headache, seizures, myasthenia, psychosis, bone marrow toxicity (including aplastic anemia), exfoliative erythroderma, exacerbation of psoriasis, elevated transaminase levels, vertigo, tinnitus, muscle weakness, nystagmus, irritability

▩ MONITORING

BASELINE: complete blood count, glucose-6-phosphate dehydrogenase, liver function tests, serum chemistry

MONTHLY FOR 3 MONTHS, THEN EVERY 4–6 MONTHS: complete blood count, liver function, serum chemistry

▩ CONTRAINDICATIONS

Hypersensitivity to drug/class, pregnancy, lactation, myasthenia gravis

▩ PREGNANCY CLASS

C

QUINUPRISTIN/DALFOPRISTIN

(Synercid® IV)

▩ INDICATIONS

- *Enterococcus faecium,* vancomycin resistant*
- *Staphylococcus aureus,* methicillin resistant^
- *Staphylococcus aureus,* methicillin sensitive*
- *Streptococcus pyogenes**

See Appendix II.

Usually effective:

- *Chlamydia* sp.
- *Clostridium,* not *difficile*
- *Legionella* sp.

- *Listeria monocytogenes*
- *Moraxella catarrhalis*
- *Mycoplasma pneumoniae*
- *Neisseria gonorrhoeae*
- *Prevotella melaninogenica*
- *Staphylococcus epidermidis*
- *Streptococcus pneumoniae*

Clinical trials lacking:

- *Clostridium difficile*
- *Haemophilus influenzae*

▓ MECHANISM OF ACTION

It inhibits bacterial protein synthesis.

▓ DOSAGE

7.5 mg/kg IV q8–12h. Infusion with central line decreases incidence of venous irritation.

▓ DRUG INTERACTIONS

INCREASED CENTRAL NERVOUS SYSTEM AND RESPIRATORY DEPRESSION: alfentanil, fentanyl

INCREASED CENTRAL NERVOUS SYSTEM DEPRESSION: benzodiazepines

INCREASED LEVELS OF: aripiprazole, bortezomib, bosentan, budesonide, buprenorphine, carbamazepine, cyclosporin, delavirdine, disopyramide, eletriptan, gefitinib, lidocaine, nevirapine, paclitaxel, protease inhibitors, quinidine, sirolimus, tacrolimus, tolterodine, vinca alkaloids, voriconazole

INCREASED MYOPATHY: statins

HYPERKALEMIA: eplerenone

ERGOT TOXICITY: ergotamine, ergot alkaloids

INCREASED QT PROLONGATION: calcium channel blockers, cisapride, pimozide

SIDE EFFECTS

COMMON: injection site reactions, nausea, vomiting, thrombophlebitis, rash, pruritus, headache, diarrhea, arthralgia, myalgia, hyperbilirubinemia

RARE: pseudomembranous colitis, superinfection

MONITORING

FREQUENTLY IF LONG-TERM USE: bilirubin

CONTRAINDICATIONS

Hypersensitivity to drug/class, cisapride/terfenadine/astemizole use, CYP 3A4 interactions

PREGNANCY CLASS

B

RANITIDINE

(Zantac® 150, 300 mg tabs; 15 mg/mL in 16 oz bottles)

INDICATIONS

- Atopic dermatitis^ (see pg. 353)
- Cronkhite-Canada syndrome+
- Duodenal ulcer, active and maintenance*
- Erosive esophagitis, treatment and maintenance*
- Gastric ulcer, benign active and maintenance*
- Gastroesophageal reflux*
- Hypersecretory syndrome*
- Psoriasis$ (see pg. 392)
- Urticaria^ (see pg. 403)
- Urticaria pigmentosa+

MECHANISM OF ACTION

It is a reversible competitive inhibitor of histamine at H_2 receptors on gastric cells.

DOSAGE

300–600 mg PO qd

DRUG INTERACTIONS

DECREASED LEVELS OF: atazanavir, cefditoran, cefpodoxime, delavirdine, enoxacin, gefitinib, iron, itraconazole, ketoconazole

INCREASED LEVELS OF: fluvastatin, triazolam

SIDE EFFECTS

COMMON: nausea, vomiting, diarrhea, constipation, abdominal pain, headache, rash, fatigue, dry mouth, myalgia, vertigo

RARE: thrombocytopenia, hepatotoxicity, malaise, dizziness, dry skin, confusion, arrhythmias, hepatitis, erythema multiforme, alopecia, anaphylaxis, aplastic anemia, pancytopenia, granulocytopenia, gynecomastia, impotence, loss of libido

MONITORING

None

CONTRAINDICATIONS

Hypersensitivity to drug/class, porphyria, impaired liver function, impaired renal function

PREGNANCY CLASS

B

RIFABUTIN

(Mycobutin® 150 mg tabs)

▓ INDICATIONS

- *Mycobacterium avium-intracellulare**
- *Mycobacterium haemophilum*⁺
- *Mycobacterium xenopi*^

See Appendix III.

▓ MECHANISM OF ACTION

It inhibits DNA-dependent RNA polymerase.

▓ DOSAGE

300 mg PO qd

▓ DRUG INTERACTIONS

DECREASED LEVELS OF RIFABUTIN: antacids, ketoconazole, pyrazinamide

INCREASED LEVELS OF RIFABUTIN: atovaquone, clarithromycin, delavirdine, fluconazole, amprenavir, indinavir, nelfinavir, ritonavir, itraconazole, ketoconazole, protease inhibitors, bactrim

DECREASED LEVELS OF: beta blockers, steroids, digoxin, disopyramide, methadone, nevirapine, warfarin, oral contraceptives, phenytoin, quinidine, sulfonylureas, tacrolimus, theophylline, sirolimus

DECREASED EFFICACY OF: cyclosporin, tocainide, alfentanil, aprepitant, aripiprazole, calcium channel blockers, bortezomib, bosentan, buprenorphine, bupropion, buspirone, benzodiazepines, caffeine, caspofungin, clozapine, disopyramide, donepezil, efavirenz, eplerenone, fentanyl, imatinib, gefitinib, lamotrigine, lovastatin, modafinil, olanzapine, paclitaxel, phenytoin, quetiapine, quinidine, repaglinide, riluzole, rofecoxib, sildenafil, terbinafine, thyroid hormone, tramadol, tricyclic antidepressants, valproic acid, zidovudine, dapsone, clozapine

INCREASED LEVELS OF: isoniazid, leflunomide, levobupivicaine

HEPATOTOXICITY: acetaminophen, halothane, isoniazid, pyrazinamide

INCREASED EFFICACY OF: clopidogrel

SIDE EFFECTS

COMMON: brown-orange urine/feces/tears/saliva/sputum/sweat, rash, nausea, vomiting, abdominal pain, headache, dyspepsia, diarrhea, yellow-orange skin, myalgia, arthralgia

RARE: neutropenia, leukopenia, thrombocytopenia, anterior uveitis (with clarithromycin), seizures, aphasia, confusion, eructation, taste changes, fever, anorexia, flatulence, myalgias, asthenia, chest pain, pain, insomnia, hepatitis, hemolysis, arrhythmias, uveitis, paresthesias

MONITORING

PERIODICALLY: complete blood count

CONTRAINDICATIONS

Hypersensitivity to drug/class, active tuberculosis, neutropenia, thrombocytopenia

PREGNANCY CLASS

B

RIFAMPIN

(Rifadin® 150, 300 mg tabs; Rimactane® 600 mg tabs)

INDICATIONS

- *Mycobacterium leprae*^
- *Mycobacterium tuberculosis**
- *Neisseria Meningitidis* prophylaxis meningitis*

See Appendix III.

▓ MECHANISM OF ACTION

It inhibits DNA-dependent RNA polymerase.

▓ DOSAGE

10 mg/kg PO/IV qd to maximum of 600 mg qd

NEISSERIA MENINGITIDIS PROPHYLAXIS MENINGITIS: 600 mg PO bid for 2 days

MYCOBACTERIUM LEPRAE
Paucibacillary: 600 mg PO monthly supervised for 6 months, with dapsone 100 mg PO qd
Multibacillary: 600 mg PO monthly supervised for 24 months, with clofazimine 300 mg PO monthly supervised, clofazimine 50 mg PO qd, and dapsone 100 mg PO qd

RENAL DOSING
Creatinine clearance (CrCl) 50–90 mL/min: 600 mg qd
CrCl 10–50 mL/min: 300–600 mg qd
CrCl < 10 mL/min: 300–600 mg qd
Continuous arteriovenous hemofiltration and chronic peritoneal dialysis: 300–600 mg qd
Hemodialysis: none

▓ DRUG INTERACTIONS

DECREASED LEVELS OF RIFAMPIN: antacids, ketoconazole, pyrazinamide

INCREASED LEVELS OF RIFAMPIN: atovaquone, clarithromycin, delavirdine, fluconazole, amprenavir, indinavir, nelfinavir, ritonavir, itraconazole, ketoconazole, protease inhibitors, bactrim

DECREASED LEVELS OF: beta blockers, steroids, digoxin, disopyramide, methadone, nevirapine, warfarin, oral contraceptives, phenytoin, quinidine, sulfonylureas, tacrolimus, theophylline, sirolimus

DECREASED EFFICACY OF: cyclosporin, tocainide, alfentanil, aprepitant, aripiprazole, calcium channel blockers, bortezomib, bosentan, buprenorphine, bupropion, buspirone, benzodiazepines, caffeine, caspofungin, clozapine, disopyramide, donepezil, efavirenz, eplerenone, fentanyl, imatinib, gefitinib, lamotrigine, lovastatin, modafinil, olanzapine, paclitaxel, phenytoin, quetiapine, quinidine, repaglinide, riluzole, rofecoxib, sildenafil, terbinafine, thyroid hormone, tramadol, tricyclic antidepressants, valproic acid, zidovudine

INCREASED LEVELS OF: isoniazid, leflunomide, levobupivicaine

HEPATOTOXICITY: acetaminophen, halothane, isoniazid, pyrazinamide

INCREASED EFFICACY OF: clopidogrel

SIDE EFFECTS

COMMON: reddish-orange body fluids, anorexia, nausea, vomiting, headache, elevated liver function test results, fatigue, drowsiness, dizziness, abdominal pain, diarrhea, pruritus, urticaria, rash, flu-like symptoms, dyspnea, ataxia, visual changes, stained contact lenses

RARE: shock, renal failure, thrombocytopenia, hepatotoxicity, hemolytic anemia, leukopenia, interstitial nephritis, disseminated intravascular coagulation, confusion, psychosis, insomnia, purpura, visual disturbances, menstrual disturbances, myopathy, sore tongue, anaphylaxis, eosinophilia, Stevens-Johnson syndrome, toxic epidermal necrolysis, edema, dyspnea

MONITORING

BASELINE, THEN MONTHLY: liver function, renal function, complete blood count

CONTRAINDICATIONS

Hypersensitivity to drug/class, impaired liver function, hepatic enzyme inducers, pregnancy

PREGNANCY CLASS

C

RISPERIDONE

(Risperdal® 1 mg/mL solution; 0.25, 0.5, 1, 2, 3, 4 mg tabs)

▓ INDICATIONS

- Delusions of parasitosis[+] (see pg. 362)
- Psychiatric dementia*
- Schizophrenia*
- Trichotillomania[+]

▓ MECHANISM OF ACTION

It antagonizes dopamine D_2 receptors and serotonin $5HT_2$ receptors.

▓ DOSAGE

Do not take with cola or tea.

PSYCHIATRIC DEMENTIA: 0.5–1.5 mg PO qd

SCHIZOPHRENIA: Start with 1–2 mg PO qd, increase by 0.5–1 mg qd for 2–7 days to maximum of 16 mg PO qd.

RENAL DOSING: 0.25–0.5 mg PO qd

HEPATIC DOSING: 0.25–0.5 mg PO qd

▓ DRUG INTERACTIONS

INCREASED QT PROLONGATION: angiotensin receptor blockers, amphotericin, antiarrhythmics class Ia/III, beta blocker/thiazide combinations, budesonide, carbonic anhydrase inhibitors, cidofovir, cisapride, systemic steroids, loop diuretics, potassium-sparing diuretics, thiazides, dolasetron, erythromycin, foscarnet, grapefruit, halothane, imatinib, mefloquine, meperidine, phenothiazines, promethazine, protease inhibitors, quinolones, quinupristin/dalfopristin, tricyclic antidepressants, ziprasidone, droperidol, pimozide, propafenone

INCREASED CENTRAL NERVOUS SYSTEM DEPRESSION: opiates, tramadol, antidepressants, antihistamine/decongestant combinations, sedating antihistamines, aripiprazole, barbiturates, droperidol, benzodiazepines, alpha-2 agonists, cetirizine, ethanol, meprobamate, metoclopramide, molindone, muscle relaxants, olanzapine, quetiapine, sedatives, thalidomide, thiothixene

INCREASED EFFECTS OF: anticholinergics, clozapine

INCREASED LEVELS OF RISPERIDONE: bupropion, clozapine, serotonin reuptake inhibitors

DECREASED EFFECTS OF: dopamine agonists

DECREASED LEVELS OF RISPERIDONE: carbamazepine, haloperidol

■ SIDE EFFECTS

COMMON: insomnia, agitation, headache, anxiety, rhinitis, constipation, nausea, vomiting, dyspepsia, dizziness, tachycardia, somnolence, increased dream activity, dry mouth, diarrhea, weight gain, visual disturbances

RARE: hypotension, syncope, extrapyramidal symptoms, tardive dyskinesia, neuroleptic malignant syndrome, hyperglycemia, diabetes mellitus, seizures, QT prolongation, priapism, stroke, transient ischemic attacks, sexual dysfunction, hyperprolactinemia, menstrual irregularities, seizures, dysphagia, thrombotic thrombocytopenic purpura

■ MONITORING

None

■ CONTRAINDICATIONS

Hypersensitivity to drug/class, prolonged QT, impaired renal or liver function, history of neuroleptic malignant syndrome, seizures, cardiac disease, cerebrovascular disease, hypotension, hypovolemia, dehydration, risk of aspiration pneumonia, pregnancy

■ PREGNANCY CLASS

C

SALICYLIC ACID

(Tinamed® 40% plaster patch, 17% corn and callus remover, 17% wart remover; Beta-Lift 2.0 peel® with 20% salicylic acid [over the counter]; Beta-Lift 3.0 peel® with 30% salicylic acid [over the counter]; Dermarest psoriasis medicated moisturizer lotion® with 2% salicylic acid [over the counter]; T-Sal maximum-strength therapeutic shampoo® with 3% salicylic acid [over the counter]; Sebulex® 2% shampoo with 2% salicylic acid in 210 mL bottles [over the counter]; Neutrogena oil-free acne wash® with 2% salicylic acid [over the counter]; Neutrogena oil-free Sunblock SPF 30® with benzophenones and cinnamates [over the counter]; Duofilm® 17% solution and 40% patch [over the counter]; Kerasal® with 5% salicylic acid and 10% urea [over the counter]. This is only a partial list.)

■ INDICATIONS

- Acne^ (see pg. 347)
- Calluses$
- Corns$
- Dermatophyte infections^
- Hyperkeratosis^
- Hyperpigmentation^
- Ichthyosis$ (see pg. 369)
- Keratoderma+
- Peels$
- Photoprotection^
- Psoriasis^ (see pg. 392)
- Seborrheic dermatitis^ (see pg. 399)
- Tinea versicolor^
- Warts^ (see pg. 406)
- Xerosis^ (see pg. 408)

■ MECHANISM OF ACTION

It is a keratolytic and comedolytic agent with anti-inflammatory effects.

■ DOSAGE

Apply qd to bid.

■ DRUG INTERACTIONS

None

■ SIDE EFFECTS

COMMON: contact dermatitis, erythema, burning

RARE: salicylate toxicity (systemic absorption), hypoglycemia

■ MONITORING

None

■ CONTRAINDICATIONS

Hypersensitivity to drug/class

■ PREGNANCY CLASS

Not applicable

SELENIUM SULFIDE

(Selsun® 2.5% lotion in 120 mL bottles, Selsun Blue® 1% shampoo [over the counter]; Exsel® 2.5% lotion in 120 mL bottles; Head and Shoulders® intensive treatment for dandruff and seborrheic dermatitis 1% shampoo [over the counter])

■ INDICATIONS

- Adjunct for tinea capitis^
- Confluent and reticulated papillomatosis of Gougerot and Carteaud (CRPGC)+
- Pityrosporum folliculitis§
- Psoriasis+ (see pg. 392)
- Seborrheic dermatitis* (see pg. 399)
- Tinea versicolor*

MECHANISM OF ACTION

It reduces epidermal and follicular epithelial corneocyte production.

DOSAGE

CRPGC: Apply qd for 5 weeks.

PSORIASIS: Apply qd to qod.

SEBORRHEIC DERMATITIS: 5–10 mL topical twice a week for 2 weeks. Leave on 2–3 min, rinse, repeat. For maintenance, use q1–4 weeks.

TINEA VERSICOLOR: Apply qd for 7 days. Leave on 10 min, rinse. For maintenance, use monthly for 3 months.

DRUG INTERACTIONS

None

SIDE EFFECTS

COMMON: skin irritation, hair loss, hair discoloration, oily scalp, dry scalp

RARE: none

MONITORING

None

CONTRAINDICATIONS

Hypersensitivity to drug, inflamed skin, pregnancy

PREGNANCY CLASS

C

SILVER SULFADIAZINE

(Silvadene® 1% cream in 20, 50, 85, 400 g jars)

▓ INDICATIONS

- Burns, second and third degree (gram-positive and -negative, including *Pseudomonas* and methicillin-resistant *Staphylococcus aureus*)*
- Infected wounds^
- Wound healing^ (see pg. 407)

▓ MECHANISM OF ACTION

It is a bactericidal agent that inhibits bacterial dihydropteroate synthetase (sulfonamide).

▓ DOSAGE

Apply qd to bid.

▓ DRUG INTERACTIONS

None

▓ SIDE EFFECTS

COMMON: pain, burning, rash, pruritus, skin necrosis, brown-gray skin discoloration, erythema

RARE: erythema multiforme, neutropenia, leukopenia, sensitization

▓ MONITORING

None

▓ CONTRAINDICATIONS

Hypersensitivity to drug/class, sulfonamide allergy, infants

PREGNANCY CLASS

B

SODIUM SULFACETAMIDE

(Rosac® 10% sodium sulfacetamide and 5% sulfur with sunscreen in 45 g tubes; Zetacet® 10% sodium sulfacetamide and 5% sulfur topical suspension in 30 g tubes, lotion in 25 g bottles, topical wash in 170.1 and 340.2 g bottles; Plexion® 10% sodium sulfacetamide and sulfur 5% cleanser in 6, 12 oz bottles, and lotion in 30, 60 g tubes; Sulfacet-R® and Sulfacet-R tint-free lotion® 10% sodium sulfacetamide and 5% sulfur lotion in 25 g bottles)

INDICATIONS

- Acne vulgaris* (see pg. 347)
- Perioral dermatitis^ with hydrocortisone
- Rosacea* (see pg. 395)
- Seborrheic dermatitis* (see pg. 399)

MECHANISM OF ACTION

It is a sulfonamide with antibacterial properties that acts as a competitive antagonist to para-aminobenzoic acid (PABA), an essential component for bacterial growth.

DOSAGE

Apply lotion qd to tid.
Wash with cleanser bid, massage into skin for 10–20 sec, then rinse.
   Sulfacet-R® lotion contains Dermik Color Blender®, which enables the patient to alter the shade of the lotion to match skin color.

DRUG INTERACTIONS

None

■ SIDE EFFECTS

COMMON: contact dermatitis, erythema, scaling, irritation

RARE: agranulocytosis, erythema multiforme, Stevens-Johnson syndrome, acute hemolytic anemia, purpura hemorrhagica, drug fever, jaundice

■ MONITORING

None

■ CONTRAINDICATIONS

Hypersensitivity to drug/class, hypersensitivity to sulfonamides, kidney disease, pregnancy

■ PREGNANCY CLASS

C

STANOZOLOL

(Winstrol® 2 mg tabs)

■ INDICATIONS

- Angioedema, hereditary* (see pg. 351)
- Behçet's disease+ (see pg. 355)
- Cryofibrinogenemia+
- Lichen sclerosus et atrophicus$ (see pg. 372)
- Lipodermatosclerosis^ (see pg. 374)
- Pityriasis rubra pilaris+ (see pg. 387)
- Protein C deficiency$
- Pruritus of primary biliary cirrhosis$ (see pg. 391)
- Rheumatoid arthritis^
- Scleroderma^ (see pg. 398)
- Urticaria, chronic^ (see pg. 403)
- Vasculitis^ (see pg. 404)

■ MECHANISM OF ACTION

It is an anabolic steroid that is a synthetic derivative of testosterone. It increases low-density lipoproteins, cholesterol, and triglycerides; decreases high-density lipoproteins; has fibrinolytic activity; and inhibits hepatic production of C1, some clotting factors, and several plasma glycoproteins.

■ DOSAGE

HEREDITARY ANGIOEDEMA: begin 2 mg PO tid. Decrease every 1–3 months to 2 mg PO qd.

■ DRUG INTERACTIONS

INCREASED RISK OF BLEEDING: anticoagulants

HYPERGLYCEMIA: insulin, oral hypoglycemics

■ SIDE EFFECTS

COMMON: virilization and menstrual irregularities in women, suppression of clotting factors, elevated liver function test results, penile enlargement, testicular atrophy and oligospermia, more frequent erections, clitoral enlargement, change in libido, insomnia, depression, nausea, vomiting, diarrhea, gynecomastia, acne, premature closure of epiphyses, edema

RARE: liver tumors, peliosis hepatis, atherosclerosis, cholestatic hepatitis and jaundice, edema with or without congestive heart failure, compromised adult stature if given to children, decreased levels of thyroxine-binding globulin and total T4, polycythemia, retention of electrolytes (sodium, potassium, chloride, phosphate, calcium), decreased glucose tolerance, increased lipoproteins (low-density lipoprotein, cholesterol, triglycerides), decreased high-density lipoprotein, increased creatinine, increased creatine phosphokinase, drug dependence/abuse

■ MONITORING

BASELINE: hemoglobin, hematocrit, liver function tests, x-rays for bone age in prepubertal children, prostate-specific antigen in men

MONTHLY: hemoglobin, hematocrit, liver function tests

EVERY 6 MONTHS: x-rays for bone age in prepubertal children

■ CONTRAINDICATIONS

Men with breast or prostate carcinoma, women with breast carcinoma and hypercalcemia, pregnancy, nephrotic syndrome, hypersensitivity to drug/class

■ PREGNANCY CLASS

X

STEROIDS, SYSTEMIC

- Betamethasone (Celestone,® Beben® 0.6 g tabs; 0.6 g/5 mL suspension)
- Cortisone (Cortone® 25 mg tabs)
- Dexamethasone (Decadron,® Dexasone,® Dexone,® Hexadrol® 0.25, 0.5, 0.75, 1, 1.5, 2, 4, 6 g tabs; 0.5 mg/5 mL solution; 0.5 mg/0.5 mL suspension)
- Fludrocortisone (Florinef® 0.1 mg tabs)
- Hydrocortisone (Cortef,® Solu-Cortef® 5, 10, 20 mg tabs; 10 mg/5 mL suspension)
- Methylprednisolone (Solu-Medrol,® Medrol,® Depo-Medrol® 2, 4, 8, 16, 24, 32 mg tabs; Dosepak, 21 4 g tabs, tapers from 24 mg to 0 mg over 7 days)
- Prednisolone (Prelone,® Pediapred® 5 mg tabs; 5 mg/5 mL solution; 15 mg/5 mL suspension)
- Prednisone (Deltasone,® Meticorten,® Pred-Pak® 45 and 79 5 mg tabs; Prednisone Intensol® 5 mg/5 mL, 5 mg/mL solution; Sterapred® 21 and 48 5 mg tabs; Sterapred DS® 21, 48, and 49 10 mg tabs; Winpred,® Metreton® 1, 2.5, 5, 10, 20, 30 g tabs)
- Triamcinolone (Aristocort,® Kenalog,® Aristospan® 4 mg tabs; 10 mg/mL, 25 mg/mL, 40 mg/mL solution)

STEROID	EQUIVALENT DOSE (mg)	ANTI-INFLAMMATORY POTENCY
Betamethasone	0.6–0.75	20–30
Cortisone	25	0.8
Dexamethasone	0.75	20–30
Hydrocortisone	20	1
Methylprednisolone	4	5
Prednisolone	5	4
Prednisone	5	4
Triamcinolone	4	5

■ INDICATIONS (ORAL UNLESS OTHERWISE INDICATED; PARTIAL LIST)

- Acne[$] (pulse with isotretinoin[+], IL[^]) (see pg. 347)
- Alopecia areata[$] (pulse[$], IL[$]) (see pg. 349)
- Annular elastolytic giant-cell granuloma (IL[+])
- Atopic dermatitis[*] (IL[$], IM[$]) (see pg. 353)
- Behçet's disease[$] (pulse[+], IL[+]) (see pg. 355)
- Benign lymphocytic infiltrate (IL[+])
- Bullous pemphigoid[*] (see pg. 355)
- Churg-Strauss syndrome[^] (see pg. 404)
- Cicatricial pemphigoid[$] (pulse with cyclophosphamide[$], IL[+]) (see pg. 356)
- Contact dermatitis[*] (IM[$]) (see pg. 357)
- Dermatitis herpetiformis[*] (see pg. 360)
- Dermatomyositis[*] (pulse[$]) (see pg. 361)
- Drug hypersensitivity reactions[*] (IM[$])
- Epidermolysis bullosa[+] (see pg. 362)
- Epidermolysis bullosa acquisita[+] (see pg. 363)
- Erythema multiforme[*] (IM[+]) (see pg. 364)
- Exfoliative dermatitis[*] (pulse[+])
- Granuloma annulare (IL[+]) (see pg. 365)
- Granulomatous cheilitis (IL[$])
- Hemangioma[$] (IL[$])
- Henoch-Schönlein purpura[^] (pulse with cyclophosphamide[$]) (see pg. 404)
- Herpes gestationis[$] (see pg. 368)
- Keloids (IL[^]) (see pg. 371)
- Keratoacanthoma, eruptive (IL[+])
- Lichen planopilaris[+] (pulse with acitretin[+]) (see pg. 371)
- Lichen planus[^] (IL[+], IM[+]) (see pg. 371)
- Lichen sclerosus et atrophicus (IL[+]) (see pg. 372)
- Linear IgA dermatosis[$] (see pg. 374)
- Lupus, discoid (IL[$]), subacute cutaneous (IL[$]), systemic[*] (pulse with cyclophosphamide for nephritis[^], pulse for cerebritis[^])
- Lymphomatoid papulosis (IL[+]) (see pg. 377)
- Melkersson-Rosenthal syndrome (IL[$])
- Mycosis fungoides[*] (IL[$], IM[$]) (see pg. 358)
- Myxoid cyst (IL[+])
- Necrobiosis lipoidica diabeticorum (IL[+]) (see pg. 381)
- Nodular fasciitis (IL[+])
- Nummular dermatitis (IM[$])
- Ofuji's papuloerythroderma[$]
- Paraneoplastic pemphigus[+] (pulse with cyclophosphamide[+]) (see pg. 382)
- Pemphigus foliaceus[*] (pulse[^]) (see pg. 383)

- Pemphigus vulgaris* (pulse^) (see pg. 385)
- Polyarteritis nodosa^ (pulse with cyclophosphamide+) (see pg. 404)
- Postherpetic neuralgia prevention$ (see pg. 389)
- Prurigo nodularis (IM$, IL$)
- Pruritic urticarial papules and plaques of pregnancy+ (see pg. 390)
- Psoriasis* (IL$, IM$) (see pg. 392)
- Psoriatic arthritis*
- Pyoderma gangrenosum$ (pulse+, IL+) (see pg. 394)
- Rheumatoid arthritis* (pulse^)
- Rheumatoid nodule (IL^)
- Sarcoidosis, cutaneous$, pulmonary^, neurologic^ (pulse neurologic$, polyneuropathy+, hypopituitarism+, IL+) (see pg. 396)
- Scar/keloid (IL^) (see pg. 371)
- Seborrheic dermatitis, severe* (see pg. 399)
- Sjögren's syndrome$ (pulse+)
- Stevens-Johnson syndrome* (pulse+) (see pg. 400)
- Sunburn$
- Sweet's syndrome$ (pulse with chlorambucil+) (see pg. 401)
- Toxic epidermal necrolysis* (pulse+) (see pg. 402)
- Urticaria* (IM$) (see pg. 403)
- Urticaria pigmentosa+ (IL+)
- Urticarial vasculitis$ (pulse with cyclophosphamide+) (see pg. 404)
- Vasculitis$ (see pg. 404)
- Vitiligo$ (pulse$, IL^) (see pg. 405)
- Weber-Christian syndrome+

▓ MECHANISM OF ACTION

They exert anti-inflammatory and immunosuppressive effects. They inhibit nuclear factor kappa B (NFkB), decreasing production of interleukin-1 (IL-1), tumor necrosis factor alpha, adhesion molecules, and growth factors. They also inhibit AP-1, which is a heterodimeric transcription factor composed of c-jun, c-fos, and activating transcription factor, thus decreasing cytokine production. They cause lymphocyte and eosinophil apoptosis. They inhibit phospholipase-A2, leading to decreased production of cyclooxygenase, prostaglandins, leukotrienes, and hydroxyeicosatetraenoic acid inflammatory mediators.

▓ DOSAGE

IL, MONTHLY
Acne, alopecia areata on face: triamcinolone 2.5 mg/mL
Keloids, alopecia areata on scalp, severe and recalcitrant lesions (requiring higher doses): triamcinolone 5–40 mg/mL

Less than 20 mg of triamcinolone does not suppress serum cortisol levels. May dilute with 0.9% sodium chloride and/or local anesthetic. Draw steroid into syringe first before adding dilutant to avoid precipitation. Inject into papillary dermis and avoid producing blanching of the skin.

IM: triamcinolone 40 mg every 3–4 weeks as needed

IV Pulse: methylprednisolone 1 g qd for 3–5 days

IV: methylprednisolone 10–100 q8h, tapering every 1–3 days

Oral: prednisone 0.5–1 mg/kg/d, depending on severity, tapering every 3–7 days

Except IL, give concomitant oral calcium with vitamin D, bisphosphonate, and H_2 blockers/proton pump inhibitors.

▓ DRUG INTERACTIONS

Decreased Levels of Steroids: barbiturates, phenytoin, ephedrine, rifampin, cholestyramine

Increased Levels of Steroids: estrogens, ketoconazole, aspirin, non-steroidal anti-inflammatory agents, macrolides

Decreased Levels of: warfarin, vaccines, antidiabetic agents, isoniazid

Increased Levels of: cyclosporin, potassium-depleting diuretics, digitalis

Hypokalemia: potassium-depleting diuretics, digitalis

Weakness in Myasthenia Gravis: anticholinesterase agents

▓ SIDE EFFECTS

IM, IV, PO, PULSE

Common: sodium retention, fluid retention, congestive heart failure, hypokalemia, hypertension, muscle weakness, steroid myopathy, osteoporosis, peptic ulcer, headache, nausea, vomiting, Cushing's disease, hyperglycemia, hyperlipidemia, weight gain, cataracts, acne, hirsutism, infection, striae, skin atrophy, glaucoma

Rare: compression fractures, avascular necrosis, pathologic fractures, pancreatitis, esophagitis, abdominal distension, impaired wound healing, petechiae/ecchymoses, facial erythema, increased sweating, decreased reaction to skin testing, convulsions, increased intracranial pressure with papilledema (pseudotumor cerebri), vertigo, menstrual irregularities, suppression of growth in children, adrenocortical and pituitary unresponsiveness, diabetes mellitus, increased insulin requirements, exophthalmos, negative nitrogen balance, bowel perforation, agitation, psychosis, opportunistic infections, hypocalcemia, fatty liver changes, depression, peripheral neuropathy, herpes infections, tuberculosis reactivation, telangiectasias, rebound poison ivy, pustular psoriasis flare, acanthosis nigricans, telogen effluvium, adrenal crisis, non-Hodgkin's lymphoma, Kaposi's sarcoma, squamous cell carcinoma of genitourinary tracts

IM (SPECIFIC)

COMMON: local atrophy, local bleeding, pain, local pigmentary changes

RARE: flushing, muscle cramps, fat necrosis, ecchymosis

IL

COMMON: pain, bleeding, atrophy, pigmentary changes

RARE: ulceration, calcification, secondary infection, granuloma formation, allergic reactions, hypothalamic-pituitary adrenal (HPA) axis suppression, hirsutism, acne, Cushing's disease, growth inhibition, syncope, blindness

▮ MONITORING (NOT IL)

BASELINE: chest x-ray, blood pressure, fasting serum glucose, eye exam, weight, electrolytes, purified protein derivative (PPD), fasting lipids

FIRST MONTH, THEN EVERY 3 MONTHS: blood pressure, fasting serum glucose, weight, electrolytes, fasting lipids

AFTER 6 MONTHS, THEN YEARLY: eye exam

If giving pulse therapy, check electrocardiogram before each daily dose; laboratory results (potassium, glucose) before and after each dose; and during infusion vital signs every 20 min, cardiac monitoring and frequent finger sticks for glucose levels.

▮ CONTRAINDICATIONS

Hypersensitivity to drug/class, systemic fungal infection, herpes simplex keratitis, psychosis/depression, peptic ulcer, hypertension, tuberculosis, diabetes mellitus, osteoporosis, glaucoma, cataracts, use of live vaccines, pregnancy

■ PREGNANCY CLASS

C

STEROIDS, TOPICAL

GROUP 1 (MOST POTENT)

- Betamethasone dipropionate, augmented (Clobevate® 0.05% gel; Diprolene® 0.05% lotion, ointment, gel)
- Clobetasol propionate (Temovate® 0.05% cream, ointment, gel, solution; Temovate E® 0.05% emollient cream; Olux® 0.05% foam)
- Diflorasone diacetate (Psorcon® 0.05% ointment)
- Halobetasol propionate (Ultravate® 0.05% cream, ointment)

GROUP 2

- Amcinonide (Cyclocort® 0.1% ointment, lotion, cream)
- Betamethasone dipropionate (Diprosone® 0.05% ointment; Maxivate® 0.05% cream, ointment)
- Desoximetasone (Topicort® 0.25% cream, ointment, gel; Topicort® 0.05% gel)
- Diflorasone diacetate (Florone,® Maxiflor® 0.05% ointment)
- Fluocinonide (Lidex® 0.05% cream, ointment, gel, solution; Lidex E® 0.05% emollient cream)
- Halcinonide (Halog® 0.1% cream, ointment, solution)

GROUP 3

- Amcinonide (Cyclocort® 0.1% lotion)
- Betamethasone dipropionate (Diprosone® 0.05% cream)
- Betamethasone valerate (Betatrex,® Valisone® 0.1% ointment)
- Diflorasone diacetate (Florone,® Maxiflor® 0.05% cream)
- Fluticasone propionate (Cutivate® 0.005% ointment)
- Mometasone furoate (Elocon 0.1% ointment)
- Triamcinolone acetonide (Aristocort,® Kenalog® 0.5% cream, ointment)

GROUP 4

- Amcinonide (Cyclocort® 0.1% cream)
- Desoximetasone (Topicort LP® 0.05% emollient cream)
- Fluocinolone acetonide (Synalar HP® 0.2% emollient cream; Synalar® 0.025% ointment)

- Flurandrenolide (Cordran® 0.05% ointment)
- Halcinonide (Halog® 0.025% cream)
- Hydrocortisone valerate (Westcort® 0.2% ointment)
- Mometasone furoate (Elocon® 0.1% cream, lotion)
- Triamcinolone acetonide (Aristocort,® Kenalog® 0.1% ointment)

GROUP 5

- Betamethasone dipropionate (Diprosone,® Maxivate® 0.05% lotion)
- Betamethasone valerate (Valisone,® Betatrex® 0.1% cream, lotion; Luxiq® 0.1% foam)
- Clocortolone pivalate (Cloderm® 0.1% cream)
- Desonide (DesOwen,® Tridesilon® 0.05% ointment)
- Fluocinolone acetonide (Synalar® 0.025% cream)
- Flurandrenolide (Cordran® 0.05% cream, lotion; Cordran® 0.025% ointment)
- Fluticasone (Cutivate® 0.05% cream)
- Hydrocortisone butyrate (Locoid® 0.1% cream, ointment, solution)
- Hydrocortisone valerate (Westcort® 0.2% cream)
- Prednicarbate (Dermatop® 0.1% cream)
- Triamcinolone acetonide (Aristocort,® Kenalog® 0.1% cream; Kenalog® 0.025% ointment, lotion)

GROUP 6

- Alclometasone dipropionate (Aclovate® 0.05% cream, ointment)
- Betamethasone valerate (Valisone® 0.01% cream)
- Desonide (DesOwen® 0.05% cream, lotion; Tridesilon® 0.05% cream)
- Fluocinolone acetonide (Synalar® 0.01% cream, solution)
- Triamcinolone acetonide (Aristocort,® Kenalog® 0.025% cream)

GROUP 7 (LEAST POTENT)

- Hydrocortisone (Hytone® 0.5, 1, 2.5% cream, ointment, lotion)

INDICATIONS (PARTIAL LIST)

- Acne$ (see pg. 347)
- Alopecia areata$ (see pg. 349)
- Atopic dermatitis* (see pg. 353)
- Behçet's disease, cutaneous$ (see pg. 355)
- Bullous pemphigoid* (see pg. 355)
- Chondrodermatitis nodularis helicis+
- Cicatricial pemphigoid$ (see pg. 356)
- Contact dermatitis* (see pg. 357)

- Cutaneous T-cell lymphoma, patch stage* (see pg. 358)
- Dermatomyositis* (see pg. 361)
- Diaper dermatitis^
- Drug reaction*
- Dyshidrotic eczema^
- Epidermolysis bullosa acquisita+ (see pg. 363)
- Erythema multiforme* (see pg. 364)
- Erythroderma$
- Granuloma annulare+ (see pg. 365)
- Herpes gestationis$ (see pg. 368)
- Jessner's lymphocytic infiltrate$
- Lichen planopilaris+ (see pg. 371)
- Lichen planus^ (see pg. 371)
- Lichen sclerosus et atrophicus$ (see pg. 372)
- Lichen simplex chronicus^ (see pg. 373)
- Linear IgA dermatosis+ (see pg. 374)
- Lupus, cutaneous* (see pg. 375)
- Lymphomatoid papulosis+ (see pg. 377)
- Morphea$ (see pg. 381)
- Necrobiosis lipoidica diabeticorum+ (see pg. 381)
- Nummular dermatitis$
- Pemphigus erythematosus+
- Pemphigus foliaceus* (see pg. 383)
- Pemphigus vulgaris* (see pg. 385)
- Pityriasis rosea+ (see pg. 387)
- Pruritic urticarial papules and plaques of pregnancy$ (see pg. 390)
- Pruritus* (see pg. 391)
- Psoriasis,* with calcipotriene ointment* (see pg. 392)
- Pyoderma gangrenosum$ (see pg. 394)
- Sarcoidosis, cutaneous+ (see pg. 396)
- Scar/keloid$ (see pg. 371)
- Seborrheic dermatitis* (see pg. 399)
- Sunburn^
- Sweet's syndrome+ (see pg. 401)
- Urticaria* (see pg. 403)
- Urticaria pigmentosa+
- Vitiligo^ (see pg. 405)
- Well's syndrome+

MECHANISM OF ACTION

They have local anti-inflammatory and antiproliferative effects and, rarely, systemic immunosuppressive effects. They inhibit production of prostaglandins, reduce sensitivity to and release of histamine, and inhibit mast cell sensitization. They induce lipocortins, vasocortin, and vasoregulin, which prevent formation of inflammatory mediators (prostaglandins, leukotrienes, and hydroxyeicosanoic acid). They inhibit nuclear factor kappa B (NFkB), decreasing production of interleukin-1, tumor necrosis factor alpha, adhesion molecules, and growth factors. They also inhibit AP-1, a heterodimeric transcription factor composed of c-jun, c-fos, and activating transcription factor, thus decreasing cytokine production. They cause lymphocyte and eosinophil apoptosis. They inhibit phospholipase-A2, which leads to decreased production of cyclooxygenase, prostaglandins, leukotrienes, and hydroxyeicosatetraenoic acid inflammatory mediators. Leukocytes have decreased ability to adhere, migrate, and phagocytize. There is also decreased production of interferon gamma, IL-2, and granulocyte-macrophage colony-stimulating factor.

■ DOSAGE

Apply qd to bid. Lowest potency for face, groin, intertriginous areas. Highest potency for 2 week or 20 g limit because of risk of systemic absorption. May compound with Orabase® for use on mucosa.

CREAM: weeping areas

FOAM: scalp or body

GEL: scalp or mucosa

LOTION: scalp or mucosa

OINTMENT: thick, lichenified, or scaly areas

SOLUTION: scalp or mucosa

■ DRUG INTERACTIONS

None

■ SIDE EFFECTS

COMMON: burning, stinging, irritation, atrophy, telangiectasias, striae, pruritus, cracking, fissuring, erythema, folliculitis, acne, perioral dermatitis, dryness, hypopigmentation

RARE: numbness, Cushing's disease, contact dermatitis, infection, miliaria, hypothalamic-pituitary adrenal (HPA) axis suppression, growth retardation in children, steroid rebound, glaucoma, cataracts, tachyphylaxis, facial hypertrichosis, genital ulceration, reactivation of Kaposi's sarcoma, rosacea, delayed wound healing

MONITORING

PERIODICALLY IF LONG-TERM USE: morning cortisol, urinary free cortisol, or ACTH stimulation test

CONTRAINDICATIONS

Hypersensitivity to drug/class, pregnancy, acute infection, infestation

PREGNANCY CLASS

C

SULFONAMIDES

Trimethoprim/sulfamethoxazole (Bactrim,® Septra® 80, 400 single-strength [SS] tabs, 160, 800 double-strength [DS] tabs, 40–200 mg/5 mL suspension [20 mL = 2 SS = 1 DS], IV), sulfadiazine (Sulfadiazine® 500 mg tabs), sulfamethoxazole (Gantanol® 500 mg tabs, 500 mg/5 mL suspension)

INDICATIONS

- *Actinomycetoma*§
- *Enterobacter* sp. (trimethoprim/sulfamethoxazole*)
- *Escherichia coli* (trimethoprim/sulfamethoxazole,* sulfamethoxazole*)
- *Haemophilus influenzae* (trimethoprim/sulfamethoxazole*)
- *Klebsiella* sp. (trimethoprim/sulfamethoxazole*)
- *Morganella morganii* (trimethoprim/sulfamethoxazole*)
- *Plasmodium falciparum,* chloroquine-resistant (sulfadiazine*)
- *Pneumocystis carinii* (trimethoprim/sulfamethoxazole*)
- *Proteus mirabilis* (trimethoprim/sulfamethoxazole*)
- *Proteus vulgaris* (trimethoprim/sulfamethoxazole*)
- *Shigella flexneri* and *sonnei* (trimethoprim/sulfamethoxazole*)
- *Streptococcus pneumoniae* (tulfamethoxazole,* trimethoprim/sulfamethoxazole*)
- *Toxoplasma gondii* (sulfadiazine*)
- *Wegener's granulomatosis*^ (see pg. 404)

See Appendix II.

Usually effective (trimethoprim/sulfamethoxazole):

- *Aeromonas* sp.
- *Brucella* sp.
- *Bulkholderia cepacia*
- *Enterococcus faecalis*
- *Francisella tularensis*
- *Legionella* sp.
- *Listeria monocytogenes*
- *Moraxella catarrhalis*
- *Neisseria meningitidis*
- *Staphylococcus aureus*, methicillin sensitive
- *Stenotrophomonas maltophilia*
- *Streptococcus*, group A, B, C, G
- *Yersinia enterocolytica*

Clinical trials lacking (trimethoprim/sulfamethoxazole):

- *Haemophilus ducreyi*
- *Neisseria gonorrhoeae*
- *Salmonella* sp.
- *Serratia marcescens*
- *Shigella* sp.
- *Staphylococcus epidermidis*

▓ MECHANISM OF ACTION

They are bacteristatic agents that inhibit bacterial dihydropteroate synthetase (sulfonamides) and bacterial dihydrofolate reductase (trimethoprim).

▓ DOSAGE

SULFAMETHOXAZOLE

1000 mg PO bid

RENAL DOSING
Creatinine clearance (CrCl) 50–90 mL/min: q12h
CrCl 10–50 mL/min and continuous arteriovenous hemofiltration (CAVH): q18h
CrCl < 10 mL/min: q24h
Hemodialysis: extra 1 g after dialysis
Chronic ambulatory peritoneal dialysis (CAPD): 1 g qd

TRIMETHOPRIM/SULFAMETHOXAZOLE

4–5 mg/kg trimethoprim IV q12h, 1–2 SS tabs PO bid, 1 DS tab PO bid

RENAL DOSING TRIMETHOPRIM
  CrCl 50–90 mL/min: 100–200 mg q12h
  CrCl 10–50 mL/min: q18h
  CrCl < 10 mL/min: q24h
  Hemodialysis: dose after dialysis
  CAVH: q18h
  CAPD: q24h

SULFADIAZINE

Toxoplasmosis, cerebral: 1–1.5 g PO q6h, with pyrimethamine and folinic acid as treatment, then 0.5–1 g PO q6h for suppression with pyrimethamine and folinic acid

▓ DRUG INTERACTIONS (SULFAMETHOXAZOLE UNLESS OTHERWISE INDICATED)

INCREASED LEVELS OF: bosentan (trimethoprim), dapsone (trimethoprim), digoxin (trimethoprim), lamivudine (trimethoprim), methotrexate, phenytoin (sulfadiazine, trimethoprim), procainamide (trimethoprim), sildenafil (trimethoprim), voriconazole (trimethoprim), warfarin, zidovudine (trimethoprim)

BLOOD DYSCRASIAS: lamotrigine (trimethoprim)

DECREASED EFFICACY OF SULFONAMIDES: ester anesthetics

BONE MARROW SUPPRESSION: mercaptopurine (trimethoprim), methotrexate, phenytoin (trimethoprim), pyrimethamine (trimethoprim)

DECREASED EFFICACY OF: oral contraceptives, cyclosporin (sulfadiazine)

INCREASED QT INTERVAL: dofetilide (trimethoprim), antipsychotics, arsenic, astemizole, chloral hydrate, cisapride, macrolides, antiarrhythmics, clindamycin, dolasetron, enflurane, fluconazole, foscarnet, halothane, isoflurane, levomethoxazole, mefloquine, octreotide, pentamidine, terfenadine, tricyclic antidepressants, vasopressin, zolmitriptan, venlafaxine

HYPOGLYCEMIA: insulin, metformin, sulfonylureas (sulfadiazine), chlorpropamide (sulfadiazine)

INCREASED LEVELS OF SULFONAMIDES: probenecid, monoamine oxidase inhibitors

INCREASED BLEEDING: warfarin

INCREASED NEPHROTOXICITY: cyclosporin

DECREASED LEVELS OF SULFONAMIDES: atovaquone

▓ SIDE EFFECTS (ONLY SULFONAMIDES UNLESS OTHERWISE INDICATED)

COMMON: nausea, vomiting, anorexia, allergic rash, hypersensitivity reactions, photosensitivity, diarrhea, dizziness, gastrointestinal upset, headache, lethargy, pruritus, taste change (trimethoprim), glossitis (trimethoprim), epigastric pain (trimethoprim)

RARE: Stevens-Johnson syndrome, toxic epidermal necrolysis, hepatic necrosis, agranulocytosis, aplastic anemia, blood dyscrasias, anaphylaxis, hepatitis, hepatotoxicity, interstitial nephritis, nephrotoxicity, pulmonary infiltrates, pseudomembranous colitis, kernicterus, aseptic meningitis, bone marrow suppression, methemoglobinemia (trimethoprim), hyperkalemia, goiter, systemic lupus, cholestatic jaundice (trimethoprim), megaloblastic anemia (trimethoprim), leukopenia (trimethoprim), thrombocytopenia (trimethoprim), seizures, hypoglycemia, elevated liver or renal function test results (trimethoprim), hyperkalemia (trimethoprim), hematuria (sulfadiazine), crystalluria (sulfadiazine)

▓ MONITORING

FREQUENTLY IF LONG-TERM USE: complete blood count, renal function and urinalysis (if renal impairment)

▓ CONTRAINDICATIONS (ONLY SULFONAMIDES, UNLESS OTHERWISE INDICATED)

Hypersensitivity to drug/class, sulfonamide allergy, pregnancy, glucose-6-phosphate dehydrogenase deficiency (trimethoprim, sulfadiazine), volume depletion (sulfadiazine), megaloblastic anemia (trimethoprim), folate deficiency (trimethoprim), neonates, lactating, bone marrow suppressants (trimethoprim), impaired liver or renal function, porphyria

PREGNANCY CLASS

C

SULFUR

(Rosac® 10% sodium sulfacetamide and 5% sulfur with sunscreen in 45 g tubes; Sulfur soap® 10% precipitated sulfur [over the counter]; Zetacet® 10% sodium sulfacetamide and 5% sulfur topical suspension in 30 g tubes, lotion in 25 g bottles, wash in 170.1 and 340.2 g bottles; Novacet® 5% lotion with 10% salicylic acid in 30, 60 mL bottles; Sulfoxyl® 2% lotion with 5% benzoyl peroxide in 59 mL bottles, 5% lotion with 10% benzoyl peroxide in 59 mL bottles; Sebulex® 2% shampoo with 2% salicylic acid in 210 mL bottles; Plexion® 5% cleanser with 10% sodium sulfacetamide in 180 and 360 mL bottles) This is only a partial list.

INDICATIONS

- Acne vulgaris^ (see pg. 347)
- Demodex^
- Dermatophyte$
- Perioral dermatitis^
- Rosacea^ (see pg. 395)
- Scabies^ (see pg. 397)
- Seborrheic dermatitis$ (see pg. 399)
- Tinea versicolor^
- Verruca$ (see pg. 406)

MECHANISM OF ACTION

It is a keratolytic agent that interacts with keratinocyte cysteine bonds.

DOSAGE

Apply qd to bid.

SCABIES: 5 – 10% sulfur in petrolatum base applied qhs for 3 nights

▨ DRUG INTERACTIONS

None

▨ SIDE EFFECTS

COMMON: odor of rotten eggs

RARE: contact dermatitis, hemolytic anemia, agranulocytosis, fever, jaundice

▨ MONITORING

None

▨ CONTRAINDICATIONS

Hypersensitivity to drug/class, hypersensitivity to sulfonamides (if combined with sodium sulfacetamide), pregnancy

▨ PREGNANCY CLASS

C

TACROLIMUS

(Protopic® 0.03% ointment in 30 g tubes, 0.1% ointment in 30, 60 g tubes; Prograf® 0.5, 1, 5 mg caps; 5 mg/mL ampules)

▨ INDICATIONS

ORAL

- Crohn's fistulas^
- Prophylaxis for liver and kidney transplant rejection*
- Psoriasis^ (see pg. 392)
- Rheumatoid arthritis^

TOPICAL

- Annular erythema[+]
- Atopic dermatitis* (see pg. 353)
- Balanitis xerotica obliterans[+]
- Bovine collagen hypersensitivity[+]
- Bullous pemphigoid[+] (see pg. 355)
- Chronic actinic dermatitis[§]
- Cicatricial pemphigoid, oral[+] (see pg. 356)
- Contact dermatitis[^] (see pg. 357)
- Crohn's disease, periostomal[§]
- Dermatomyositis[+] (see pg. 361)
- Dyshidrotic hand eczema[^]
- Erosive lichen planus[§] (see pg. 371)
- Graft-versus-host disease, chronic (see pg. 365)
- Granuloma annulare[+] (see pg. 365)
- Hailey-Hailey disease[+] (see pg. 367)
- Ichthyosis linearis circumflexa[+]
- Lichen amyloidosis[+] (see pg. 350)
- Lichen sclerosus et atrophicus, anogenital[§] (see pg. 372)
- Lichen striatus[+]
- Lupus, discoid[+] (see pg. 375)
- Necrobiosis lipodica diabeticorum[+] (see pg. 381)
- Netherton's syndrome[+]
- Ocular pemphigoid and pemphigus[+] (see pg. 356)
- Pityriasis lichenoides chronica[+] (see pg. 386)
- Pityriasis lichenoides et varioliformis acuta[+] (see pg. 386)
- Plasmacytosis, cutaneous[+]
- Psoriasis,[^] face and intertriginous,[§] pustular[+] (see pg. 392)
- Pyoderma gangrenosum[^] (see pg. 394)
- Reticula erythematous mucinosis[+]
- Rosacea, erythrodermic,[§] papulopustular[§] (see pg. 395)
- Sarcoidosis, cutaneous[+] (see pg. 396)
- Seborrheic dermatitis[§] (see pg. 399)
- Vitiligo[^] (see pg. 405)

MECHANISM OF ACTION

Like cyclosporin, it has the structure of a macrolide antibiotic. It inhibits the activation of helper T cells by binding to the intercellular protein FKBP2, inhibiting calcineurin. This ultimately inhibits the dephosphorylation and translocation of the nuclear factor of activated T cells, a nuclear component of gene transcription for the formation of lymphokines (interleukin-2, interferon gamma). It also inhibits the production of interleukin-8.

▪ DOSAGE

ORAL
   Liver transplant: Start 0.1–0.15 mg/kg/d PO divided into bid.
   Kidney transplant: Start 0.03–0.05 mg/kg/d PO divided into bid.
   Rheumatoid arthritis: 1–3 mg PO qd
   Crohn's fistulas: 0.2 mg/kg PO qd
   Psoriasis: Start 0.05 mg/kg/d, increasing by 0.05 mg every 3 weeks to 0.15 mg/kg/d.

TOPICAL: Apply qd to bid.

▪ DRUG INTERACTIONS (ORAL)

INCREASED LEVELS OF TACROLIMUS: diltiazem, nicardipine, nifedipine, verapamil, clotrimazole, ketoconazole, itraconazole, fluconazole, clarithromycin, erythromycin, troleandomycin, cisapride, metoclopramide, bromocriptine, cimetidine, cyclosporin, danazol, methylprednisolone, protease inhibitors

DECREASED LEVELS OF TACROLIMUS: carbamazepine, phenobarbital, phenytoin, rifabutin, rifampin

HYPERKALEMIA: potassium-sparing diuretics

RENAL DYSFUNCTION: aminoglycosides, amphotericin, cisplatin, cyclosporin

▪ SIDE EFFECTS

ORAL

COMMON: headache, tremors, diarrhea, hypertension, constipation, infection, abdominal pain, insomnia, nausea, renal dysfunction, paresthesias, dizziness, vomiting, dyspepsia, chest pain, hypophosphatemia, hypomagnesemia, edema, anemia, leukopenia, asthenia, fever, back pain, cough, arthralgia, rash, pruritus

RARE: hyperglycemia, hyperlipidemia, elevated liver function test results, anaphylaxis, thrombocytopenia, seizures, malignancy, myocardial hypertrophy, hyperkalemia, nephrotoxicity

COMMON: burning, erythema, allergic reaction, skin infection, hyperesthesia, acne, folliculitis, rash, urticaria, tingling

RARE: herpes simplex/zoster infection, eczema herpeticum, flu-like symptoms, headaches, alcohol intolerance

■ MONITORING (ORAL)

BASELINE: renal function, magnesium, complete blood count, electrolytes, phosphate, glucose, blood pressure

MONTHLY: renal function, magnesium, blood pressure

■ CONTRAINDICATIONS

Hypersensitivity to drug/class (oral and topical), hypersensitivity to poly-oxyl-60 hydrogenated castor oil (oral and topical), live vaccines should be avoided (oral), herpes simplex/zoster infection (topical), sun exposure (topical), pregnancy (oral and topical)

■ PREGNANCY CLASS

C

TAZAROTENE

(Tazorac® 0.04% cream in 15, 60 g tubes, gel in 30, 100 g tubes, 0.1% cream in 15, 30 g tubes, gel in 30, 100 g tubes; Avage® 0.1% cream in 30 g tubes)

■ INDICATIONS

- Acanthosis nigricans+ (see pg. 347)
- Acne vulgaris* (see pg. 347)
- Basal cell carcinoma$ (see pg. 354)
- Confluent and reticulated papillomatosis of Gougerot and Carteaud+

- Cutaneous T-cell lymphoma, patch/plaque§ (see pg. 358)
- Darier's disease^{+} (see pg. 359)
- Elastosis perforans serpiginosa^{+}
- Follicular dyskeratosis^{+}
- Ichthyoses, congenital§ (see pg. 369)
- Keratoderma blenorrhagicum^{+}
- Keratosis pilaris§
- Lentigo maligna^{+}
- Lichen planus, oral$^{\wedge}$ (see pg. 371)
- Lupus, discoid^{+} (see pg. 375)
- Photodamage$^{\wedge}$
- Psoriasis* (see pg. 392)
- Pyogenic granuloma–like lesions^{+}
- Seborrheic keratosis$^{\wedge}$
- Spiny keratoderma^{+}
- Steroid-induced epidermal atrophy$^{\wedge}$
- Warty dyskeratoma^{+}

■ MECHANISM OF ACTION

It is a retinoid that binds to retinoic acid receptors on keratinocytes to modify gene expression, with resultant cellular proliferation and differentiation.

■ DOSAGE

Apply qd to bid.

■ DRUG INTERACTIONS

Other retinoids should not be used.

INCREASED PHOTOSENSITIVITY: photosensitizers

■ SIDE EFFECTS

COMMON: pruritus, burning, stinging, erythema, worsening psoriasis, irritation, skin pain, rash, desquamation, contact dermatitis, fissuring, dryness, edema, discoloration, photoallergy/phototoxicity

RARE: teratogenicity

▨ MONITORING

None

▨ CONTRAINDICATIONS

Hypersensitivity to drug/class, pregnancy, avoid sunlight

▨ PREGNANCY CLASS

X

TERBINAFINE

(Lamisil® 250 mg tabs prescription; 1% cream, spray, solution [over the counter])

▨ INDICATIONS

- Aspergillosis$
- Black piedra+
- Candidiasis, cutaneous (topical,$ oral^)
- Chromomycosis$
- Majocchi's granuloma+
- Onychomycosis* (oral)
- Sporotrichosis, cutaneous$
- Tinea capitis^ (oral)
- Tinea corporis, cruris, pedis^ (oral and topical)
- Tinea imbricata^

See Appendix I.

▨ MECHANISM OF ACTION

It inhibits squalene epoxidase, thus reducing fungal cell membrane ergosterol synthesis.

▮ DOSAGE

ASPERGILLOSIS: 5–15 mg/kg/d PO for 3–5 months

BLACK PIEDRA: 250 mg PO qd for 6 weeks

CANDIDIASIS, CUTANEOUS: topical applied bid for 4 weeks, or 500 mg PO qd for 3 weeks

CHROMOMYCOSIS: 500 mg PO qd for 8–12 months

ONYCHOMYCOSIS: 250 mg PO qd for 6 weeks for fingernails, 12 weeks for toenails

SPOROTRICHOSIS: 250 mg PO bid for 8 weeks

TINEA CAPITIS: 250 mg PO qd for 4 weeks for *Trichophyton tonsurans* and 4–8 weeks for *Microsporum canis*

TINEA CORPORIS, CRURIS, PEDIS: 250 mg PO qd for 2 weeks; topical applied bid for 4 weeks

TINEA IMBRICATA: 250 mg PO qd for 4 weeks

See Appendix I.

▮ DRUG INTERACTIONS (ORAL)

INCREASED LEVELS OF: aripiprazole, atomoxetine, flecainide, propafenone, theophylline, tricyclic antidepressants

INCREASED LEVELS OF TERBINAFINE: cimetidine

DECREASED LEVELS OF: codeine, cyclosporin

DECREASED LEVELS OF TERBINAFINE: rifampins

INCREASED QT PROLONGATION: thioridazine

▮ SIDE EFFECTS

ORAL

COMMON: headache, rash, diarrhea, dyspepsia, elevated transaminases, taste changes, pruritus, nausea, abdominal pain, flatulence, urticaria, visual changes, constipation

Rare: Stevens-Johnson syndrome, toxic epidermal necrolysis, subacute cutaneous lupus, neutropenia, hepatotoxicity, hepatic failure, erythema multiforme, anaphylaxis, thrombocytopenia, malaise, fatigue, arthralgia, myalgia, hair loss, vomiting, acute generalized exanthematous pustulosis

TOPICAL

Common: irritation, burning, tingling, pruritus

Rare: none

MONITORING (ORAL)

Baseline: complete blood count, liver function

After 6 Weeks: liver function

CONTRAINDICATIONS

Oral: hypersensitivity to drug/class, pregnancy, children, impaired liver or renal function

Topical: hypersensitivity to drug/class

PREGNANCY CLASS

B

TETRACYCLINES

Doxycycline (Doryx® 50, 100 mg caps; Periostat® 20 mg caps; Vibramycin® 50, 100 mg caps, IV), minocycline (Minocin® 50, 100 mg caps; 50 mg/5 mL suspension; Vectrin® 50, 100 mg caps), tetracycline (Achromycin V® 250, 500 mg caps; Sumycin® 250, 500 mg caps, 125 mg/5 mL suspension)

INDICATIONS

- *Acinetobacter* sp.*
- Acne* with Periostat® therapy^ (see pg. 347)

- *Actinomyces israelii**
- *Bacillus anthracis**
- *Bacteroides fragilis* (tetracycline*)
- *Bartonella bacilliformis**
- *Borrelia recurrentis**
- *Brucella* sp.*
- *Calymmobacterium granulomatis**
- *Campylobacter fetus**
- *Chlamydia psittaci**
- *Chlamydia trachomatis**
- *Clostridium,* not *difficile**
- *Confluent and reticulated papillomatosus of Gougerot and Carteaud* (minocycline+)
- *Enterobacter aerogenes**
- *Enterococcus faecalis* (tetracycline*)
- Epidermolysis bullosa, Weber-Cockayne syndrome (tetracycline)^ (see pg. 362)
- *Escherichia coli**
- *Foreign body granuloma* (minocycline+)
- *Francisella tularensis**
- *Fusobacterium fusoformis**
- *Haemophilus ducreyi**
- *Haemophilus influenzae**
- *Herellea* sp. (tetracycline*)
- *Klebsiella* sp.*
- *Listeria monocytogenes**
- *Mima* sp. (tetracycline*)
- *Mycobacterium fortuitum* (doxycycline$)
- *Mycobacterium marinum* (minocycline*)
- *Mycoplasma pneumoniae**
- *Neisseria gonorrhoeae**
- *Neisseria meningitidis,* carriers (minocycline*)
- Pemphigus foliaceus, with niacinamide 1.5 g PO qd (tetracycline)+ (see pg. 383)
- *Plasmodium falciparum* prophylaxis (doxycycline*)
- *Rickettsia* sp.*
- *Shigella* sp.*
- *Streptococcus pneumoniae**
- *Streptococcus pyogenes* (tetracycline*)
- *Treponema pallidum**
- *Treponema pertenue**
- *Ureaplasma urealytica* (doxycycline*)
- *Vibrio cholerae**
- *Yersinia pestis**

See Appendix II.

Usually effective (not tetracycline):

- *Aeromonas* sp.
- *Chlamydia* sp.
- *Legionella* sp.
- *Moraxella catarrhalis*
- *Neisseria meningitidis* (doxycycline)
- *Peptostreptococcus* sp.
- *Prevotella melaninogenica*
- *Staphylococcus aureus,* methicillin sensitive (minocycline)
- *Vibrio vulnificus*

Clinical trials lacking (not tetracycline):

- *Bacteroides fragilis*
- *Burkholderia cepacia* (minocycline)
- *Pseudomonas aeruginosa* (minocycline)
- *Salmonella* sp.
- *Staphylococcus aureus,* methicillin sensitive (doxycycline)

MECHANISM OF ACTION

They are bacteriostatic agents that inhibit bacterial protein synthesis.

DOSAGE

DOXYCYCLINE

BACTERIAL INFECTION: 100 mg PO/IV bid

ACNE/ROSACEA: 20 mg PO bid (Periostat® for rosacea), 100 mg PO qd to bid

TETRACYCLINE

BACTERIAL INFECTION: 1–2 g PO divided bid to qid

ACNE: 250–500 mg PO bid

EPIDERMOLYSIS BULLOSA, WEBER-COCKAYNE SYNDROME: 1500 mg PO qd

PEMPHIGUS FOLIACEUS: 500 mg PO tid with niacinamide 1.5 g PO qd

RENAL DOSING
Creatinine clearance (CrCl) 50–90 mL/min: q8–12h
CrCl 10–50 mL/min: q12–24h
CrCl < 10 mL/min: q24h

MINOCYCLINE

BACTERIAL INFECTION: 200 mg IV once, then 100 mg IV q12h, or 100 mg PO bid

ACNE/ROSACEA: 50 mg PO bid

MYCOBACTERIUM MARINUM: 100 mg PO bid for 6–8 weeks

DRUG INTERACTIONS

DECREASED EFFICACY OF TETRACYCLINES: antacids, bismuth, calcium, iron, multivitamins, didanosine, magnesium, molindone, quinapril

DECREASED EFFICACY OF: oral contraceptives

DECREASED LEVEL OF: atovaquone

INCREASED LEVELS OF: digoxin, lithium, warfarin

PSEUDOTUMOR CEREBRI: isotretinoin

SIDE EFFECTS

COMMON: dyspepsia, nausea, vomiting, anorexia, diarrhea, photosensitivity, stomatitis, candidiasis, discolored teeth (<8 years old), esophagitis, phlebitis (IV), lightheadedness, dizziness, vertigo, ataxia, headache, tinnitus, drowsiness

RARE: pseudotumor cerebri (with isotretinoin), neutropenia, thrombocytopenia, hepatotoxicity, Jarisch-Herxheimer reaction (when treating *Treponema pallidum*), superinfection, pseudomembranous colitis, increased intracranial pressure (infants), skeletal retardation (infants)

MONITORING

None

CONTRAINDICATIONS

Hypersensitivity to drug/class, pregnancy, children, impaired liver or renal function

PREGNANCY CLASS

D

THALIDOMIDE

(Thalomid® 50, 100, 200 mg caps)

INDICATIONS

- Actinic prurigo$
- Aphthous stomatitis, oral and esophageal in AIDS^ (see pg. 352)
- Behçet's disease^ (see pg. 355)
- Bullous pemphigoid⁺ (see pg. 355)
- Cicatricial pemphigoid⁺ (see pg. 356)
- Cutaneous lymphoid hyperplasia⁺
- Erythema multiforme, chronic/recurrent$ (see pg. 364)
- Erythema nodosum leprosum*
- Graft-versus-host disease, chronic$ (see pg. 365)
- Granulomatous cheilitis⁺
- Jessner's lymphocytic infiltrate^
- Kaposi's sarcoma in AIDS$ (see pg. 370)
- Langerhans cell histiocytosis⁺
- Lichen planus, erosive⁺ (see pg. 371)
- Lupus, discoid$, profundus⁺, subacute cutaneous$ (see pg. 375)
- Multicentric reticulohistiocytosis⁺
- Palmoplantar pustulosis⁺
- Postherpetic neuralgia⁺ (see pg. 389)
- Prurigo nodularis$
- Pruritus, chronic$, uremic^ (see pg. 391)
- Pyoderma gangrenosum⁺ (see pg. 394)
- Sarcoidosis, cutaneous$ (see pg. 396)
- Schnitzler's syndrome⁺
- Scleromyxedema⁺
- Weber-Christian disease⁺

█ MECHANISM OF ACTION

It is an immunomodulatory agent that inhibits tumor necrosis factor alpha production and down-regulates selected cell-surface adhesion molecules involved in leukocyte migration and phagocytosis. It also inhibits monocyte phagocytosis. It leads to decrease in T helper cells and a concomitant increase in T suppressor cells. It suppresses interleukin-12 and interferon gamma while increasing interleukin-4 and -5 production. It antagonizes histamine, acetylcholine, prostaglandins, and serotonin. It inhibits angiogenesis and proliferation of abnormal neural tissue.

█ DOSAGE

APHTHAE IN AIDS: 200 mg PO qd

APHTHAE IN BEHÇET'S DISEASE: 100 mg PO qd

BEHÇET'S DISEASE: 400 mg PO qd

BULLOUS PEMPHIGOID: 100 mg PO qd

CICATRICIAL PEMPHIGOID: 100 mg PO qd

ERYTHEMA MULTIFORME, CHRONIC/RECURRENT: 100 mg PO qd

ERYTHEMA NODOSUM LEPROSUM: 100–400 mg PO qhs for 2 weeks or until symptoms improve, then decrease by 50 mg/d every 2–4 weeks

GRAFT-VERSUS-HOST DISEASE: 800–1600 mg PO qd

GRANULOMATOUS CHEILITIS: 100 mg PO qd

JESSNER'S LYMPHOCYTIC INFILTRATE: 100 mg PO qd

KAPOSI'S SARCOMA IN AIDS: 200–1000 mg PO qd

LANGERHANS CELL HISTIOCYTOSIS: 100 mg PO qd

LICHEN PLANUS: 200 mg PO qd

LUPUS, DISCOID: 50–300 mg PO qd

LUPUS, PROFUNDUS: 200 g PO bid

LUPUS, SUBACUTE CUTANEOUS: 50–100 mg PO qd

PRURIGO NODULARIS: 50–300 mg PO qd

PRURITUS, CHRONIC: 200 mg PO qd

PYODERMA GANGRENOSUM: 100 mg PO qd

SARCOIDOSIS, CUTANEOUS: 50–200 mg PO qd

SCHNITZLER'S SYNDROME: 100 mg PO qd

WEBER-CHRISTIAN DISEASE: 300 mg PO qd

Must give only 1 month supply at a time. Men and women must use effective contraception 1 month before starting treatment and 1 month after completing treatment. Man must wear a condom when having sex with a woman of childbearing age even if he has had a vasectomy. Woman who has not had a hysterectomy or who has not been postmenopausal for at least 24 months is considered a woman of childbearing age. In the United States, prescriber must be registered in the STEPS program (1-888-423-5436).

DRUG INTERACTIONS

INCREASED CENTRAL NERVOUS SYSTEM DEPRESSION OR PSYCHOMOTOR IMPAIRMENT: opiates, propoxyphene combination, tramadol, antidepressant, antihistamine with or without decongestant, antipsychotics, barbiturates, benzodiazepines, cetirizine, chlorpheniramine, hydrocodone, dronabinol, ethanol, meperidine, promethazine, meprobamate, muscle relaxants, opiate agonists/antagonists, phenothiazines, sedative-hypnotics, tricyclic antidepressants

INCREASED RISK OF NEPHROTOXICITY IN MULTIPLE MYELOMA PATIENTS: zoledronic acid

SIDE EFFECTS

COMMON: drowsiness, somnolence, dizziness, hypotension, rash, diarrhea, fever, chills, headache, increased appetite, weight gain, dry mouth, confusion, photosensitivity, abdominal pain, asthenia, back pain, facial edema, infection, anorexia, constipation, flatulence, increased liver function tests, nausea, oral moniliasis, tooth pain, anemia, edema, paresthesias, pruritus, sweating, peripheral neuropathy

RARE: birth defects (if woman is pregnant), peripheral neuropathy, neutropenia, hypertension, bradycardia, Stevens-Johnson syndrome/toxic epidermal necrolysis, seizures, amnesia, mood changes, increased HIV viral load, hyperlipidemia, albuminuria, hematuria, impotence, lymphadenopathy, agitation, nervousness, pharyngitis, rhinitis, sinusitis, acne, vertigo, tremor

MONITORING

BASELINE: serum pregnancy test 24 h before starting treatment

WEEKLY FOR FIRST MONTH: serum pregnancy test

MONTHLY (OR EVERY 2 WEEKS IF IRREGULAR MENSTRUAL CYCLE): serum pregnancy test

CONTRAINDICATIONS

Hypersensitivity to drug/class, pregnancy, neuritis/peripheral neuropathy, absolute neutrophil count <750, congestive heart failure, hypotension, seizures, hypothyroid, significant renal or hepatic failure, toxic epidermal necrolysis

PREGNANCY CLASS

X

THIABENDAZOLE

(Mintezol® 500 mg/5 mL suspension in 120 mL bottle, 500 mg chewable tabs)

INDICATIONS

- Ascariasis (*Ascaris lumbricoides*)*
- Chromomycosis$
- Cutaneous larva migrans (*Ancylostoma braziliense*)*
- Dracunculiasis^
- Enterobiasis (*Enterobius vermicularis*)*
- Pediculosis capitis$

- Scabies[§] (see pg. 397)
- Strongyloidiasis (*Strongyloides stercoralis*)[*]
- Tinea capitis/corporis[^]
- Tinea nigra palmaris[+]
- Trichinosis (*Trichinella spiralis*)[*]
- Trichuriasis (*Trichuris trichiura*)[*]
- Uncinariasis (*Necator americanus, Ancylostoma duodenale*)[*]
- Visceral larva migrans (*Toxocara cati* and *canis*)[*]

MECHANISM OF ACTION

It inhibits the helminth-specific enzyme fumarate reductase.

DOSAGE

Take after meals. Maximum of 3 g/d.

ASCARIASIS, ENTEROBIASIS, UNCINARIASIS: 25 mg/kd PO bid for 2 days (maximum 3 g/d)

CHROMOMYCOSIS: 25 mg/kg/d PO for 6 weeks to 22 months

CUTANEOUS LARVA MIGRANS: 25 mg/kg PO bid for 2–5 days (maximum 3 g/d), or topically tid for 15 days

DRACUNCULIASIS: 25 mg/kg PO bid for 3 days (maximum 3 g/d)

HELMINTHIC INFECTIONS: 25 mg/kg PO bid for 2 days, 7–10 days if hyper-infection (maximum 3 g/d)

PEDICULOSIS CAPITIS: 20 mg/kg PO bid for 1 day, then repeat in 10 days

SCABIES: Apply 10% suspension topically bid for 5 days.

TINEA CORPORIS/CAPITIS: Apply 10% cream tid until clinically clear.

TINEA NIGRA PALMARIS: Apply topically bid for 2 weeks.

TRICHINOSIS: 25 mg/kg PO bid for 2–4 days (maximum 3 g/d)

VISCERAL LARVA MIGRANS: 25 mg/kg PO bid for 5–7 days (maximum 3 g/d)

▨ DRUG INTERACTIONS

INCREASED LEVELS OF: theophylline

▨ SIDE EFFECTS

COMMON: anorexia, nausea, vomiting, headache, somnolence, numbness, tinnitus, blurred vision, yellow vision, dry mouth, diarrhea, malodorous urine, rash, pruritus, dizziness

RARE: anaphylaxis, Stevens-Johnson syndrome, jaundice, hepatic dysfunction, erythema multiforme, seizures, hallucinations, leukopenia, nephrotoxicity, enuresis, hematuria, leukopenia, hyperglycemia, hypotension, altered mental status

▨ MONITORING

None

▨ CONTRAINDICATIONS

Hypersensitivity to drug/class, pregnancy, pinworm prophylaxis, malnutrition, anemia, impaired liver function, impaired renal function, volume depletion

▨ PREGNANCY CLASS

C

THIOGUANINE

(Tabloid® 40 mg tabs)

▨ INDICATIONS

- Acute nonlymphocytic leukemias*
- Chronic lymphocytic leukemia*
- Hodgkin's lymphoma*

- Hypereosinophilic syndrome[+] (see pg. 368)
- Multiple myeloma[*]
- Psoriasis[$] (see pg. 392)
- Waldenström's macroglobulinemia[+]

MECHANISM OF ACTION

It leads to feedback inhibition of de novo purine synthesis, inhibits purine nucleotide interconversions, and incorporates into DNA and RNA, which blocks synthesis and utilization of purine nucleotides.

DOSAGE

PSORIASIS: 80–100 mg PO twice a week, increasing by 20 mg every 2–4 weeks, to maintenance dose of 120 mg PO twice a week to 160 mg PO 3 times a week

HYPEREOSINOPHILIC SYNDROME: 100 mg/m^2 qd with cytarabine

DRUG INTERACTIONS

COMPLETE CROSS-RESISTANCE: mercaptopurine

ESOPHAGEAL VARICES, ELEVATED LIVER FUNCTION TEST RESULTS: busulfan

INHIBITED THIOPURINE METHYL TRANSFERASE (TPMT) ENZYME: sulfa-salazine, mesalazine, olsalazine

SIDE EFFECTS

COMMON: myelosuppression, hyperuricemia, nausea, vomiting, anorexia, stomatitis

RARE: intestinal necrosis and perforation, hepatitis, hepatomegaly, jaundice, veno-occlusive liver disease, esophageal varices, biliary stasis, fever, infection.

▩ MONITORING

BASELINE: complete blood count, liver function, bilirubin

WEEKLY AT BEGINNING OF THERAPY (WHILE INCREASING DOSE), THEN MONTHLY: complete blood count, liver function, bilirubin

▩ CONTRAINDICATIONS

Cross-resistance to mercaptopurine, hypersensitivity to drug/class, pregnancy

▩ PREGNANCY CLASS

D

TOLNAFTATE

(Tinactin® 1% cream, powder, solution [over the counter])

▩ INDICATIONS

- Tinea corporis*
- Tinea cruris*
- Tinea pedis*

See Appendix I.

▩ MECHANISM OF ACTION

It inhibits fungal sterol biosynthesis by inhibiting squalene epoxidase.

▩ DOSAGE

Apply bid for 2–3 weeks, may need up to 4–6 weeks.

▩ DRUG INTERACTIONS

None

■ SIDE EFFECTS

COMMON: irritation, pruritus

RARE: contact dermatitis, burning, pain

■ MONITORING

None

■ CONTRAINDICATIONS

Hypersensitivity to drug/class, pregnancy

■ PREGNANCY CLASS

C

TRETINOIN

(Retin A® 0.025% gel in 15, 45 g tubes; 0.025, 0.05, 0.1% cream in 20, 45 g tubes; 0.05% solution in 28 mL bottle; Retin A micro® 0.04, 0.1% gel in 20, 45 g tubes; Renova® 0.05% cream in 20, 40, 60 g tubes; Avita® 0.025% gel and cream in 20, 45 g tubes; Altinac® 0.025, 0.05, 0.1% cream in 20, 45 g tubes)

■ INDICATIONS

- Acne vulgaris* (see pg. 347)
- Alopecia areata with intralesional triamcinolone$ (see pg. 349)
- Anhidrotic ectodermal dysplasia with vellus hair cysts+
- Atrophoderma vermiculatum+
- Basal cell carcinoma$ (see pg. 354)
- Bateman's actinic purpura^
- Confluent and reticulated papillomatosis of Gougerot and Carteaud+
- Darier's disease+ (see pg. 359)
- Dysplastic nevi^
- Erythrokeratoderma variabilis+
- Fox-Fordyce disease+

- Granulation tissue formation$
- Hypertrophic scars$
- Ichthyosis$ (see pg. 369)
- Keloids$ (see pg. 371)
- Keratoderma$
- Kyrle's disease+
- Lichen planus, oral^ (see pg. 371)
- Lichen sclerosus et atrophicus$ (see pg. 372)
- Lupus, cutaneous+ (see pg. 375)
- Melasma^
- Miliaria osteoma cutis+
- Molluscum contagiosum$ (see pg. 380)
- Morphea+ (see pg. 381)
- Necrobiosis lipoidica diabeticorum+ (see pg. 381)
- Nevoid hyperkeratosis of nipple+
- Oral leukoplakia^
- Oral mucositis prophylaxis in bone marrow transplants^
- Photodamage^
- Porokeratosis+
- Premalignant lesions^
- Premalignant and malignant lesions in transplants^
- Prevention of steroid atrophy^
- Psoriasis$ (see pg. 392)
- Reactive perforating collagenosis+
- Squamous cell carcinoma$ (see pg. 400)
- Systemic sclerosis+ (see pg. 398)
- Verruca vulgaris^ (see pg. 406)
- Vitiligo in conjunction with clobetasol+ (see pg. 405)

▓ MECHANISM OF ACTION

It modifies abnormal follicular keratinization, which promotes detachment of cornified cells and enhances shedding of corneocytes from the follicle. It also increases the mitotic activity of follicular epithelia, which increases the turnover of corneocytes. It modulates the proliferation and differentiation of epidermal cells by activation of retinoic acid receptors, which alters gene expression.

▓ DOSAGE

Apply small amount qhs. Use of sunscreen and sun avoidance are recommended.

▦ DRUG INTERACTIONS

INCREASED RISK OF SKIN DRYNESS: tretinoin, sulfur, benzoyl peroxide, isotretinoin

▦ SIDE EFFECTS

COMMON: peeling, erythema, edema, blistering

RARE: none

▦ MONITORING

None

▦ CONTRAINDICATIONS

Hypersensitivity to drug/class, pregnancy

▦ PREGNANCY CLASS

C

TRIFLURIDINE

(Viroptic® 1% ophthalmic solution, can be compounded into 0.5% ointment)

▦ INDICATIONS

- Herpes simplex keratitis*
- Herpes simplex keratoconjunctivitis*
- HIV-associated acyclovir-resistant mucocutaneous herpes simplex^

▦ MECHANISM OF ACTION

It is a fluorinated pyrimidine nucleoside that inhibits viral DNA synthesis.

DOSAGE

KERATOCONJUNCTIVITIS/KERATITIS: 1 drop each eye q2h to maximum of 9 drops qd until complete re-epithelialization, then treat for 7 more days with 1 drop q4h to each eye to a maximum of 5 drops qd. If no improvement is seen after 7 days or complete re-epithelialization is not achieved after 14 days, treatment should be discontinued.

MUCOCUTANEOUS HERPES SIMPLEX: Compound with white petrolatum to make 0.5% ointment. Apply ointment qd to wounds.

DRUG INTERACTIONS

None

SIDE EFFECTS

COMMON: burning, edema, superficial punctate keratitis, irritation, hyperemia, increased intraocular pressure

RARE: epithelial keratopathy

MONITORING

None

CONTRAINDICATIONS

Hypersensitivity to drug/class, pregnancy

PREGNANCY CLASS

C

ULTRAVIOLET A-1

INDICATIONS

- Atopic dermatitis^ (see pg. 353)
- Cutaneous T-cell lymphoma, stage Ib-III$ (see pg. 358)
- Dyshidrotic eczema^
- Lichen planus$ (see pg. 371)
- Lupus*, cutaneous^ (see pg. 375)
- Pityriasis lichenoides$ (see pg. 386)
- Polymorphous light eruption^
- Psoriasis^ (see pg. 392)
- Scleroderma, localized$, systemic$, acrosclerosis$ (see pg. 398)
- Urticaria pigmentosa^
- Vitiligo^ (see pg. 405)

MECHANISM OF ACTION

It inhibits T-cell activation through suppression of ICAM-1 and induction of epidermal cell apoptosis. In addition to decreasing keratinocyte production and Langerhans cell function, it also affects dermal fibroblasts, dendritic cells, endothelial cells, mast cells, and T cells.

DOSAGE

Weekly

ACROSCLEROSIS OF SCLERODERMA: 4 times a week

URTICARIA PIGMENTOSA, DYSHIDROTIC ECZEMA, LICHEN PLANUS: 5 times a week

DRUG INTERACTIONS

Increases photosensitization potential of medications.

SIDE EFFECTS

COMMON: sunburn, blisters, skin cancers, pruritus, xerosis

MONITORING

None

CONTRAINDICATIONS

Photosensitivity, melanoma, skin cancers

PREGNANCY CLASS

Not applicable

ULTRAVIOLET B

INDICATIONS

- Atopic dermatitis^ (narrow band^) (see pg. 353)
- Eosinophilic folliculitis$
- Epidermolysis bullosa acquisita+ (see pg. 363)
- Graft-versus-host disease$ (see pg. 365)
- Hand dermatitis^
- Ichthyosis linearis circumflexa+
- Lichen planus$ (narrow band$) (see pg. 371)
- Macular amyloid+ (see pg. 350)
- Mycosis fungoides Ia, Ib$ (see pg. 358)
- Papuloerythroderma of Ofuji$
- Papulopruritic eruption of HIV$
- Pityriasis lichenoides$ (see pg. 386)
- Pityriasis rosea^ (see pg. 387)
- Pityriasis rubra pilaris$ (see pg. 387)
- Polymorphous light eruption^ (narrow band$)
- Prurigo nodularis (narrow band$ with thalidomide)
- Pruritus, hemodialysis$, polycythemia vera$, HIV$, breast cancer (narrow band+) (see pg. 391)
- Psoriasis^ (narrow band^) (see pg. 392)
- Reticular erythematous muciosis+
- Seborrheic dermatitis$ (narrow band$) (see pg. 399)

- Skin hardening for actinic prurigo$^\$$, hydroa vacciniforme$^+$ (narrow band$^\$$), solar urticaria$^+$ (narrow band$^+$) (see pg. 403), porphyria$^\$$ (see pg. 388), polymorphous light eruption (narrow band$^\$$)
- Subcorneal pustular dermatosis$^+$
- Urticaria, chronic$^\$$ (see pg. 403)
- Vitiligo$^\wedge$ (narrow band$^\$$, narrow band with calcipotriene$^+$) (see pg. 405)

MECHANISM OF ACTION

It inhibits cell proliferation in the epidermis, suppresses the immune system by inhibiting Langerhans cells, and induces epidermal T-cell apoptosis.

DOSAGE

Qd to weekly

DRUG INTERACTIONS

Increased photosensitivity

SIDE EFFECTS

COMMON: sunburn, skin cancers, xerosis, pruritus

MONITORING

None

CONTRAINDICATIONS

Photosensitivity, melanoma, invasive skin cancers

PREGNANCY CLASS

Not applicable

UREA

(Carmol 40® cream with 40% urea; Carmol 20® cream with 20% urea [over the counter]; Carmol 10® cream with 10% urea [over the counter]; Carmol deep cleansing shampoo® with 10% urea in 240 mL bottles [over the counter]; Kerasal® with 5% salicylic acid and 10% urea [over the counter]) This is only a partial list.

▨ INDICATIONS

- Atopic dermatitis^ (see pg. 353)
- Calluses$
- Dystrophic nails^
- Ichthyosis^ (see pg. 369)
- Keratoderma$
- Keratosis pilaris$
- Nail avulsion$ (with 40% urea)
- Xerosis^ (see pg. 408)

▨ MECHANISM OF ACTION

It is an antimicrobial agent, a protein solvent, and a denaturant. It enhances penetration of topical medications and increases water absorption into the skin.

▨ DOSAGE

Apply qd to bid.

▨ DRUG INTERACTIONS

None

▨ SIDE EFFECTS

COMMON: stinging, burning, irritation, erythema

▨ MONITORING

None

CONTRAINDICATIONS

Hypersensitivity to drug/class

PREGNANCY CLASS

Not applicable

VALACYCLOVIR

(Valtrex® 500, 1000 mg tabs)

INDICATIONS

- Cytomegalovirus (CMV) prophylaxis in bone marrow transplant and solid organ transplant^
- CMV prophylaxis in HIV^
- Episodic herpes labialis^
- Herpes labialis suppression^
- Herpes simplex prophylaxis after laser resurfacing^
- Herpes zoster*
- Herpes zoster ophthalmicus^
- Primary and recurrent herpes simplex*
- Recurrent erythema multiforme+ (see pg. 364)
- Suppression and episodic treatment for herpes simplex in HIV^
- Varicella^

MECHANISM OF ACTION

It is the valine ester of acyclovir, with increased bioavailability. It requires phosphorylation by viral thymidine kinase to activate. It inhibits viral DNA polymerase and thus DNA synthesis.

DOSAGE

CMV PROPHYLAXIS IN BONE MARROW TRANSPLANT AND SOLID ORGAN TRANSPLANT: 2 g PO qid

CMV PROPHYLAXIS IN HIV: 2 g PO qid

Episodic Herpes Labialis: 2 g PO bid for 1 day

Herpes Labialis Suppression: 500 mg PO qd

Herpes Simplex Prophylaxis after Laser Resurfacing: 500 mg PO bid for 14 days

Herpes Zoster: 1000 mg PO q8h for 7 days

Herpes Zoster Ophthalmicus: 1 g PO tid for 7 days

Primary Genital Herpes: 1000 mg PO q12h for 10 days

Recurrent Genital Herpes: 500 mg PO q12h for 5 days

Suppression and Episodic Treatment for Herpes Simplex in HIV: 500 mg PO bid, 1000 mg PO bid for 5 days

Suppressive Genital Herpes: 500–1000 mg PO q12h

Varicella: 1 g PO tid for 7 days

Renal Dosing
   Creatinine clearance (CrCl) 50–90 mL/min: 1 g PO q8h
   CrCl 10–50 mL/min: 1 g PO q12h–q24h
   CrCL < 10 mL/min: 500 mg PO q24h
   Hemodialysis: 500 mg PO q24h after dialysis
   Continuous ambulatory peritoneal dialysis: 500 mg PO q24h
   Continuous arteriovenous hemofiltration: 1g PO q12h–q24h

▓ DRUG INTERACTIONS

Decreased Rate of Conversion of Drug to Acyclovir: cimetidine, probenecid

▓ SIDE EFFECTS

Common: headache, nausea, vomiting, dizziness, abdominal pain, dysmenorrhea, arthralgia, depression, pruritus, rash, urticaria, confusion, agitation, hallucinations

Rare: thrombocytopenia, aplastic anemia, leukopenia, anaphylaxis, renal failure, hypertension, facial edema, tachycardia, elevated liver function test results, mania, hepatitis, elevated creatinine levels

▒ MONITORING

None

▒ CONTRAINDICATIONS

Hypersensitivity to drug/class or acyclovir

▒ PREGNANCY CLASS

B

VANCOMYCIN

(Vancocin® 125, 250 mg caps, 500 mg/6 mL suspension, IV)

▒ INDICATIONS

- *Clostridium difficile** (oral only)
- *Enterococcus faecalis**
- *Staphylococcus aureus,* methicillin resistant* (IV)
- *Staphylococcus epidermidis**
- *Streptococcus bovis**
- *Streptococcus viridans**

See Appendix II.

Usually effective:

- *Actinomyces* sp.
- *Clostridium,* not *difficile*
- *Listeria monocytogenes*
- *Staphylococcus aureus,* methicillin sensitive
- *Staphylococcus epidermidis*
- *Streptococcus pneumoniae*

Clinical trials lacking:

- *Enterococcus faecium*

▦ MECHANISM OF ACTION

It inhibits bacterial cell wall and RNA synthesis.

▦ DOSAGE

1 g IV q12h (peak 25–40 µg/mL, trough 5–10 µg/mL)

RENAL DOSING
   Creatinine clearance (CrCl) 10–50 mL/min: 1 g IV q14–96h
   CrCl < 10 mL/min, hemodialysis, and chronic ambulatory peritoneal dialysis (CAPD): 1 g IV q4–7d
   Continuous arteriovenous hemofiltration (CAVH): 500 mg IV q24–48h

▦ DRUG INTERACTIONS

NEPHROTOXICITY: adefovir, aminoglycosides, carboplatin, cidofovir, cisplatin, tenofovir, zoledronic acid

OTOTOXICITY: carboplatin, cisplatin

LACTIC ACIDOSIS: metformin, sulfonylureas

PROLONGED NEUROMUSCULAR BLOCKADE: nondepolarizing neuromuscular blockers

INCREASED LEVELS OF: adefovir, tenofovir, cidofovir

▦ SIDE EFFECTS

COMMON: red-man syndrome, chills, fever, nausea, vomiting, tinnitus, superinfection, urticaria, rash, phlebitis

RARE: neutropenia, anaphylaxis, Stevens-Johnson syndrome, toxic epidermal necrolysis, thrombocytopenia, nephrotoxicity, ototoxicity

▦ MONITORING

FREQUENTLY IF LONG-TERM USE: complete blood count, renal function

■ CONTRAINDICATIONS

Hypersensitivity to drug/class, impaired liver or renal function, hearing loss, nephrotoxic agents, pregnancy

■ PREGNANCY CLASS

C

VINCRISTINE

(Oncovin® 1, 2, 5 mg vials)

■ INDICATIONS

- Acute leukemias*
- Bullous pemphigoid+ (see pg. 355)
- Castleman's disease+
- Hemangioma with Kasabach-Merritt syndrome$
- Hodgkin's lymphoma*
- Hypereosinophilic syndrome+ (see pg. 368)
- Idiopathic thrombocytopenic purpura$
- Kaposi's sarcoma$
- Langerhans cell histiocytosis$
- Metastatic melanoma^ (see pg. 378)
- Neuroblastoma*
- Pemphigus vulgaris+ (see pg. 385)
- Postherpetic neuralgia^ (see pg. 389)
- Primary amyloidosis$ (see pg. 350)
- Rhabdomyosarcoma*
- Thrombotic thrombocytopenic purpura^
- Waldenström's macroglobulinemia$
- Wilms' tumor*

■ MECHANISM OF ACTION

It inhibits microtubule production in mitotic spindle, which arrests dividing cells in metaphase.

▤ DOSAGE

HEMANGIOMA: 1–2 mg/m^2 IV weekly for 2–6 weeks

HEPATIC DOSING: decrease dose by 50% if direct bilirubin > 3 mg/dL

▤ DRUG INTERACTIONS

INCREASED RISK OF IMMUNOSUPPRESSION: alefacept

INCREASED TOXICITY OF VINCRISTINE: azole antifungals, clarithromycin, cyclosporin, diltiazem, efavirenz, erythromycin, fluvoxamine, imatinib, nefazodone, protease inhibitors, quinupristin/dalfopristin, verapamil

INCREASED BONE MARROW SUPPRESSION: bone marrow suppressants, rituximab, zidovudine

DECREASED LEVELS OF VINCRISTINE: bosentan

ANTAGONISTIC EFFECTS: colony-stimulating factors

INCREASED NEUROTOXICITY: interferon alpha

BRONCHOSPASM: mitomycin

▤ SIDE EFFECTS

COMMON: alopecia, constipation, anorexia, fatigue, paresthesias, urinary retention, diarrhea, dizziness, hyperuricemia, nausea, vomiting, nystagmus, thrombophlebitis, foot/wrist drop, ataxia, weakness, blood pressure changes, electrolyte disorders, decreased deep tendon reflexes

RARE: myelosuppression, peripheral neuropathy, paralytic ileus, intestinal obstruction, intestinal necrosis, cranial nerve palsy, ototoxicity, loss of deep tendon reflexes, neuromuscular impairment, seizures, neurotoxicity, anaphylaxis, bronchospasm, myocardial infarction, syndrome of inappropriate antidiuretic hormone secretion, infertility, extravasation necrosis, tumor lysis syndrome, uric acid nephropathy

▤ MONITORING

BASELINE/PRIOR TO INFUSION: white blood cells, platelets, uric acid

FREQUENTLY DURING FIRST 3 TO 4 WEEKS OF TREATMENT: uric acid

CONTRAINDICATIONS

Hypersensitivity to drug/class, acute bacterial infection, demyelinating disorders/Charcot-Marie-Tooth disease, intrathecal administration, intestinal obstruction, paralytic ileus, pregnancy, lactation, bone marrow suppression, neuropathy, neuromuscular disease, use of neurotoxic agents, pulmonary disease, liver impairment, avoid extravasation, use of medications that interact with cytochrome P450 CYP 3A, use of live vaccines

PREGNANCY CLASS

D

VORICONAZOLE

(Vfend® 50, 200 mg tabs, 40 mg/mL suspension, IV)

INDICATIONS

- *Aspergillus fumigatus**
- Esophageal candidiasis*
- *Fusarium* sp.*
- *Monosporium apiospermum**

See Appendix I.

MECHANISM OF ACTION

It is a triazole antifungal that inhibits fungal cytochome P450–mediated 14-α-lanosterol demethylase, necessary for fungal ergosterol synthesis of fungal cell walls.

DOSAGE

ESOPHAGEAL CANDIDIASIS: 400 mg PO q12h for 2 doses, then 200 mg PO q12h for at least 14 days, and continued for 7 days after clinical recovery. If <40 kg, 200 mg PO q12h for 2 doses, then 100 mg PO q12h.

ASPERGILLUS FUMIGATUS, MONOSPORIUM APIOSPERMUM, FUSARIUM SP.: loading dose of 6 mg/kg IV q12h for 2 doses, then maintenance dose of

4 mg/kg IV q12h or 200 mg PO q12h. If <40 kg, 100 mg PO q12h maintenance dose until clear.

CIRRHOSIS (CHILD-PUGH CLASSIFICATION A OR B): normal loading dose, half the maintenance dose

CIRRHOSIS (CHILD-PUGH CLASSIFICATION C OR CREATININE CLEARANCE < 50 ML/MIN): only if benefits outweigh risks

Correct hypokalemia, hypomagnesemia, or hypocalcemia before administering.

DRUG INTERACTIONS

PROLONGED QT INTERVAL: terfenadine, astemizole, cisapride, pimozide, quinidine

INCREASED LEVELS OF: sirolimus, efavirenz, rifabutin, ergots, omeprazole, protease inhibitors, nonnucleoside reverse transcriptase inhibitors

DECREASED LEVELS OF VORICONAZOLE: rifampin, carbamazepine, barbiturates, ritonavir, efavirenz, rifabutin, phenytoin, protease inhibitors, nonnucleoside reverse transcriptase inhibitors

INCREASED LEVELS OF VORICONAZOLE: sirolimus, tacrolimus, terfenadine, astemizole, cisapride, coumadin, benzodiazepines, calcium channel blockers, pimozide, quinidine, ergots, cyclosporin, statins, sulfonylureas, vinca alkaloids

SIDE EFFECTS

COMMON: blurred vision, photophobia, photosensitivity, fever, rash, nausea, vomiting, diarrhea, headache, sepsis, edema, abdominal pain, elevated liver function tests, respiratory problems

RARE: hepatitis, cholestasis, hepatic failure, visual loss, decreased color perception, flushing, sweating, tachycardia, chest pain, dyspnea, pruritus, hypo-/hypertension, vasodilation, jaundice, dry mouth, thrombocytopenia, anemia, pancytopenia, leukopenia, hypokalemia, hypomagnesemia, hypocalcemia, hyperbilirubinemia, hallucinations, dizziness, renal failure/elevated creatinine levels, ascites, asthenia, cellulitis, infections, arrhythmias, congestive heart failure, pulmonary embolus, discoid lupus, erythema multiforme, Stevens-Johnson syndrome, toxic epidermal necrolysis, fixed drug eruption, herpes simplex virus, psoriasis, urticaria, angioedema, alopecia

■ MONITORING

BASELINE AND DURING COURSE OF TREATMENT: renal function, liver function, bilirubins

■ CONTRAINDICATIONS

Hypersensitivity to drug/class, terfenadine, astemizole, cisapride, pimozide, quinidine, sirolimus, rifampin, carbamazepine, barbiturates, ritonavir, efavirenz, rifabutin, ergots, galactose intolerance, arrhythmias, hypokalemia, hypomagnesemia, hypocalcemia, fructose intolerance, sucrase-isomaltase deficiency, glucose-galactose malabsorption, creatinine clearance < 50 mL/min, cirrhosis (Child-Pugh C), pregnancy

■ PREGNANCY CLASS

D

Appendix I
Treatments for Fungal Infections

■ ASPERGILLOSIS, BRONCHOPULMONARY

FIRST CHOICE: steroids

ALTERNATIVE: itraconazole 200 mg PO qd to bid for 8 months

■ ASPERGILLOSIS, SINUSITIS

FIRST CHOICE: steroids and surgical débridement

ALTERNATIVE: itraconazole 200 mg PO bid for 12 months

▓ ASPERGILLOSIS, ASPERGILLOMA

Itraconazole 200 mg PO qd for 3 months

▓ ASPERGILLOSIS, INVASIVE

FIRST CHOICE: amphotericin 1 mg/kg IV qd for total of 2–2.5 g, then itraconazole 200 mg PO bid; or caspofungin 70 mg IV first day, then 50 mg IV qd; or voriconazole 6 mg/kg IV q12h for 2 doses, then 4 mg/kg IV q12h or 200 mg PO q12h

ALTERNATIVE: itraconazole 200 mg PO tid for 4 days, then 200 mg PO bid

▓ BLASTOMYCOSIS

FIRST CHOICE: itraconazole 200–400 mg PO qd for 6 months; or amphotericin 0.7–1 mg/kg/d IV for total of 1.5 g

ALTERNATIVE: fluconazole 400–800 mg PO qd for 8 months

▓ CANDIDIASIS, BLOOD, NOT NEUTROPENIC, NOT HIV

FIRST CHOICE: fluconazole 400 mg IV qd for 7 days, then 400 mg PO qd for 14 days; or amphotericin 0.5–0.6 mg/kg/d IV for total of 5–7 mg/kg

ALTERNATIVE: amphotericin 0.8–1 mg/kg/d IV or fluconazole 800 mg PO/IV qd

▓ CANDIDIASIS, BLOOD, NEUTROPENIC, STABLE

FIRST CHOICE: fluconazole 400 mg IV/PO qd until neutropenia resolves; or amphotericin 0.5–0.6 mg/kg/d IV to total dose of 5–7 mg/kg, then fluconazole 400 mg PO qd until neutropenia resolves

ALTERNATIVE: caspofungin 70 mg IV first day, then 50 mg IV qd; or voriconazole 6 mg/kg IV q12h for 2, then 4 mg/kg IV q12h or 200 mg PO q12h

▓ CANDIDIASIS, BLOOD, UNSTABLE OR METSATIC

FIRST CHOICE: amphotericin 0.8–1 mg/kg/d IV with or without flucytosine 37.5 mg/kg PO q6h; or fluconazole 400–800 mg IV qd

ALTERNATIVE: Ablecet® 5 mg/kg/d IV to total of 1.1 g; or caspofungin 70 mg IV first day, then 50 mg IV qd; or voriconazole 6 mg/kg IV q12h for 2, doses, then 4 mg/kg IV q12h or 200 mg PO q12h

CANDIDIASIS, CHRONIC MUCOCUTANEOUS

Ketoconazole 400 mg PO qd for 3–9 months

CANDIDIASIS, CUTANEOUS

Ketoconazole 400 mg PO qd for 14 days; or nystatin or azole antifungals 3–4 times a day for 14 days

CANDIDIASIS, ENDOCARDITIS

FIRST CHOICE: amphotericin 0.6 mg/kg/d IV for 7 days, then 0.8 mg/kg IV qod for 6–10 weeks after surgery

ALTERNATIVE: fluconazole 200–400 mg IV qd if valves not replaced

CANDIDIASIS, THRUSH

FIRST CHOICE: fluconazole 200 mg once or 100 mg PO qd for 5–14 days; or itraconazole 200 mg PO qd for 7 days

ALTERNATIVE: nystatin lozenges qid for 14 days, or clotrimazole troches 5 times a day for 14 days

CANDIDIASIS, HIV STOMATITIS/ESOPHAGITIS/VAGINITIS

FIRST CHOICE: fluconazole 200 mg PO first day, then 100 mg PO qd for 14 days; or itraconazole 200 mg PO qd for 14 days; or caspofungin 70 mg IV first day, then 50 mg IV qd

ALTERNATIVE: fluconazole 400–800 mg PO qd to bid; or itraconazole 100–200 mg PO bid; or amphotericin 0.5 mg/kg/d IV; or voriconazole 6 mg/kg IV q12h for 2 doses, then 4 mg/kg IV q12h or 200 mg PO q12h (or 400 mg PO q12h for 2 doses, then 200 mg PO q12h)

▪ CANDIDIASIS, PERITONITIS

FIRST CHOICE: flucytosine 2 g PO first day, then 1 g PO qd with fluconazole 200 mg PO qd for 4–6 weeks

ALTERNATIVE: amphotericin IP 1.5 mg/L dialysis fluid for 4–6 weeks

▪ CANDIDIASIS, CYSTITIS

FIRST CHOICE: fluconazole 200 mg PO first day, then 100 mg PO qd for 4 days

ALTERNATIVE: amphotericin bladder irrigation 5 mg/100 mL H_2O at 42 mL/h for 1–2 days, or 0.3 mg/kg IV once

▪ CANDIDIASIS, VAGINAL

FIRST CHOICE: fluconazole 150 mg PO once; or itraconazole 200 mg PO bid for 1 day

ALTERNATIVE: topical vaginal imidazoles

▪ CHROMOMYCOSIS

FIRST CHOICE: surgery

ALTERNATIVE: itraconazole 100 mg PO qd for 18 months

▪ COCCIDIODOMYCOSIS, HIV-POSITIVE WITH PULMONARY OR DISSEMINATED

MILD/MODERATE: itraconazole 200 mg PO bid for 3–12 months; or fluconazole 400 mg PO qd for 3–12 months

SEVERE: amphotericin 0.6–1 mg/kg/d IV for 7 days, then 0.8 mg/kg IV qod to total of 2.5 g, then fluconazole or itraconazole as above

▨ COCCIDIODOMYCOSIS, MENINGITIS

FIRST CHOICE: fluconazole 400–800 mg PO qd indefinitely

ALTERNATIVE: amphotericin as for pulmonary coccidiodomycosis plus 0.1–0.3 mg qd intrathecal

▨ CRYPTOCOCCOSIS, NOT MENINGEAL, NOT HIV

FIRST CHOICE, MILD: fluconazole 400 mg PO/IV qd for 2–6 months

FIRST CHOICE, SEVERE: amphotericin 0.5–0.8 mg/kg/d IV until response, then fluconazole 400 mg PO qd for 8–10 weeks

ALTERNATIVE: itraconazole 200–400 mg PO qd for 6–12 months; or amphotericin 0.3 mg/kg/d IV with flucytosine 37.5 mg/kg PO q6h for 6 weeks

▨ CRYPTOCOCCOSIS, MENINGEAL

Amphotericin 0.5–0.8 mg/kg/d IV plus flucytosine 37.5 mg/kg PO q6h until afebrile and culture negative, then fluconazole 200 mg PO qd; or fluconazole 400 mg PO qd for 8–10 weeks

▨ CRYPTOCOCCOSIS, HIV

FIRST CHOICE: amphotericin 0.7–1 mg/kg/d/ IV plus flucytosine 25 mg/kg PO q6h for 2 weeks, then fluconazole 400 mg PO qd for 10 weeks, then 200 mg PO qd indefinitely

ALTERNATIVE: fluconazole 400 mg PO qd for 6–10 weeks; or liposomal amphotericin 5 mg/kg/d for 2 weeks, then fluconazole as above; or amphotericin lipid complex 5 mg/kg/d IV for 2 weeks, then 3 times a week for 4 weeks, then fluconazole as above

▨ DERMATOPHYTE

ONYCHOMYCOSIS
Fingernail: terbinafine 250 mg PO qd for 6 weeks; or pulse itraconazole 200 mg PO bid for 7 days, off for 21 days, then 200 mg PO bid for 7 more days (or 200 mg PO qd for 3 months); or fluconazole 150–300 mg PO weekly for 3–6 months.

Toenail: terbinafine 250 mg PO qd for 12 weeks; or itraconazole 200 mg PO qd for 3 months; or fluconazole 150–300 mg PO weekly for 6–12 weeks

TINEA CAPITIS
First choice: terbinafine 250 mg PO qd for 4 weeks *Trichophyton tonsurans,* 4–8 weeks *Microsporum canis.*
Alternative: itraconazole 3–5 mg/kg/d for 30 days; or fluconazole 8 mg/kg weekly for 8–12 weeks; or griseofulvin 500 mg PO qd for 4–6 weeks

TINEA CORPORIS, CRURIS, PEDIS
First choice: butenafine or terbinafine topical bid for 2–3 weeks
Alternative: terbinafine 250 mg PO qd for 2 weeks; or ketoconazole 200 mg PO qd for 4 weeks; or fluconazole 150 mg weekly for 2–4 weeks; or griseofulvin 500 mg PO qd for 4–6 weeks

TINEA VERSICOLOR
First choice: ketoconazole 400 mg PO once or topical qd for 2 weeks
Alternative: fluconazole 400 mg PO once; or itraconazole 400 mg PO qd for 3–7 days; or selenium sulfide 2.5% shampoo, lather and leave on 10 min qd for 7 days (or 3–5 times a week for 2–4 weeks)

▓ *FUSARIUM*

First choice: voriconazole 6 mg/kg IV q12h for 2, then 4 mg/kg IV q12h or 200 mg PO q12h
Alternative: amphotericin 1–1.2 mg/kg IV

▓ HISTOPLASMOSIS, IMMUNOCOMPETENT

MILD: none

MODERATE: itraconazole 200 mg PO qd for 9 months

SEVERE: amphotericin 0.5–1 mg/kg/d IV for 7 days, then 0.8 mg/kg IV

▓ HISTOPLASMOSIS, IMMUNOCOMPROMISED

FIRST CHOICE: amphotericin 0.5–1 mg/kg/d IV for 7 days, then 0.8 mg/kg IV qod to total of 10–15 mg/kg, then itraconazole 200 mg PO qd

ALTERNATIVE, NOT FOR MENINGITIS: itraconazole 300 mg PO bid for 3 days, then 200 mg PO bid for 12 weeks, then 200 mg PO qd

MUCORMYCOSIS

Amphotericin 0.8–1.5 mg/kg/d IV, then qod when improving, to total of 2.5–3 g

PARACOCCIDIOIDOMYCOSIS

FIRST CHOICE: itraconazole 200 mg PO qd for 6 months; or ketoconazole 400 mg PO qd for 6–18 months

ALTERNATIVE: amphotericin 0.4–0.5 mg/kg/d IV to total of 1.5–2.5 g

LOBOMYCOSIS

Surgery, clofazimine, or amphotericin

PENICILLIOSIS

FIRST CHOICE: amphotericin 0.5–1 mg/kg/d for 2 weeks, then itraconazole 400 mg PO qd for 10 weeks, then 200 mg PO qd indefinitely

ALTERNATIVE: itraconazole 200 mg PO tid for 3 days, then 200 mg PO bid for 12 weeks, then 200 mg PO qd indefinitely

PHAEOHYPHOMYCOSIS

Surgery and itraconazole 400 mg PO qd for 6 months

PSEUDALLESCHERIA BOYDII

Surgery and itraconazole 200 mg PO bid until resolution

SPOROTRICHOSIS, CUTANEOUS/LYMPHOCUTANEOUS

FIRST CHOICE: itraconazole 100–200 mg PO qd for 3–6 months (then 200 mg PO bid indefinitely if HIV positive)

ALTERNATIVE: fluconazole 400 mg PO qd for 6 months; or super saturated potassium iodide (SSKI) 40–50 drops tid for 3–6 months (SSKI 1 g in 100 mL H_2O)

▨ SPOROTRICHOSIS, DISSEMINATED/MENINGEAL

Amphotericin 0.5 mg/kg/d IV to total of 1–2 g, then itraconazole 200 mg PO bid or fluconazole 800 mg PO qd

▨ SPOROTRICHOSIS, OSTEOARTICULAR/PULMONARY

Itraconazole 300 mg PO bid for 6–12 months (then 200 mg PO bid indefinitely if HIV positive)

Appendix II
Treatments for Bacterial Infections

Parentheses indicate second-line treatment.

▨ *ACINETOBACTER BAUMANNII*

Imipenem, meropenem, fluoroquinolone plus amikacin or ceftazidime, (ampicillin/sulbactam)

▨ *ACTINOMYCES ISRAELII*

Ampicillin, penicillin G, (soxycycline, ceftriaxone)

▨ *BACILLUS ANTHRACIS*

Ciprofloxacin, doxycycline, (penicillin G, amoxicillin)

▨ *BACTEROIDES FRAGILIS*

Metronidazole, (clindamycin)

■ *BARTONELLA HENSELAE, B. QUINTANA*

Doxycycline or erythromycin for bacillary angiomatosis, azithromycin for cat scratch, (clarithromycin, ciprofloxacin)

■ *BORRELIA BURGDORFERI*

Doxycycline, ceftriaxone, cefuroxime, amoxicillin, (penicillin G, ceftazidime)

■ *CHLAMYDIA PNEUMONIAE*

Doxycycline, (erythromycin, fluoroquinolone)

■ *CHLAMYDIA TRACHOMATIS*

Doxycycline, azithromycin, (azithromycin, ofloxacin)

■ *CLOSTRIDIUM DIFFICILE*

Metronidazole, (vancomycin PO)

■ *ENTEROBACTER CLOACA*

Imipenem, meropenem, fourth-generation penicillins plus aminoglycosides, (piperacillin/tazobactam, ticarcillin/clavulanate, ciprofloxacin)

■ *ENTEROCOCCUS FAECALIS*

Penicillin G, ampicillin, (vancomycin), add gentamicin for endocarditis

■ *ENTEROCOCCUS FAECIUM*

No good treatment

■ *ENTEROCOCCUS FAECIUM,* VANCOMYCIN RESISTANT

Quinupristin/dalfopristin, linezolid

■ ESCHERICHIA COLI

Amoxicillin/clavulanate, ampicillin/sulbactam, ticarcillin/clavulanate, piperacillin/tazobactam, fluoroquinolones, cephalosporin, trimethoprim/sulfamethoxazole, aminoglycosides, imipenem, meropenem

■ FRANCISELLA TULARENSIS

Gentamicin, tobramycin, (doxycycline, ciprofloxacin)

■ GARDNERELLA VAGINALIS

Metronidazole, (clindamycin)

■ HAEMOPHILUS DUCREYI

Azithromycin, ceftriaxone, (erythromycin, ciprofloxacin)

■ HAEMOPHILUS INFLUENZAE

Cefotaxime, ceftriaxone, amoxicillin/clavulanate, ampicillin/sulbactam, trimethoprim/sulfamethoxazole, second- or third-generation cephalosporin, (meropenem, imipenem, fluoroquinolones)

■ HELICOBACTER PYLORI

Clarithromycin and amoxicillin, (tetracycline and metronidazole)

■ KLEBSIELLA PNEUMONIAE

Third-generation cephalosporin, fluoroquinolone, (ticarcillin/clavulanate, ampicillin/sulbactam, piperacillin/tazobactam, aminoglycosides)

■ LEGIONELLA PNEUMOPHILA

Fluoroquinolone, azithromycin, erythromycin with or without rifampin, linezolid, (clarithromycin)

LISTERIA MONOCYTOGENES

Ampicillin, (trimethoprim/sulfamethoxazole)

MORAXELLA CATARRHALIS

Amoxicillin/clavulanate, trimethoprim/sulfamethoxazole, second- or third-generation cephalosporin, (azithromycin, clarithromycin)

MORGANELLA MORGANII

Imipenem, meropenem, third- or fourth-generation cephalosporin, fluoroquinolone, (aztreonam, amoxicillin/clavulanate, ampicillin/sulbactam, piperacillin/tazobactam, ticarcillin/clavulanate)

MYCOPLASMA PNEUMONIAE

Erythromycin, clarithromycin, fluoroquinolone, azithromycin, (doxycycline)

NEISSERIA GONORRHOEAE

Ceftriaxone, cefixime, cefpodoxime, (fluoroquinolones)

NEISSERIA MENINGITIDIS

Penicillin G, (ceftriaxone, cefuroxime, cefotaxime)

PASTEURELLA MULTOCIDA

Penicillin G, ampicillin, amoxicillin, (doxycycline, amoxicillin/clavulanate, trimethoprim/sulfamethoxazole, second-generation cephalosporin)

PROTEUS MIRABILIS

Ampicillin, (trimethoprim/sulfamethoxazole)

PROTEUS VULGARIS

Third-generation cephalosporin, fluoroquinolone, (aminoglycosides)

■ *PROVIDENCIA STUARTII*

Amikacin, third-generation cephalosporin, fluoroquinolones (trimethoprim/sulfamethoxazole)

■ *PSEUDOMONAS AERUGINOSA*

Fourth-generation penicillins, third-generation cephalosporins, imipenem, meropenem, tobramycin, ciprofloxacin, aztreonam, (cefipime)

■ *RICKETTSIAE SP.*

Doxycycline, (chloramphenicol)

■ *SALMONELLA TYPHI*

Fluoroquinolone, ceftriaxone, (trimethoprim/sulfamethoxazole, amoxicillin, chloramphenicol, azithromycin)

■ *SERRATIA MARCESCENS*

Imipenem, meropenem, third-generation cephalosporin, fluoroquinolones, (aztreonam, gentamicin)

■ *SHIGELLA DYSENTERIAE*

Fluoroquinolones, azithromycin, (trimethoprim/sulfamethoxazole, ampicillin)

■ *STAPHYLOCOCCUS AUREUS,* METHICILLIN SENSITIVE

Oxacillin, nafcillin, (first-generation cephalosporins, clindamycin)

■ *STAPHYLOCOCCUS AUREUS,* METHICILLIN RESISTANT

Vancomycin, (linezolid, quinupristin/dalfopristin, trimethoprim/sulfamethoxazole), daptomycin

▨ *STAPHYLOCOCCUS AUREUS,* VANCOMYCIN RESISTANT

Linezolid, quinupristin/dalfopristin, daptomycin

▨ *STAPHYLOCOCCUS EPIDERMIDIS*

Vancomycin with or without rifampin, (trimethoprim/sulfamethoxazole with or without rifampin, fluoroquinolone with or without rifampin)

▨ *STREPTOCOCCUS PNEUMONIAE*

Penicillin G, vancomycin, third-generation fluoroquinolones, (amoxicillin, many others)

▨ *STREPTOCOCCUS PYOGENES* GROUP A, B, C, G

Penicillin G or V, (macrolides)

▨ *VIBRIO CHOLERAE*

Doxycycline, fluoroquinolone, (bactrim)

▨ *YERSINIA ENTEROCOLITICA*

Trimethoprim/sulfamethoxazole, fluoroquinolone, (third-generation cephalosporin, aminoglycosides)

▨ *YERSINIA PESTIS*

Gentamicin, tobramycin, (chloramphenicol, doxycycline, ciprofloxacin)

Appendix III
Treatments for Mycobacterial Infections

▉ *MYCOBACTERIUM TUBERCULOSIS*

PROPHYLAXIS

FIRST CHOICE: isoniazid 5 mg/kg PO qd (maximum 300 mg qd) for 9 months

ALTERNATIVE: isoniazid by directly observed therapy (DOT) 15 mg/kg twice a week for 9 months, or rifampin 600 mg PO qd with pyrazinamide 15–20 mg/kg PO qd for 2 months, or rifampin 600 mg PO twice a week with pyrazinamide 50 mg/kg PO twice a week for 2–3 months, or rifampin 600 mg PO qd for 4 months

PURIFIED PROTEIN DERIVATIVE (PPD)-POSITIVE

FIRST CHOICE: isoniazid 5 mg/kg PO qd (maximum 300 mg qd) for 12 months

PPD-POSITIVE AND ISONIAZID RESISTANCE LIKELY

FIRST CHOICE: rifampin 600 mg PO qd with pyrazinamide 15–20 mg/kg PO qd for 2 months, or rifampin 600 mg PO qd for 4 months

PPD-POSITIVE AND ISONIAZID AND RIFAMPIN RESISTANCE LIKELY

FIRST CHOICE: pyrazinamide 25–30 mg/kg PO qd to maximum of 2 g qd with ethambutol 15–25 mg/kg PO qd for 6–12 months

ALTERNATIVE: pyrazinamide 25 mg/kg PO qd with levofloxacin 500 mg PO qd or ofloxacin 400 mg PO bid for 6–12 months

PULMONARY

ISONIAZID RESISTANCE < **4%:** isoniazid 5 mg/kg PO qd with rifampin 10 mg/kg PO qd (or rifabutin 5 mg/kg PO qd) with pyrazinamide 15–30 mg/kg PO qd for 2 months. Then continue isoniazid with rifampin (or rifabutin) at same dose for 4 more months.

ISONIAZID RESISTANCE NOT KNOWN, COMPLIANT: isoniazid 5 mg/kg PO qd with rifampin 10 mg/kg PO qd (or rifabutin 5 mg/kg PO qd) with pyrazinamide 15–30 mg/kg PO qd with ethambutol 15–25 mg/kg PO qd (or streptomycin 15 mg/kg PO qd) for 2 months. Then continue isoniazid with rifampin (or rifabutin) at same dose for 4 more months.

ISONIAZID RESISTANCE NOT KNOWN, NONCOMPLIANT, DIRECTLY OBSERVED THERAPY (DOT): isoniazid 15 mg/kg PO 3 times a week with rifampin 10 mg/kg PO twice a week (or rifabutin 5 mg/kg PO qd) with pyrazinamide 50–70 mg/kg PO qd with ethambutol 25–30 mg/kg PO qd (or streptomycin 25–30 mg/kg PO qd) for 6 months. Then isoniazid and rifampin (or rifabutin) at same dose for 4 more months.

ISONIAZID RESISTANCE: rifampin 10 mg/kg PO qd (or rifabutin 5 mg/kg PO qd) with ethambutol 15–25 mg/kg PO qd with pyrazinamide 15–30 mg/kg PO qd for 18 months

RIFAMPIN RESISTANCE: isoniazid 5 mg/kg PO qd with ethambutol 15–25 mg/ kg PO qd with pyrazinamide 15–30 mg/kg PO qd for 18 months

ISONIAZID AND RIFAMPIN RESISTANCE: isoniazid 5 mg/kg PO qd with rifampin 10 mg/kg PO qd (or rifabutin 5 mg/kg PO qd) with pyrazinamide 15–30 mg/kg PO qd with ethambutol 15–25 mg/kg PO qd (or streptomycin 25–30 mg/kg PO qd) with amikacin with ciprofloxacin/gatifloxacin/ levofloxacin

EXTRAPULMONARY

Isoniazid 5 mg/kg PO qd with rifampin 10 mg/kg PO qd (or rifabutin 5 mg/ kg PO qd) with pyrazinamide 15–30 mg/kg PO qd for 2 months. Then isoniazid with rifampin (or rifabutin) at same dose for 4–10 more months.

MENINGITIS

Isoniazid 5 mg/kg PO qd with rifampin 10 mg/kg PO qd with pyrazinamide 15–30 mg/kg PO qd with ethambutol 15–25 mg/kg PO qd for 12 months

PREGNANCY

Isoniazid 5 mg/kg PO qd with rifampin 10 mg/kg PO qd with ethambutol 15–25 mg/kg PO qd for 9 months

HIV POSITIVE

Isoniazid 5 mg/kg PO qd with rifampin 10 mg/kg PO qd (or rifabutin 5 mg/kg PO qd) with pyrazinamide 15–30 mg/kg PO qd for 2 months.

Then isoniazid with rifampin (or rifabutin) at same dose for 4 more months. Add nelfinavir or indinavir.

■ *MYCOBACTERIUM BOVIS*

Isoniazid 5 mg/kg PO qd with rifampin 10 mg/kg PO qd with ethambutol 15–25 mg/kg PO qd for 9–12 months

■ *MYCOBACTERIUM AVIUM-INTERCELLULARE*

IMMUNOCOMPETENT

FIRST CHOICE: clarithromycin 500 mg PO bid (or azithromycin 600 mg PO qd) with ethambutol 25 mg/kg PO qd for 2 months, then 15 mg/kg PO qd with rifampin 600 mg PO qd (or rifabutin 300 mg PO qd) until cultures negative for 1 year. May add streptomycin 15 mg/kg PO qd or amikacin or clofazimine 100–200 mg PO qd for severe disease.

ALTERNATIVE: clarithromycin with ethambutol with rifabutin at above doses for 24 months

IMMUNOCOMPROMISED

PRIMARY PROPHYLAXIS: azithromycin 1200 mg PO every week or clarithromycin 500 mg PO bid
Alternative: rifabutin 300 mg PO qd or azithromycin 1200 mg PO every week with rifampin 300 mg PO qd

TREATMENT: clarithromycin 500 mg PO bid (or azithromycin 600 mg PO qd) with ethambutol 15–25 mg/kg PO qd with rifabutin 300 mg PO qd
Alternative: The above regimen with more: ciprofloxacin 750 mg PO bid, ofloxacin 400 mg PO bid, or amikacin 7.5–15 mg/kg IV qd. If patient receiving protease inhibitors, can use clarithromycin 500 mg PO bid (or azithromycin 600 mg PO qd) with ethambutol 15–25 mg/kg PO qd.

POST-TREATMENT SUPPRESSION: clarithromycin 500 mg PO bid (or azithromycin 600 mg PO qd) with ethambutol 15 mg/kg PO qd
Alternative: clarithromycin 500 mg PO bid (or azithromycin 600 mg PO qd) with rifabutin 300 mg PO qd

■ *MYCOBACTERIUM CHELONAE*

FIRST CHOICE: clarithromycin 500 mg PO bid for 6 months

ALTERNATIVE: amikacin 7.5 mg/kg IV q12 hours

▓ *MYCOBACTERIUM FORTUITUM*

Regimen not defined. Amikacin with cefoxitin with probenecid for 2–6 weeks, then trimethoprim/sulfamethoxazole or doxycycline for 2–6 months.

▓ *MYCOBACTERIUM HAEMOPHILUS*

Regimen not defined. Clarithromycin with rifabutin.

ALTERNATIVE: ciprofloxacin with rifabutin with clarithromycin

▓ *MYCOBACTERIUM GENAVENSE*

Regimen not defined. Two or more of the following: ethambutol, rifampin, rifabutin, clofazimine, clarithromycin.

▓ *MYCOBACTERIUM GORDONAE*

Regimen not defined. Rifampin with ethambutol with kanamycin (or ciprofloxacin)

▓ *MYCOBACTERIUM KANSASII*

Isoniazid 30 mg PO qd with rifampin 600 mg PO qd with ethambutol 25 mg/kg PO qd for 2 months, then 15 mg/kg PO qd for 18 months

▓ *MYCOBACTERIUM MARINUM*

Clarithromycin 500 mg PO bid, or minocycline 100–200 mg PO qd, or doxy-cycline 100–200 mg PO qd, or trimethoprim/sulfamethoxazole 160/800 mg PO bid, or rifampin and ethambutol for 3 months

▓ *MYCOBACTERIUM SCROFULACEUM*

Regimen not defined. Clarithromycin with clofazimine, with or without ethambutol.

▓ *MYCOBACTERIUM ULCERANS*

FIRST CHOICE: rifampin 10 mg/kg PO qd with amikacin 7.5 mg/kg IM bid for 4–6 weeks

ALTERNATIVE: ethambutol 15–25 mg/kg PO qd with trimethoprim/sulfamethoxazole 160/800 mg PO tid for 4–6 weeks

▓ *MYCOBACTERIUM XENOPI*

Regimen not defined. Macrolide with rifampin (or rifabutin) with ethambutol, with or without streptomycin.

▓ *MYCOBACTERIUM LEPRAE*

PAUCIBACILLARY

Dapsone 100 mg PO qd with rifampin (supervised) 600 mg PO monthly for 6 months

MULTIBACILLARY

FIRST CHOICE: dapsone 100 mg PO qd with clofazimine 50 mg PO qd with rifampin 600 mg PO monthly (supervised) with clofazimine 300 mg PO monthly (supervised) for 24 months

ALTERNATIVE: ethionamide 250 mg PO qd or prothionamide 375 mg PO qd (or clofazimine)

GENERAL REFERENCES

Bolognia JL, Jorizzo JL, Rapini RP. *Dermatology.* Philadelphia: C.V. Mosby/Elsevier Ltd., 2003.

Freedberg IM, Eisen AZ, Wolff K, Austen KF, Goldsmith LA, Katz SI (eds.). *Fitzpatrick's Dermatology in General Medicine,* 6th ed. New York: McGraw-Hill, 2003.

Gilbert DN, Moellering RC, Sande MA. *The Sanford Guide to Antimicrobial Therapy.* Hyde Park, Vermont: Antimicrobial Therapy, 2003.

Physicians' Desk Reference, 55th ed. Montvale, NJ: Medical Economics, 2001.

Wolverton SE. *Comprehensive Dermatologic Drug Therapy.* Philadelphia: W. B. Saunders, 2001.

Section 2

Dermatologic Conditions

ACANTHOSIS NIGRICANS

▨ DEFINITION

Acanthosis nigricans is most commonly found in association with obesity, but can be a cutaneous marker, most commonly of insulin resistance and less frequently of malignancy. It is recognized clinically by hyperpigmented, hyperkeratotic, verrucous plaques that bestow a velvety texture on involved skin (neck/axillae), typically symmetric in distribution.

Associated syndromes: Hyper Androgenism, Insulin Resistance, Acanthosis Nigricans (HAIR-AN), Beare-Stevenson, Crouzon, Lawrence-Seip.

Schwartz RA. *J Am Acad Dermatol*. 1994; 31: 1.

▨ TREATMENT OPTIONS

- Ammonium lactate[+]
- Calcipotriene[+]
- Continuous-wave CO_2 laser[+]
- Cyproheptadine[+]
- Dermabrasion[+]
- Etretinate[+]
- Fish oil[+]
- Isotretinoin[+]
- Ketoconazole, oral[+]
- Nicotinic acid[+]
- Palliative radiotherapy[+] (malignancy associated)
- PUVA[+]
- Salicylic acid[+]
- Tazarotene[+]
- Treatment of underlying cause[$]
- Tretinoin, topical[+]
- Weight loss[$]

ACNE

▨ DEFINITION

Acne is a self-limited disease, seen primarily in adolescents, involving the sebaceous follicles. Most cases are pleomorphic, presenting with a variety of lesions consisting of comedones, papules, pustules, nodules, and, as a seque-lae, pitted or hypertrophic scars. It is a process that involves the pilosebaceous unit.

Guy R. *J Invest Dermatol.* 1996; 106: 76.

▣ TREATMENT OPTIONS

- Adapalene*
- Adapalene gel and clindamycin gel*
- Aluminum chloride^
- Azelaic acid*
- Azithromycin$
- Benzoyl peroxide*
- Benzoyl peroxide and clindamycin, topical*
- Cimetidine+
- Clindamycin, topical*
- Clofazimine+ (acne conglobata and fulminans)
- Erythromycin, topical*
- Gentamicin, topical^ (*Pseudomonas aeruginosa* grown on culture)
- Isotretinoin (nodulocystic acne)
- Metronidazole, topical^
- Periostat® ^
- Salicylic acid^
- Sodium sulfacetamide*
- Steroids, topical$, intralesional^, oral$, pulse+ (with isotretinoin)
- Sulfur^
- Tazarotene*
- Tetracyclines*
- Tretinoin, topical*

ACTINIC KERATOSES

▣ DEFINITION

Actinic keratoses are cutaneous neoplasms consisting of proliferations of cytologically aberrant epidermal keratinocytes that develop in response to prolonged exposure to ultraviolet radiation.

Cockerell CJ. *J Am Acad Dermatol.* 2000; 42: S11.

▨ TREATMENT OPTIONS

- Acitretin[^]
- Adapalene[^]
- Cryotherapy[^]
- Curettage and dessication[$]
- Dermabrasion[$]
- Diclofenac/hyaluronic acid gel[*]
- Excision[$]
- Fluorouracil, topical[*]
- Glycolic aid peels[^]
- Imiquimod[$]
- Interferon alpha 2B, intralesional[^], and topical[^]
- Interferon beta, intralesional[+]
- Jessner's peels[^]
- Photodynamic therapy with topical aminolevulinic acid (ALA)[^]
- Salicylic acid peels[$]
- Tretinoin, topical with[^] or without[$] fluorouracil
- Trichloracetic acid peels[^]

ALOPECIA AREATA

▨ DEFINITION

Alopecia areata is a nonscarring alopecia postulated to be an organ-specific autoimmune disease. In affected areas, anagen is abruptly terminated prematurely and affected hairs move prematurely into telogen, with resultant hair shedding. "Exclamation point" hairs may be present at the periphery of areas of hair loss.

Madani S. *J Am Acad Dermatol.* 2000; 42: 549.

▨ TREATMENT OPTIONS

- Anthralin[$]
- Cyclosporin[$]
- Imiquimod[+]
- Mechlorethamine[$]
- Minoxidil, topical[^], oral[$]
- PUVA[^]
- Squaric acid[^]

- Steroids, oral[§], pulse[§], intralesional[§], topical[§]
- Tacrolimus, topical[+]
- Tretinoin, topical with intralesional triamcinolone[§]

AMYLOIDOSIS

▓ DEFINITION

Amyloidosis refers to several diseases that have in common the abnormal extracellular deposition of amyloid, a fibrillar proteinaceous material, in tissues. Amyloidosis may be classified into two main groups: systemic (generalized, with involvement of several organ systems) and cutaneous. In the systemic group, there are several types: primary, reactive, heredo-familial, and organ limited (localized), in which deposits are limited to a single organ, such as the skin, endocrine glands, or brain. The three major forms of primary cutaneous amyloidosis are macular (confluent or rippled hyperpigmentation, often on the upper arm or back), lichen (hyperpigmented papules, often on the extensor surfaces of the extremities and back), and nodular (waxy nodules).

Skinner M. *Am J Med.* 1996; 100: 290.

▓ TREATMENT OPTIONS

- Chloroquine[§] (secondary to rheumatoid arthritis)
- CO_2 laser[+] (lichen, macular)
- Colchicine[§] (primary, familial Mediterranean, secondary)
- Cyclophosphamide[+] (lichen, macular)
- Cyclosporin[+] (lichen, macular)
- Dermabrasion[§] (lichen, macular)
- Dimethyl sulfoxide[§] (lichen, macular)
- Melphalan + prednisone[^] (primary)
- Melphalan + prednisone + colchicine[^] (primary)
- Melphalan[^] (primary)
- PUVA[§] (lichen, macular)
- Stem cell transplantation[^] (primary)
- Steroids, topical[§] (lichen, macular)
- Systemic retinoids[§] (lichen, macular)
- Tacrolimus topical[§] (lichen, macular)
- Thalidomide[§]
- UVB[§] (lichen, macular)
- Vincristine[§] (primary)

ANDROGENIC ALOPECIA

▦ DEFINITION

MALE ANDROGENETIC ALOPECIA

Male androgenic alopecia is commonly called male pattern baldness, characterized by several patterns of hair loss, most commonly frontal recession and vertex thinning. It is related to dihydrotestosterone (DHT) and believed to be inherited in an autosomal dominant and/or polygenic fashion.

Rebora A. *Arch Dermatol.* 2001; 137: 943.

FEMALE ANDROGENETIC ALOPECIA

Female pattern hair loss occurring with hyperandrogenemia is called female androgenetic alopecia. Most patients do not show excess androgens but, rather, exhibit an increased sensitivity to normal androgen levels. When there is no evidence of hyperandrogenemia and the presentation is associated with increased hair shedding, the diagnoses of both telogen effluvium hair loss and female pattern alopecia are made, and treatment may be more challenging.

Price VH. *J Am Acad Dermatol.* 2000; 43: 768.

▦ TREATMENT OPTIONS

- Antiandrogens (flutamide^, cyproterone^)
- Cimetidine$
- Finasteride* (for men)
- Hair transplantation*
- Minoxidil* (5% solution for men* and for women^, 2% solution for women*)

ANGIOEDEMA

▦ DEFINITION

Hereditary angioedema is a dominantly inherited disorder characterized by recurrent attacks that involve the skin and mucous membranes of the respiratory and gastrointestinal tracts. There are two types: one with low levels of functional C1 esterase inhibitor and one with normal levels of dysfunctional C1 esterase inhibitor. Acquired angioedema with depletion of C1 esterase inhibitor has two forms. One is associated with malignant disorders (B-cell lymphomas) and autoantibody to paraproteins. The second form is associated with an autoantibody directed against the C1 esterase inhibitor molecule.

Markovich SN. *Ann Intern Med.* 2000; 132: 144.

▦ TREATMENT OPTIONS

- Aminocaproic acid^ (hereditary)
- C1 inhibitor concentrate* (C1 esterase inhibitor deficiency)
- Cyproheptadine*
- Danazol* (hereditary)
- Fresh-frozen plasma$ (C1 esterase inhibitor deficiency)
- Hydroxychloroquine+ (C1 esterase inhibitor deficiency)
- Stanozolol* (hereditary)
- Tranexamic acid^ (hereditary and non-hereditary)

APHTHOUS STOMATITIS

▦ DEFINITION

Recurrent aphthous stomatitis are the most common oral ulcerative condition and are likely to be a multifactorial disorder influenced by a host of predisposing factors, including trauma, hematinic deficiencies, hormonal fluctuations, psychological stress, infectious agents, food hypersensitivities, genetic factors, HIV infection, and gluten-sensitive enteropathy. There are three types of ulcers: minor, major, and herpetiform (unrelated to herpes infection).

Porter SR. *Clin Dermatol.* 2000; 18: 569.

▦ TREATMENT OPTIONS

- Colchicine^
- Cyclosporin^
- Dapsone^
- Etanercept+
- Interferon alpha 2B^

- Lidocaine, topical[+] (pain relief)
- Magic mouthwash[+]
- Methotrexate[$]
- Pentoxifylline[$]
- Steroids, topical[^], oral[$], inhaled, intralesional
- Sucralfate, topical[^]
- Thalidomide[^]

ATOPIC DERMATITIS

DEFINITION

Atopic dermatitis is a chronically relapsing skin disease that occurs most commonly during early infancy and childhood. It is frequently associated with elevated serum IgE levels and a personal or family history of atopic dermatitis (allergic rhinitis and/or asthma). Atopic dermatitis is characterized by a proliferation of Th2 cells, which stimulate IL-4, IL-5, IL-6, and IL-10 production.

Nghiem P. *J Am Acad Dermatol.* 2002; 46: 228.

TREATMENT OPTIONS

- Antihistamines (cetirizine[^], loratadine[^], desloratadine[^], fexofenadine[^], hydroxyzine[^], diphenhydramine[^], cyproheptadine[^], doxepin oral[^]/topical*)
- Avoidance of trigger factors
- Azathioprine[^]
- Chloroquine[$]
- Coal tar[^]
- Cyclosporin[^]
- Emollients[$]
- Hydroxychloroquine[+]
- Interferon alpha 2A[^], 2B[^]
- Interferon gamma[^]
- Intravenous immunoglobulin[^]
- Methotrexate[$]
- Mycophenolate mofetil[$]
- Photopheresis[+]
- Pimecrolimus, topical*
- PUVA[^]

- Quinacrine$ (with giardiasis)
- Ranitidine^
- Steroids, topical*, oral*, intralesional$, intramuscular$
- Tacrolimus, topical*
- Urea^
- UVA^
- UVB^, UVB narrow band$
- Vitamin B$_{12}$ cream^

BASAL CELL CARCINOMA

▦ DEFINITION

Basal cell carcinoma (BCC) is a malignant neoplasm derived from nonkeratinizing cells in the basal layer of the epidermis. If left untreated, BCC can become invasive and may result in substantial tissue damage. Metastasis is a rare event. An early onset of multiple basal cell carcinomas is a hallmark of Gorlin syndrome (BCC nevus syndrome). The PTCH gene is mutated in patients with Gorlin syndrome and thus strongly linked to development of BCC.

Johnson RL. *Science*. 1996; 272: 1668.

▦ TREATMENT OPTIONS

Destructive or surgical treatments are the most commonly employed.
- Cidofovir$
- Curettage and desiccation
- Excision
- Fluorouracil, topical* (superficial)
- Imiquimod, superficial^, nodular^
- Interferon alpha 2A$, 2B^
- Interferon gamma^
- Ionizing radiation (XRT)
- Liquid nitrogen
- Mohs micrographic surgery
- Photodynamic therapy with intravenous verteporfin^
- Tazarotene$
- Tretinoin, topical$

BEHÇET'S DISEASE

▨ DEFINITION

Behçet's disease is a complex multisystem disease of unknown etiology characterized clinically by oral aphthae (minor, major, or herpetiform) present at least three times in a 12 month period, genital aphthae, arthritis, cutaneous lesions (erythema nodosum–like, papulopustular), and ocular (anterior uveitis, posterior uveitis, or retinal vasculitis), gastrointestinal and neurological manifestations. Positive pathergy test results and HLA-B51 are also associated.

Ghate JV. *J Am Acad Dermatol.* 1999; 40: 1.

▨ TREATMENT OPTIONS

- Azathioprine^
- Chlorambucil, cutaneous^, ocular$
- Colchicine^
- Cyclophosphamide$
- Cyclosporin topical+, systemic^
- Dapsone^
- Etanercept^
- Infliximab$
- Interferon alpha 2A^, 2B^
- Intravenous immunoglobulin+
- Methotrexate+
- Mycophenolate mofetil+
- Pentoxifylline+
- Stanazolol+
- Steroids, topical$, oral^, pulse+, intralesional+
- Thalidomide^

BULLOUS PEMPHIGOID

▨ DEFINITION

Bullous pemphigoid (BP) is a subepidermal blistering skin disease, usually occurring in the elderly, characterized by large, tense blisters and the immunopathologic findings of C3 and IgG at the epidermal basement membrane zone. All BP patients have autoantibodies against the BPAG1 (230-kDa) and BPAG2 (180-kDa) molecules localized in the hemidesmosome.

Joly P. *N Engl J Med.* 2002; 346: 321.

▩ TREATMENT OPTIONS

- Azathioprine$
- Chlorambucil$
- Cyclophosphamide$
- Cyclosporin$
- Dapsone$
- Intravenous immunoglobulin$
- Methotrexate$
- Mycophenolate mofetil+
- Nicotinamide and tetracycline^
- Photopheresis+
- Pimecrolimus, topical+
- Plasma exchange^
- Steroids, oral*, topical*
- Tacrolimus, topical+
- Thalidomide+
- Vincristine+

CICATRICIAL PEMPHIGOID

▩ DEFINITION

Cicatricial pemphigoid is a rare chronic autoimmune subepithelial blistering disease characterized by erosive lesions of mucous membranes and skin that result in scarring. Lesions commonly involve the oral mucosa and the conjunctivae. Nasopharyngeal, laryngeal, esophageal, genital, and rectal mucosae may also be affected. Autoantigens identified in cicatricial pemphigoid target BPAG2, laminin-5 (alpha-3 subunit), integrin (beta-4 subunit), M168, and type VII collagen.

Fleming TE. *J Am Acad Dermatol.* 2000; 43: 571.

▓ TREATMENT OPTIONS

- Azathioprine[^]
- Cyclophosphamide[^]
- Cyclosporin[+]
- Dapsone[$]
- Etanercept[+]
- Intravenous immunoglobulin[$]
- Minocycline[$], with nicotinamide[$]
- Mycophenolate mofetil[$]
- Steroids, oral[$], pulse with cyclophosphamide[$], topical[$], intralesional[+]
- Sulfapyridine[$]
- Tacrolimus, topical for oral lesions[+], ocular lesions[+]
- Tetracycline[+], with nicotinamide[+]
- Thalidomide[+]

CONTACT DERMATITIS

▓ DEFINITION

Allergic contact dermatitis (ACD) is a pruritic, eczematous reaction. Acute ACD and many cases of chronic ACD are well demarcated and localized to the site of contact with the allergen. The prototypic reactions are ACD due to poison ivy and nickel. Patch testing remains the gold standard for accurate and consistent diagnosis.

Boffa MJ. *Contact Derm.* 1995; 33: 149.

▓ TREATMENT OPTIONS

- Avoidance of allergen
- Barrier creams
- Bexarotene topical for hand dermatitis[^]
- Pimecrolimus, topical[$]
- PUVA cream[^]
- Steroids, oral[*], intramuscular[$], topical[*]
- Tacrolimus, topical[^]
- UVA[^]

CUTANEOUS T-CELL LYMPHOMA

■ DEFINITION

The term *cutaneous T-cell lymphoma* (CTCL) describes a heterogeneous group of neoplasms of skin-homing T cells that show considerable variation in clinical presentation, histological appearance, immunophenotype, and prognosis. Mycosis fungoides and Sezary's syndrome represent more than 60% of CTCL. The skin-homing T cells of CTCL are best delineated from other T cells by a unique cell-surface receptor called cutaneous lymphocyte-associated antigen (CLA).

■ STAGING SYSTEM FOR CTCL

T (skin)	T1	Patch, plaque <10%
	T2	Patch, plaque >10%
	T3	Tumors
	T4	Generalized erythroderma
N (nodes)	N0	Clinically uninvolved
	N1	Enlarged, histologically uninvolved
	N2	Clinically uninvolved, histologically involved
	N3	Enlarged and histologically involved
M (viscera)	M0	No involvement
	M1	Involvement
B (blood)	B0	No circulating Sezary cells (<5%)
	B1	Circulating Sezary cells (>5%)
IA	T1, N0, M0	
IB	T2, N0, M0	
IIA	T1-2, N1, M0	
IIB	T3, N0-1, M0	
IIIA	T4, N0, M0	
IIIB	T4, N1, M0	
IVA	T1-4, N2-3, M0	
IVB	T1-4, N0-3, M1	

Willemze R. *Blood.* 1997; 90: 354.

■ TREATMENT OPTIONS

- Acitretin^, with interferon alpha^
- Alemtuzumab$
- Alitretinoin$
- Atorvastatin$ (with bexarotene)

- Bexarotene, topical (IA*, IB*, 2A$), oral*
- Calcipotriene[+]
- Carmustine (BCNU®)$
- Chlorodeoxyadenosine (Cladribine®)$
- CHOP (cyclophosphamide, doxorubicin, vincristine, prednisone)$
- COP (cyclophosphamide, vincristine, prednisone)$
- Cyclophosphamide*
- Cyclosporin with cyclophosphamide/doxorubicin/vincristine/prednisone for subcutaneous childhood CTCL[+]
- Denileukin diftitox*
- Doxil®$
- Etoposide (VP16)^
- Imiquimod[+] (IA)
- Interferon alpha 2A^, 2B$
- Isotretinoin$, with interferon alpha$
- Mechlorethamine$, with electron beam^
- Methotrexate$
- Pentostatin^
- Peripheral blood stem cell transplantation$
- Photodynamic therapy with topical aminolevulinic acid (ALA) for stage IB, 2B, CD30 positive anaplastic large-cell lymphoma[+]
- Photopheresis*
- PUVA*
- PUVA (bath) with oral bexarotene[+]
- Steroids, topical* (patch)
- Tazarotene gel for patch/plaque stage$
- Total body electron beam$, with mechlorethamine^
- UVA* (IB-III)
- UVB$ (IA, IB), narrow band$
- X-ray radiation$

DARIER-WHITE DISEASE

▨ DEFINITION

Darier-White disease (DWD) is an autosomal dominant disorder with altered keratinization of the epidermis, nails, and mucous membranes. Mutations in a sarcoplasmic endoreticulum Ca^{2+}-ATPase isoform-2 (SERCA2) cause all cases of DWD. The gene defect is ATP-2A2.

Sakuntabhai A. *Nature Genet.* 1999; 21: 271.

▨ TREATMENT OPTIONS

- Acitretin$
- Adapalene+
- CO_2 laser+
- Cyclosporin+
- Emollients$
- Fluorouracil, topical+
- Isotretinoin$
- Keratolytics+
- Steroids, oral+, topical+
- Tazarotene+
- Tretinoin, topical+

DERMATITIS HERPETIFORMIS

▨ DEFINITION

Dermatitis herpetiformis (DH) is characterized by an intensely itchy, chronic papulovesicular eruption that usually is distributed symmetrically on extensor surfaces. Most patients have an associated gluten-sensitive enteropathy (GSE) that is usually asymptomatic and is probably related to the IgA deposits found in the skin of these patients. It is known that patients with both DH and GSE have antibodies to transglutaminases, which are thought to be the major autoantigens in these diseases.

Sardy M. *J Exp Med.* 2002; 195: 1.

▨ TREATMENT OPTIONS

- Cholestyramine+
- Colchicine+
- Dapsone*
- Gluten-free diet^
- Methotrexate+
- Steroids, oral*
- Sulfapyridine$
- Sulfasalazine+
- Tetracycline and nicotinamide+

DERMATOMYOSITIS

■ DEFINITION

Dermatomyositis is a disease of presumed autoimmune pathogenesis that is manifested by a symmetric proximal, extensor, inflammatory myopathy and a characteristic cutaneous eruption. The rash is photodistributed, violaceous, and poikilodermatous, favoring the scalp, periocular and extensor skin sites with Gottron's papules, and nailfold telangiectasias. Muscle enzyme levels (aldolase, creatine kinase) may be elevated and autoantibodies (Jo-1, Mi-2, PL-7) may be present.

Jorizzo JL. *Arch Dermatol.* 2002; 138: 114.

■ TREATMENT OPTIONS

- Azathioprine[$]
- Chlorambucil[+]
- Chloroquine[$]
- Colchicine[+]
- Cyclophosphamide, lung involvement[$]
- Cyclosporin[$]
- Dapsone[+]
- Diltiazem[+] (calcinosis cutis)
- Fludarabine[$]
- Hydroxychloroquine[$], with quinacrine[+]
- Intravenous immunoglobulin[^]
- Methotrexate[^]
- Mycophenolate mofetil[+]
- Steroids, oral[*], topical[*], pulse[$]
- Tacrolimus, topical[+]
- Thalidomide[+]

DYSESTHESIA/DELUSIONS OF PARASITOSIS

▨ DEFINITION

"Delusions of parasitosis" falls under the classification of a primary psychiatric disorder. It is a disorder in which patients have the false and fixed belief that they are infested by parasites in the absence of any objective evidence of infestation. Patients may experience sensation of biting, crawling, or stinging. The condition needs to be distinguished from substance-induced formication (cocaine). Most commonly seen in middle-aged women.

Zomer SF. *Br J Dermatol.* 1998; 138: 1030.

▨ TREATMENT OPTIONS

- Capsaicin^
- Doxepin, topical[$]
- Lidocaine, topical[$]
- Pimozide[$]
- Risperidone[$]

EPIDERMOLYSIS BULLOSA

▨ DEFINITION

Inherited epidermolysis bullosa (EB) encompasses many clinically distinctive disorders that share three major features: genetic transmission, mechanical fragility of the skin, and blister formation. There are three major forms of inherited EB—simplex (keratins 5 and 14, plectin), junctional (laminin-5, α-6-β-4-integrin) and dystrophic (type VII collagen)—which differ in the ultrastructural site in the skin within which blisters form.

Fine JD. *J Am Acad Dermatol.* 2000; 42: 1051.

TREATMENT OPTIONS

- Aluminum chloride[+]
- Apligraf[®$]
- Avoid trauma and infection
- Cyproheptadine[^]
- Epidermal autografts[$]
- Glutaraldehyde[+]
- Isotretinoin[+]
- Mupirocin[$]
- Orcel[®*]
- Phenytoin[$]
- Steroids, oral[+], topical[$]
- Tetracycline for Weber-Cockayne variant of Epidermolysis Bullosa Simplex[^]

EPIDERMOLYSIS BULLOSA ACQUISITA

DEFINITION

Epidermolysis bullosa acquisita (EBA) is a rare, acquired, subepidermal bullous disease associated with autoimmunity to type VII collagen, the major component of the anchoring fibrils of the dermal-epidermal junction. EBA is characterized by acral blisters that heal with atrophic scarring, milia, and hyper- or hypopigmentation localized to trauma-prone surfaces, especially the elbows, knees, and dorsa of the hands. Mucous membrane involvement is variable. Direct Immunofluorescence (DIF) shows a linear deposit of IgG along the basement membrane. Salt–split skin preparations of perilesional skin show the immune deposits typically located on the dermal side of the cleavage.

Fine JD. *N Engl J Med.* 1995; 333: 1475.

TREATMENT OPTIONS

- Azathioprine[+]
- Chlorambucil[+]
- Colchicine[+]
- Cyclophosphamide[+]
- Cyclosporin[+]
- Daclizumab[+]

- Dapsone[+]
- Gold[+]
- Intravenous immunoglobulin[+]
- Methotrexate[+]
- Mycophenolate mofetil[+]
- Photopheresis[+]
- PUVA[+]
- Steroids, oral[+], topical[+]
- UVB[+]

ERYTHEMA MULTIFORME

■ DEFINITION

Erythema multiforme is a self-limited, usually mild, relapsing exanthematous reaction of the skin that is etiologically most often related to recurrent herpes simplex virus infection. It is clinically characterized by acrally distributed, target-shaped plaques, and patients frequently present with mucous membrane lesions.

Assier H. *Arch Dermatol.* 1995; 131: 539.

■ TREATMENT OPTIONS

- Acyclovir[^]
- Azathioprine[$]
- Cimetidine[+]
- Intravenous immunoglobulin[$]
- Mycophenolate mofetil[+]
- Steroids, oral[*], topical[*], intramuscular[+]
- Thalidomide[$]
- Valacyclovir[+]

GRAFT-VERSUS-HOST DISEASE

DEFINITION

Graft-versus-host disease (GVHD) is induced by donor immunocompetent T-cells transferred into allogeneic hosts incapable of rejecting them. The sources of the T cells include primarily peripheral blood stem cell and bone marrow transplants and, infrequently, unirradiated blood products, solid organ transplants, and maternal-fetal lymphocyte engraftment. There are two major forms of GVHD—acute and chronic—originally defined on the basis of time of presentation. Chronic GVHD of the skin is divided into lichenoid and sclerodermoid forms.

Aractingi S. *Arch Dermatol.* 1998; 134: 602.

TREATMENT OPTIONS

- Azathioprine[$]
- Clofazimine[$]
- Cyclosporin[^]
- Daclizumab[*]
- Etretinate[$]
- Hydroxychloroquine[+]
- Infliximab[$]
- Intravenous immunoglobulin[*]
- Methotrexate[^]
- Mycophenolate mofetil[+]
- Photopheresis[$]
- PUVA[$]
- Tacrolimus, topical[$], oral[^]
- Thalidomide[$]
- UVB[$]

GRANULOMA ANNULARE

DEFINITION

Granuloma annulare is a benign, usually self-limited dermatosis of unknown cause, characterized by necrobiotic dermal papules that often assume an annular configuration. Clinical variants include localized, generalized, micropapular, nodular, perforating, patch, and subcutaneous forms. There is a rare association with lymphoma and diabetes mellitus.

Fayyazi A. *Arch Dermatol Res.* 2000; 292: 384.

▓ TREATMENT OPTIONS

- Chlorambucil§
- Chloroquine§
- Clofazimine[+]
- CO_2 laser[+]
- Cryosurgery§
- Cyclosporin[+]
- Dapsone[+]
- Hydroxychloroquine§
- Imiquimod[+]
- Interferon alpha[+] (in a patient with hepatitis C)
- Isotretinoin[+]
- Nicotinamide[+]
- Pentoxifylline[+]
- PUVA§
- Steroids, intralesional§, topical[+]
- Tacrolimus, topical[+]
- UVA§

GROVER'S DISEASE

▓ DEFINITION

Grover's disease (transient acantholytic dermatosis) is a polymorphic, pruritic, papulovesicular dermatosis of the trunk and proximal extremities characterized histologically by acantholysis resembling Darier's disease, Hailey-Hailey disease, Pemphigus Vulgaris, and spongiotic dermatitis. Exacerbating factors include friction, heat, sweating, and sunlight exposure.

Chalet M. *Arch Dermatol.* 1997; 113: 431.

▥ TREATMENT OPTIONS

- Calcipotriene[+]
- Isotretinoin[+]
- PUVA[+]
- Steroids, topical[§], oral[§]

HAILEY-HAILEY DISEASE

▥ DEFINITION

Hailey-Hailey disease, or familial benign pemphigus, is a rare blistering disorder characterized by recurrent vesicles and erosions, particularly involving flexural areas. Lesions are frequently precipitated by friction and infection with various bacteria, yeasts, and viruses. The major underlying pathologic process is acantholysis. It has been established that the genetic abnormality lies in ATP2C1, which encodes an adenosine triphosphate–powered calcium pump.

Hu Z. *Nat Genet.* 2000; 24: 61.

▥ TREATMENT OPTIONS

- Botox®
- Calcipotriene[+]
- Cyclosporin, topical[+]
- Dapsone[+]
- Dermabrasion[§]
- Erbium:YAG laser[+]
- Etretinate[+]
- Methotrexate[+]
- Short-pulse CO_2 laser[+]
- Steroids, oral[§], topical[§]
- Tacalcitol[+]
- Tacrolimus, topical[+]
- Wide excision and grafting[+]

HERPES GESTATIONIS (PEMPHIGOID GESTATIONIS)

▓ DEFINITION

Pemphigoid gestationis (PG) is a rare, pruritic, polymorphic, inflammatory, subepidermal, bullous dermatosis of pregnancy and the postpartum period. IgG1 (the HG factor) and IgG3 are the major subclasses of immunoglobulin that target the BPAG2 (BP180 or type XVII collagen). However, the heavy deposition of C3 at the basement membrane zone of skin is the diagnostic hallmark.

Chimanovitch I. *J Invest Dermatol.* 1999; 109: 140.

▓ TREATMENT OPTIONS

- Cyclophosphamide[+] (with antiphospholipid antibody syndrome)
- Cyclosporin[+]
- Dapsone[+]
- Gold[+]
- Intravenous immunoglobulin[+]
- Methotrexate[+]
- Plasmapheresis[+]
- Pyridoxine[+]
- Steroids, oral[$], topical[$]
- Tetracycline[+]

HYPEREOSINOPHILIC SYNDROME

▓ DEFINITION

The hypereosinophilic syndrome is a multisystem process characterized by peripheral blood eosinophilia and infiltration of eosinophils into many organs, including the skin. Cutaneous involvement occurs in more than 50% of patients as pruritic, macular, papular, or nodular lesions over the trunk and extremities or as urticaria or angioedema. A variant with mucosal ulcers carries an unusually grave prognosis. Criteria for the diagnosis include (1) persistent blood eosinophil counts greater than 1500/mm^3 for more than

6 months, (2) failure to diagnose parasitic, allergic, or other known causes of eosinophilia, and (3) presumptive signs and symptoms of organ involvement. Serum eosinophilic major basic protein levels are usually elevated, and eosinophils are hypodense, implying a more activated state. The cause of death is most commonly congestive heart failure.

Gleich GJ. *Lancet.* 2002; 359: 1577.

▓ TREATMENT OPTIONS

- Cyclophosphamide[+]
- Cyclosporin[+]
- Dapsone[+]
- Etoposide (VP16)[+]
- Hydroxyurea[$]
- Imatinib[$]
- Interferon alpha 2A[+], 2B[$]
- Intravenous immunoglobulin[+]
- PUVA[+]
- Steroids, oral[$]
- Thioguanine[+]
- Vincristine[+]

ICHTHYOSIS

▓ DEFINITION

Ichthyoses are disorders of cornification with abnormal differentiation and desquamation of the epidermis. They represent a large clinically and etiologically heterogeneous group that shares generalized scaling of the skin. Clinical features, inheritance, and structural and biochemical abnormalities help to differentiate these disorders.

Irvine AD. *Br J Dermatol.* 1999; 140: 815.

▓ TREATMENT OPTIONS

- Acitretin[$]
- Ammonium lactate[*]
- Calcipotriene[^] (X-linked and congenital)

- Emollients
- Isotretinoin[$]
- Methotrexate[+] (bullous and nonbullous congenital ichthyosiform erthyroderma)
- Salicylic acid[$]
- Tretinoin, topical[$]
- Urea[^]

KAPOSI'S SARCOMA

DEFINITION

In Kaposi's sarcoma, a virally induced human herpesvirus-8 (HHV-8) is the suspected agent. Kaposi's sarcoma is a multifocal systemic disease with four principal clinical variants: (1) chronic or classic, (2) African endemic, (3) iatrogenic in immunocompromised patients, and (4) AIDS-related epidemic. Cutaneous lesions present as variably distributed pink patches, blue-violet to black nodules or plaques, and polyps, depending on clinical variant and stage.

Antman K. *N Engl J Med.* 2000; 342: 1027.

TREATMENT OPTIONS

- Alitretinoin[*]
- Chlorambucil[$]
- Cryotherapy[^]
- Doxil®
- Etoposide[$]
- Gemcitabine[$]
- Highly active antiretroviral therapy[$]
- Interferon alpha, 2A[*], 2B[*]
- Paclitaxel[$]
- Pulse dye laser[$], Nd:YAG laser[$], CO_2 laser[+]
- Radiation[^]
- Reduce immunosuppression[$]
- Shark cartilage[+]
- Thalidomide[$]
- Vinblastine, intralesional[$]
- Vincristine/doxorubicin[$]
- Vincristine/doxorubicin/bleomycin[^]

KELOID

▣ DEFINITION

Keloids are abnormal growths of fibrous tissue following cutaneous injury that grow beyond the site of the original injury. They express increased levels of the gli-1 protein, an oncogene product, and contain tenascin C, a protein associated with inflammation and wound healing.

Kim A. *J Am Acad Dermatol.* 2001; 45: 707.

▣ TREATMENT OPTIONS

- Cryotherapy[+]
- Excision[$]
- Fluorouracil, intralesional[$]
- Imiquimod[$]
- Interferon alpha 2B[^] with surgery[$], monotherapy
- Interferon gamma[^]
- Methotrexate[+]
- Pulse dye laser[^], CO_2 laser[$], Nd:YAG laser[$], argon laser[$]
- Radiation[$]
- Silicone sheets[$]
- Steroids, intralesional[^], topical[$]
- Tacrolimus, topical[+]
- Tretinoin, topical[$]

LICHEN PLANUS

▣ DEFINITION

Lichen planus is an idiopathic inflammatory disease of the skin, hair, nails, and mucous membranes that clinically manifests with flat-topped violaceous pruritic, polygonal papules and plaques that favor the wrists, forearms, genitalia, distal lower extremities, and presacral area. Clinical variants include annular, bullous, hypertrophic, linear, ulcerative, and lichen planopilaris.

Spandau U. *J Invest Dermatol.* 1998; 111: 1003.

▓ TREATMENT OPTIONS

- Acitretin^
- Azathioprine⁺
- Becaplermin⁺ (ulcerated variant)
- Chloroquine⁺ (for oral involvement)
- Cyclosporin⁺ (lichen planopilaris⁺)
- Excimer 308 nm laser$ (for oral involvement)
- Griseofulvin$
- Hydroxychloroquine$ (for oral involvement)
- Isotretinoin (for oral involvement$, for cutaneous involvement⁺)
- Methotrexate⁺
- Mycophenolate mofetil⁺ (for oral involvement)
- Photopheresis$ (erosive variant)
- Pimecrolimus⁺
- PUVA$
- Steroids, oral^, topical^, intralesional⁺, intramuscular⁺
- Tacrolimus, topical$ (for oral involvement)
- Thalidomide⁺ (erosive variant)
- Tretinoin, topical^ (for oral involvement)
- UVA$
- UVB$

LICHEN SCLEROSUS ET ATROPHICUS

▓ DEFINITION

Lichen sclerosus et atrophicus is a chronic inflammatory disease that preferentially affects the anogenital region, although any cutaneous site may be affected. Pruritus is the most frequent symptom, and the major clinical signs are pallor, atrophy, fissures, and foci of hyperkeratosis. Blisters rarely occur. Given the increased risk of developing squamous cell carcinoma, patients require long-term evaluation.

Powell JJ. *Lancet.* 1999; 353: 1777.

▓ TREATMENT OPTIONS

- Acitretin^
- Calcipotriene⁺
- Chloroquine⁺

- Hydroxychloroquine[+]
- Penicillin[+]
- Photodynamic therapy[$]
- PUVA[$]
- Stanozolol[$]
- Steroids, intralesional[+], topical[$], oral[+]
- Tacrolimus, topical for body[$], topical for vulvar lesions[+], anogenital[$]
- Testosterone topical[^] (for use in normoandrogenic women)
- Tretinoin[+]
- UVA[+]

LICHEN SIMPLEX CHRONICUS

DEFINITION

Lichen simplex chronicus is a disorder resulting from excessive scratching of the skin, most frequently seen in adults over age 60. The lesions are characterized as hyperpigmented, lichenified, leathery plaques, often seen on the posterior neck, extensor surfaces of the forearms and lower legs, and the genital region.

Koo J., in *Dermatology,* by Bolognia J et al. Mosby 2003; 8: 117.

TREATMENT OPTIONS

- Antihistamines[$]
- Botox®[$]
- Capsaicin[+]
- Doxepin, topical[+]
- Emollients
- Rule out psychological issues
- Steroids, topical[^], intralesional[^]
- Tacrolimus, topical[$]

LINEAR IgA BULLOUS DERMATOSIS

▨ DEFINITION

Linear IgA bullous dermatosis (LABD) is a rare immune-mediated blistering skin disease that is defined by the presence of homogeneous linear deposits of IgA at the cutaneous basement membrane. The childhood form is frequently termed *chronic bullous disease of childhood*. In adults, it can be drug induced (ie, vancomycin). In LABD patients, the IgA antibody was found to react against a 97 kDa antigen that represents a cleaved ectodomain of BPAG2 (BP180).

Zone JJ. *J Invest Dermatol.* 1996; 106: 1277.

▨ TREATMENT OPTIONS

- Colchicine[+]
- Cyclophosphamide[+]
- Cyclosporin[+]
- Dapsone[$]
- Dapsone with mycophenolate mofetil[+]
- Erythromycin[+]
- Intravenous immunoglobulin[+]
- Mycophenolate mofetil[+]
- Steroids, oral[$], topical[+]
- Sulfapyridine and intravenous immunoglobulin[+]
- Tetracycline and nicotinamide[$]

LIPODERMATOSCLEROSIS

▨ DEFINITION

Lipodermatosclerosis is an acute or chronic form of lower-extremity panniculitis that results from venous insufficiency. This leads to decreased venous return and sludging of the blood in the lobular capillaries, resulting in pannicular ischemia, fat necrosis, and fibrosis. In the acute phase, there is pain, warmth, erythema, scale, and some induration. In the chronic phase, there is marked sclerosis of the dermis and subcutis, with hyperpigmentation due to hemosiderin deposition. The lower leg often assumes an "inverted champagne bottle" appearance.

Kirsner RS. *J Am Acad Dermatol.* 1993; 28: 623.

▓ TREATMENT OPTIONS

- Elastic compression stockings^
- Oxandrolone+
- Stanozolol^

LUPUS ERYTHEMATOSUS

▓ DEFINITION

Lupus erythematosus (LE) is a multisystem disorder that prominently affects the skin. Cutaneous lesions are a source of disability and, on many occasions, an indicator of internal disease. There are several variants of cutaneous lupus, defined in part by the location and depth of the inflammatory infiltrate. Histologically systemic lupus erythematosus (SLE) involves primarily the epidermis and upper dermis and is associated with systemic disease. Subacute cutaneous lupus erythematosus (SCLE) involves primarily the epidermis and upper dermis and is associated with anti-Ro autoantibodies and photosensitivity. Discoid lupus erythematosus (DLE) involves the epidermis, upper and lower dermis, and adnexal structures and frequently scars.

Callen JP. *Lupus.* 1997; 6: 203.

▓ TREATMENT OPTIONS

LUPUS, BULLOUS

- Cyclosporin+
- Dapsone$
- Methotrexate+
- Steroids, oral$

LUPUS, DISCOID

- Acitretin[$]
- Azathioprine[+]
- Clofazimine[$]
- Cryotherapy[+]
- Danazol[+]
- Dapsone[+]
- Hydroxychloroquine[^], with quinacrine[$]
- Imiquimod[+]
- Interferon alpha 2A[$], 2B[$]
- Isotretinoin[$]
- Methotrexate[$]
- Mycophenolate mofetil[+]
- Photopheresis[+]
- Quinacrine[^]
- Steroids, intralesional[$], topical[$], oral[$]
- Sunscreen[$]
- Tacrolimus, topical[+]
- Tazarotene[+]
- Thalidomide[$]

LUPUS, HYPERTROPHIC

- Acitretin[+]
- Erbium: YAG laser[+]
- Isotretinoin[+]
- Steroids, intralesional[$]
- Thalidomide[+]
- Tretinoin, topical[+]

LUPUS, PANNICULITIS

- Azathioprine[+]
- Chloroquine[+]
- Cyclophosphamide[+]
- Cyclosporin[+]
- Dapsone[+]
- Hydroxychloroquine[+]
- Quinacrine[+]
- Steroids, oral[$], topical[+]
- Thalidomide[+]

LUPUS, SUBACUTE

- Acitretin$^\$$
- Dapsone$^+$
- Interferon alpha 2A$^\$$
- Isotretinoin$^\$$
- Methotrexate$^\$$
- Mycophenolate mofetil$^+$
- Photopheresis$^+$
- Quinacrine$^+$
- Steroids, intralesional$^\$$, topical$^+$, oral$^\$$
- Thalidomide$^\$$

LUPUS, SYSTEMIC

- Azathioprine$^\wedge$
- Bone marrow transplants$^\$$
- Chlorambucil, nephritis$^\wedge$
- Chloroquine*
- Cyclophosphamide, renal$^\wedge$, lung/ocular/cerebral$^\$$
- Cyclosporin$^\$$
- Danazol$^\$$ (thrombocytopenia)
- Hydroxychloroquine*
- Intravenous immunoglobulin$^\$$
- Leflunomide$^\$$
- Methotrexate$^\wedge$
- Mycophenolate mofetil$^\$$
- Photopheresis$^\$$
- Quinacrine$^\wedge$
- Steroids, oral*, pulse for nephritis and cerebritis$^\wedge$
- UVA$^+$

LYMPHOMATOID PAPULOSIS

▦ DEFINITION

Lymphomatoid papulosis (LyP) is a chronic, recurrent, self-healing papu-lonecrotic or papulonodular skin disease with histologic features suggestive of a (CD30-positive) malignant lymphoma. The typical skin lesions in LyP are red-brown papules and nodules that may develop central hemorrhage, necro-sis, and crusting and subsequently spontaneously disappear within 3–8 weeks. Three histologic types of LyP have been described: type A Reed-Sternberg–like

CD30-positive T cells, type B cerebriform nuclei CD30-negative T cells, and type C large CD30-positive T cells.

Willemze R. *Blood*. 1997; 90: 354.

■ TREATMENT OPTIONS

- Bexarotene, topical[$], oral[+]
- Carmustine[$]
- Etoposide[+]
- Mechlorethamine[$]
- Methotrexate[$]
- Photopheresis[+]
- PUVA[$]
- Steroids, intralesional[+], topical[+]
- Total skin electron beam[$]

MELANOMA

■ DEFINITION

Melanoma results from the malignant transformation of melanocytes. Melanocytes are derived from the neural crest and produce melanin. During embryonic life, precursor cells known as melanoblasts migrate to the basal-cell layer of the epidermis and, less frequently, to the dermis and sebaceous glands. Melanoma can arise from melanocytes located in these sites and from altered melanocytes called nevus cells in certain precursor lesions.

Rigel DS. *Skin Cancer Found J.* 2001; 19: 13.

■ STAGING

IA	Tumor <1 mm without ulceration
	Clark II/III
	No lymph node involvement or metastasis
IB	Tumor <1 mm with ulceration, or tumor 1.01–2 mm without ulceration
	Clark IV/V
	No lymph node involvement or metastasis
IIA	Tumor 1.01–2 mm with ulceration, or tumor 2.01–4 mm without ulceration
	No lymph node involvement or metastasis

IIB	Tumor 2.01–4 mm with ulceration, or tumor >4 mm without ulceration No lymph node involvement or metastasis
IIC	Tumor >4 mm with ulceration No lymph node involvement or metastasis
IIIA	Tumor any thickness without ulceration 1–3 positive lymph nodes Micrometastasis
IIIB	Tumor any thickness without ulceration, 1–3 positive lymph nodes, macrometastasis Tumor any thickness with ulceration, 1–3 positive lymph nodes, micrometastasis Tumor any thickness without ulceration, 2–3 positive lymph nodes, In transit metastasis, no lymph node metastasis
IIIC	Tumor any thickness with ulceration, 1–3 positive lymph nodes, macrometastasis Tumor any thickness, 4 or more lymph node metastasis or matted lymph nodes or in transit metastasis with metastatic lymph nodes
IV	Tumor any thickness, Any number of lymph nodes involved, any type of metastasis

Balch CM. *J Clin Oncol.* 2001; 19: 3635.

DEPTH	CLARK LEVEL	ANATOMIC LEVEL	5 YEAR SURVIVAL
In situ	I	Epidermis	100%
<0.75 mm	II	Papillary dermis	97%
0.76–1.5 mm	III	Papillary-reticular dermis	92%
1.51–4 mm	IV	Reticular dermis	76–62%
>4 mm	V	Subcutaneous tissue	52%
>8 mm			32%

Current AAD guidelines.

DEPTH	SURGICAL MARGINS	SENTINEL LYMPH NODE BIOPSY
In situ	0.5 cm	No
<1 mm	1 cm	No
1–2 mm	1 cm	Yes
>2 mm	2 cm	No

If the patient is asymptomatic, physical exam is normal, and melanoma is ≤4 mm; no workup is needed. Otherwise the workup is based on clinical findings and depth >4 mm (chest radiograph, CT scans, complete blood count, liver function tests, lactic dehydrogenase).

Current AAD guidelines.

▦ TREATMENT OPTIONS

Surgical treatment is the preferred modality.

- Azelaic acid[$]
- Excision with appropriate margins, with or without sentinel lymph node biopsy
- Hydroxyurea[*]
- Imiquimod with or without metastasis[+], amelanotic lentigo maligna[+], lentigo maligna[+]
- Interferon alpha 2B[*]
- Interferon gamma[^]
- Melphalan[^] (metastasis)
- Radiation and chemotherapy for palliation in metastasis
- Tazarotene gel for lentigo maligna[+]
- Vincristine[^] (metastasis)

MOLLUSCUM CONTAGIOSUM

▦ DEFINITION

Molluscum contagiosum (MC) is a common benign viral infection of the skin and mucous membranes that generally affects children. Transmission is via skin-to-skin contact and, less commonly, fomites. In adults MC may be transmitted sexually. Widespread large and occasionally deforming lesions may be seen in AIDS patients. MC lesions are firm, umbilicated, pearly papules with a waxy surface, can occur anywhere in the skin surface but are most common in the skin folds and the genital region. MC is a member of the *Molluscipox* genus of Poxviridae.

Skinner RB. *Pediatr Dermatol.* 2000; 17: 420.

▦ TREATMENT OPTIONS

- Cantharidin[$]
- Cidofovir[$]
- Cimetidine[$]
- CO_2 laser[+]
- Cryotherapy[^]
- Curettage[$]
- Imiquimod[$]
- Pulse dye laser[$]

MORPHEA

▨ DEFINITION

Morphea is a clinically distinct inflammatory disease, primarily of the dermis and subcutaneous fat, that ultimately leads to scarlike sclerosis. The sclerosis may extend deeply into the fat or underlying structures, causing disability. Active lesions may have a lilac border, while inactive lesions often become hyperpigmented. Morphea may be associated with lichen sclerosus et atrophicus. There is no associated systemic disease.

Mayes MD. *Semin Cutan Med Surg.* 1998; 17: 22.

▨ TREATMENT OPTIONS

- Calcipotriene[$]
- Chloroquine[+]
- Hydroxychloroquine[+]
- Methotrexate[$]
- Penicillin[+]
- Photodynamic therapy[+]
- Photopheresis[+]
- PUVA[$]
- Steroids, topical[$], oral[+], intralesional[+]
- Tretinoin, topical[+]
- UVA[$]

NECROBIOSIS LIPOIDICA DIABETICORUM

▨ DEFINITION

Necrobiosis lipoidica diabeticorum (NLD) is characterized by well-circumscribed, hard, depressed, waxy, plaques with violaceous to red-brown, palpable peripheral rims and yellow-brown atrophic centers that contain teleangiectasias. The most common site is the shins. Ulceration can occur following trauma. The proportion of patients with diabetes mellitus and NLD varies from 14 to 65%, and the pathogenesis is unknown.

O'Toole EA. *Br J Dermatol.* 1999; 140: 283.

TREATMENT OPTIONS

- Becaplermin^ (for ulcers)
- Benzoyl peroxide[+]
- Clofazimine[+]
- Cyclosporin[+]
- Granulocyte-macrophage colony–stimulating factor[+]
- Mycophenolate mofetil[+]
- Niacinamide[+]
- Pentoxifylline[+]
- PUVA[+]
- Stanozolol[+]
- Steroids, intralesional[+], topical[+], oral[+]
- Tacrolimus, topical[+]
- Tretinoin, topical[+]

PARANEOPLASTIC PEMPHIGUS

DEFINITION

Paraneoplastic pemphigus is an autoimmune disorder that is almost invariably linked to an underlying lymphoproliferative disorder. The most commonly associated neoplasms are non-Hodgkin's lymphoma (42%), chronic lymphocytic leukemia (CLL) (29%), Castleman's disease (10%), malignant and benign thymomas (6%), and reticulum cell sarcoma (6%). The most constant clinical feature of paraneoplastic pemphigus is the presence of intractable stomatitis. Cutaneous lesions are quite polymorphic and may appear as erythematous macules, flaccid blisters and erosions, tense blisters, erythema multiforme–like lesions, and lichenoid eruptions. Pathogenic antibodies in this disease are directed toward intercellular (plakins) and basement membrane (BPAg1) antigens.

Nousari HC. *N Engl J Med.* 1999; 340: 1406.

TREATMENT OPTIONS

- Cyclosporin^
- Mycophenolate mofetil[+]
- Plasmapheresis[+]
- Rituximab[+]
- Steroids, oral[+], pulse with cyclophosphamide[+]

- Tacrolimus, topical[+] (oral mucosa)
- Treatment of underlying malignancy

PARAPSORIASIS, SMALL PLAQUE

DEFINITION

Parapsoriasis is a group of disorders characterized by a persistent, scaling, inflammatory cutaneous eruption. Two clinicopathologic features set the parapsoriasis group apart from other purely inflammatory dermatoses: (1) the relationship to malignant lymphoproliferative lesions and (2) the coexistence and/or overlapping of entities, including small-plaque parapsoriasis, large-plaque parapsoriasis, and pityriasis lichenoides. There is a predominance of CD4+ T cells in the infiltrate, and a dominant T-cell clonality is demonstrable in many cases.

Rook AH. *Blood*. 1999; 94: 902.

TREATMENT OPTIONS

- Antihistamines[+]
- Bexarotene, topical[$]
- Carmustine (BCNU®)[$]
- Coal tar[+]
- Mechlorethamine (nitrogen mustard)[$]
- PUVA[$]
- Steroids, topical[$]
- Tacrolimus, topical[+]
- UVB[$]

PEMPHIGUS FOLIACEUS

DEFINITION

Pemphigus foliaceus is an autoimmune blistering disease of the skin characterized histologically by superficial intraepidermal blisters due to acantholysis (separation of epidermal cells from each other) in the granular layer and immunopathologically by in-vivo bound and circulating IgG (anti–desmoglein-1 antibodies) directed against the cell surface of keratinocytes. Patients with pemphigus foliaceus have only cutaneous involvement, with flaccid blisters and crusts. Pemphigus erythematosus and fogo selvagem represent localized and endemic variants, respectively.

Jolles S. *Clin Exp Dermatol.* 2001; 26: 127.

▣ TREATMENT OPTIONS

- Azathioprine[^]
- Chlorambucil[$]
- Cyclophosphamide[$]
- Dapsone[$]
- Intravenous immunoglobulin[$]
- Methotrexate[+]
- Mycophenolate mofetil[$]
- Niacinamide with tetracycline[+]
- Rituximab[+]
- Steroids, oral[*], topical[*], pulse[^]

PEMPHIGUS, IgA

▣ DEFINITION

IgA pemphigus represents a group of autoimmune intraepidermal blistering diseases presenting with a vesiculopustular eruption, neutrophilic infiltration of the skin, and in-vivo bound and circulating IgA autoantibodies against the surface of keratinocytes. Two distinct types of IgA pemphigus have been described: subcorneal pustular dermatosis (SPD) and intraepidermal neutrophilic. Patients with both types present with flaccid vesicles or pustules on either erythematous or normal skin. The most common sites are the axilla and the groin. Mucous membrane involvement is rare. IgA autoantibodies in the SPD type were shown to recognize desmocollin-1.

Nishikawa T. *Clin Dermatol.* 2000; 18: 315.

■ TREATMENT OPTIONS

- Acitretin[+]
- Colchicine[+]
- Dapsone[+]
- Etretinate[+]
- Isotretinoin[+]
- Methotrexate[+]
- PUVA[+]
- Sulfapyridine[+]

PEMPHIGUS VULGARIS

■ DEFINITION

Pemphigus vulgaris is an autoimmune blistering disease of the skin and mucous membranes characterized histologically by intraepidermal blisters due to acantholysis (separation of epidermal cells from each other) just above the basal layer and immunopathologically by in-vivo bound and circulating IgG (anti–desmoglein-3 antibodies), directed against the cell surface of keratinocytes. Patients with pemphigus vulgaris frequently have mucosal membrane erosions, and more than half also have cutaneous flaccid blisters and erosions. Pemphigus vegetans is a vegetative variant of pemphigus vulgaris.

Enk AK. *Arch Dermatol.* 1999; 135: 54.

■ TREATMENT OPTIONS

- Azathioprine[$]
- Chlorambucil[$]
- Cyclophosphamide[$]
- Cyclosporin[^]
- Dapsone[$]
- Hydroxychloroquine[+]
- Intravenous immunoglobulin[$]
- Methotrexate[$]
- Mycophenolate mofetil[$]
- Photopheresis[+]
- Plasmapheresis[^]
- Quinacrine[$]
- Rituximab[+]

- Steroids, oral*, pulse^, topical*
- Tacrolimus, topical for body⁺, topical for ocular⁺
- Vincristine⁺

PITYRIASIS LICHENOIDES

▒ DEFINITION

Pityriasis lichenoides (PL) is an uncommon, idiopathic, acquired dermatosis. Based on differences in morphology and temporal evolution and course of the disorder, acute (pityriasis lichenoides et varioliformis acuta, or PLEVA) and chronic (pityriasis lichenoides chronica, or PLC) variants have been identified. PL is characterized by evolving groups of erythematous, scaly papules that may either persist for weeks to months (PLC) or erupt and recur in acute exacerbations, often accompanied by vesiculopustules, ulcerations, hemorrhage, and crusting (PLEVA). PLUH is the rare ulceronecrotic hypercaute variant of PLEVA.

Pinton PC. *J Am Acad Dermatol.* 2002; 47: 410.

PITYRIASIS LICHENOIDES CHRONICA

- Cyclosporin⁺
- PUVA⁺
- Steroids, topical$
- Tacrolimus, topical⁺
- UVA$
- UVB$

PITYRIASIS LICHENOIDES ET VARIOLIFORMIS ACUTA

- Coal tar⁺
- Erythromycin$
- Methotrexate$
- PUVA$
- Steroids, topical$, oral⁺
- Tacrolimus, topical⁺
- Tetracycline$
- UVA$
- UVB$

PITYRIASIS ROSEA

DEFINITION

Pityriasis rosea is an acute, self-limited papulosquamous skin eruption with a distinctive and constant course. The initial lesion ("herald patch") is a primary plaque that is followed after 1–2 weeks by a generalized secondary rash with a typical truncal distribution along the lines of cleavage ("Christmas tree") and lasting for about 6 weeks. Less common variants include inverse, vesicular, purpuric, and pustular.

Sharma PK. *J Am Acad Dermatol.* 2000; 42: 241.

TREATMENT OPTIONS

- Antihistamines[+]
- Emollients[+]
- Erythromycin[^]
- Steroids, topical[+]
- UVB[^]

PITYRIASIS RUBRA PILARIS

DEFINITION

Pityriasis rubra pilaris is a group of chronic disorders characterized by follicular papules on an erythematous base and a coalescence of orange-red plaques. The disease also displays islands of sparing and an orange-red waxy keratoderma of the palms and soles. Both familial and acquired forms of the disorder have been described; the classical adult form is the most common. The classical types typically resolve in 1.5–3 years. Histologically there is alternating vertical and horizontal parakeratosis.

Kirby B. *Br J Dermatol.* 2000; 142: 376.

TREATMENT OPTIONS

- Acitretin[$]
- Azathioprine[+]

- Calcipotriene[+]
- Cyclosporin[+]
- Danazol[+]
- Isotretinoin[$]
- Methotrexate[$]
- PUVA[+]
- Stanozolol[+]
- UVA[+]
- UVB[$]

PORPHYRIA

DEFINITION

The porphyrias are caused by deficiencies of enzymes involved in the heme biosynthesis metabolism. Seven types of porphyria are now recognized; they include acute (aminolevulinic acid dehydratase [ALA-D] deficient, acute intermittent, variegate, and hereditary coproporphyria) and nonacute (porphyria cutanea tarda [PCT], erythropoietic protoporphyria [EPP], and congenital erythropoietic porphyria [CEP]). The cutaneous signs include blistering, skin fragility, and erosion in light-exposed sites. Milia, hypertrichosis, hyperpigmentation, scarring alopecia, and sclerodermoid induration may also be present. Cutaneous features are not seen in acute intermittent and ALA-D–deficient porphyria.

Mustajoki P. *Arch Intern Med.* 1993; 153: 2004.

TREATMENT OPTIONS

- Acetylcysteine[+] (EPP)
- Antihistamines[$] (EPP)
- Beta carotene (EPP)[^], (CEP)[+]
- Bone marrow transplantation[+] (CEP)
- Carbohydrates[$] (acute porphyrias)
- Chloroquine (PCT)[^], (CEP)[+]
- Cholestyramine[$] (EPP)
- Colchicine (PCT)[^], (CEP)[+]
- Desferroxamine[$] (PCT)
- Erythropoietin[$] (PCT)
- Heme arginate[^] (acute porphyrias)
- Hydroxychloroquine[^] (PCT)

- Interferon⁺ (PCT)
- Luteinizing hormone–releasing hormone agonists⁺ (acute porphyrias)
- Liver transplantation$ (EPP)
- Narrow-band UVB$ (EPP)
- Phlebotomy^ (PCT)
- PUVA$ (EPP)
- Red blood cell transfusions$ (CEP)
- Splenectomy$ (CEP)
- Tin-protoporphyrins^ (acute porphyrias)
- Vitamin C (PCT)$, (EPP)^
- Vitamin E (CEP)$, (PCT)$

POSTHERPETIC NEURALGIA

DEFINITION

Postherpetic neuralgia (PHN) is a complication of herpes zoster character-ized by pain that persists after the rash has healed. Inflammation in the skin triggers nociceptive signals that further amplify cutaneous pain. Damage to neurons in the spinal cord, ganglion, and peripheral nerve is important in the pathogenesis of PHN. The anatomic and functional changes responsible for PHN appear to be established early in the course of herpes zoster.

Kost RG. *N Engl J Med.* 1996; 335: 32.

TREATMENT OPTIONS

- Acyclovir, valcyclovir, famciclovir^ (shortens the course of the disease)
- Adriamycin, intraneural$
- Amitriptyline^
- Capsaicin*
- Gabapentin^
- Lidocaine, topical^
- Narcotics (morphine$, oxycodone^, tramadol^)
- Nerve blocks$
- Nortriptyline^
- Steroids, oral$ (prevention), intrathecal⁺
- Thalidomide⁺
- Vincristine^

PRURIGO NODULARIS

▨ DEFINITION

Prurigo nodularis is an alteration in the skin that results from repetitive rubbing, scratching, and picking due a variety of pruritogenic stimuli. Clinically prurigo nodularis appears as dome-shaped nodules that often have an eroded surface with scale and crusts. Eosinophils, which contain eosinophil cationic protein and eosinophil-derived neurotoxin, are increased in the dermis.

Stander S. *J Am Acad Dermatol.* 2001; 44: 471.

▨ TREATMENT OPTIONS

- Antihistamines
- Calcipotriene
- Capsaicin[$]
- Clofazimine[+]
- Cryotherapy[$]
- Cyclosporin[+]
- Naltrexone[$]
- PUVA[+]
- Steroids, intramuscular[$], intralesional[$], topical[$]
- Thalidomide[$]
- UVA[$]
- UVB[+]

PRURITIC URTICARIAL PAPULES AND PLAQUES OF PREGNANCY

▨ DEFINITION

Pruritic urticarial papules and plaques of pregnancy (PUPPP) is a common, intensely pruritic dermatosis that usually occurs late in the third trimester and typically affects primigravidas. Clinically it is characterized by the onset of tiny erythematous papules on the abdomen, frequently beginning in the striae distensae but soon coalescing to form large erythematous plaques centered around the umbilicus. The onset of PUPPP in the immediate postpartum period is rare, it tends not to recur in subsequent pregnancies, and it is not associated with fetal involvement.

Kroumpouzos G. *J Am Acad Dermatol.* 2001; 45: 1.

▒ TREATMENT OPTIONS

- Antihistamines[+]
- Steroids, oral[+], topical[$]

PRURITUS

▒ DEFINITION

Pruritus (itching) is the predominant symptom of skin disease and can best be defined indirectly as a sensation that leads to a desire to scratch. Pruritus in disease states may originate in the skin (pruritoceptive) or in the central and/or peripheral nervous system (neuropathic or neurogenic). Mediators can act both peripherally (histamine) and centrally (opioid peptides).

Caterina MJ. *Nature.* 1997; 389: 816.

▒ TREATMENT OPTIONS

- Capsaicin[^] (psoriasis)
- Cetirizine[^] (burn, mosquito bite)
- Cholestyramine (polycythemia vera, sickle cell disease, dermatitis herpetiformis, porphyria)[+], (cholestasis, cholestasis of pregnancy, uremia, hepatic failure)[^]
- Cyproheptadine[^] (histaminic)
- Danazol[$] (myelodysplastic syndrome)
- Diphenhydramine[^] (histaminic, morphine)
- Doxepin, oral[^] (HIV, allergic), topical[^] (atopic)
- Gabapentin[+] (brachoradial pruritus)
- Hydroxyzine[*]
- Lidocaine, topical[$] (burn)
- Loratadine[^] (mosquito bite)
- Menthol lotion[^]
- Naloxone[^] (cholestasis)
- Naltrexone[^] (cholestasis, uremia)

- Stanozolol$ (primary biliary cirrhosis)
- Steroids, topical*
- Strontium^
- Tacalcitol$
- Thalidomide^ (chronic, uremic)
- Treatment of underlying cause
- UVB$ (hemodialysis, HIV, polycythemia vera, cholestasis)

PSORIASIS

DEFINITION

Psoriasis is a chronic relapsing erythrosquamous disease of the skin characterized by variable clinical features. The morphology of the skin lesions varies considerably. Psoriasis vulgaris is the most common type, with circular, scaly, silvery plaques predominant on the elbows, knees, lower back, and umbilical area. Guttate psoriasis presents with papules that are often confined to the trunk and proximal extremities. Psoriatric erythroderma involves the entire body. Psoriasis may also present with localized (Acrodermatitis Continua of Hallopeau) or generalized (Von Zumbusch) pustular forms. Psoriatic arthritis is the major associated systemic manifestation. Psoriasis is a genetically inherited disease, and a number of candidate genes have been identified. The underlying pathophysiology of psoriasis involves epidermal proliferation and differentiation, angiogenesis, and a stimulated cellular immune system.

Gottlieb A. *J Am Acad Dermatol.* 2000; 42: 428.

TREATMENT OPTIONS

- Acitretin*
- Adalimumab^
- Alefacept*
- Anthralin*
- Azathioprine$
- Bexarotene oral$
- Calcipotriene*
- Calcipotriene with diprolene*
- Cetirizine^
- Coal tar*
- Colchicine$
- Cyclosporin*
- Denileukin diftitox$

- Efalizumab*
- Etanercept*
- Excimer 308 nm laser, body$, scalp+
- Hydroxyurea^
- Infliximab^
- Interferon gamma^
- Intravenous immunoglobulin+
- Isotretinoin^
- Leflunomide$
- Mechlorethamine$^, with UVB
- Methotrexate*
- Mycophenolate mofetil$
- Paclitaxel$
- Photopheresis+
- Pimecrolimus^
- PUVA, systemic^, topical^
- PUVA, topical with narrow-band UVB^
- Ranitidine$
- Salicylic acid^
- Selenium sulfide+
- Steroids, oral*, topical*, intralesional$, intramuscular$
- Tacalcitol^
- Tacrolimus, topical for body^, topical for face and intertriginous$, oral^
- Tazarotene*
- Thioguanine$
- Tretinoin, topical$
- UVA^
- UVB^

PSORIASIS, PUSTULAR

TREATMENT OPTIONS:

- Acitretin^
- Clofazimine$
- Colchicine+
- Cyclosporin$
- Granulocyte and monocyte adsorption apheresis+
- Infliximab+
- Methotrexate$
- PUVA$
- PUVA, systemic$, topical$
- Tacrolimus topical+

PYODERMA GANGRENOSUM

▨ DEFINITION

Pyoderma gangrenosum (PG) is a rare, destructive inflammatory skin disease in which a painful nodule or pustule breaks down to form a progressively enlarged ulcer. There are five subtypes: bullous, ulcerative, vegetative, pustular, and periostomal. Lesions may occur either in absence of any apparent underlying disorder or in association with a systemic disease, such as ulcerative colitis, Crohn's disease, polyarthritis, and gammopathies. Some cases may be associated with malignacy (eg, acute myelogenous leukemia). PG has occurred as a side effect of treatment with granulocyte-macrophage colony–stimulating factor or interferon-α2b and in cases in which interleukin-8 is overexpressed in the tissue.

Ho VC. *Mayo Clin Proc.* 1996; 71: 1182.

▨ TREATMENT OPTIONS

- Apligraf[®,+]
- Azathioprine[+]
- Becaplermin[+]
- Benzoyl peroxide[+]
- Chlorambucil[$]
- Clofazimine[$]
- Colchicine[+]
- Cyclophosphamide[$]
- Cyclosporin[$]
- Dapsone[$]
- Etanercept[$]
- Hydroxyurea[+]
- Infliximab[$]
- Intravenous immunoglobulin[+]
- Maggots[+]
- Mechlorethamine[+]
- Melphalan[+]
- Methotrexate[+]
- Minocycline[$]
- Mycophenolate mofetil[+]
- Potassium iodide[+]
- Steroids, oral[$], topical[$], pulse[+], intralesional[+]
- Tacrolimus, topical[^]
- Thalidomide[$]

REITER'S SYNDROME

▨ DEFINITION

Reiter's syndrome is a characteristic clinical triad, consisting of urethritis, conjunctivitis, and arthritis, that usually develops several weeks after infection of the gastrointestinal or urinary tract with certain microorganisms (*Shigella flexneri, Salmonella* spp., *Yersinia* spp., *Ureaplasma urealyticum, Borrelia burgdorferi*). The most common cutaneous findings are circinate balanitis, keratoderma blenorrhagicum, and painless mucosal ulcers of the tongue, palate, buccal mucosa, and lips. The disease occurs chiefly in young men of HLA-B27 genotype.

Toivanen A. *Drugs*. 2001; 61: 343.

▨ TREATMENT OPTIONS

- Acitretin[+]
- Cyclosporin[+]
- Etretinate[+]
- Infliximab[+]
- Ketoconazole[+]
- Methotrexate[+]
- Steroids, oral[$], topical[+]

ROSACEA

▨ DEFINITION

Rosacea is a centrofacial disease principally localized on the nose, cheeks, chin, forehead, and glabella. The hallmarks of rosacea are livid red erythema and telangiectasias preceded by episodes of flushing, papules, and pustules. Comedones are notably absent. Granulomatous changes can emerge in later stages. Rhynophyma (bulbous nose) is the ultimate presentation.

Maddin S. *J Am Acad Dermatol*. 1999; 40: 961.

▓ TREATMENT OPTIONS

- Azelaic acid^
- Benzoyl peroxide^
- Benzoyl peroxide gel and clindamycin gel^
- Clindamycin, topical^
- Doxycycline/minocycline*
- Erythromycin, topical$
- Isotretinoin (papulopustular)+, (granulomatous)^
- Metronidazole, topical*
- Permethrin^ (papulopustular)
- Sodium sulfacetamide*
- Sulfur^
- Tacrolimus, topical$
- Tetracycline$
- Tretinoin^

SARCOIDOSIS

▓ DEFINITION

Sarcoidosis is a systemic granulomatous disorder of unknown etiology with a predilection for involvement of the lungs, liver, lymph nodes, skin, and eyes. Cutaneous manifestations are seen in up to one-third of patients and may be the first clinical sign of the disease. It usually presents with red-brown to violaceous papules and plaques, most often on the face, lips, neck, upper back, and extremities. Many variants exist, including subcutaneous, lupus pernio, and ulcerative.

English JC. *J Am Acad Dermatol.* 2001; 44: 725.

▓ TREATMENT OPTIONS

- Allopurinol+
- Azathioprine$
- Chlorambucil$
- Chloroquine (lung)$, (cutaneous)^
- Clofazimine+ (laryngeal)
- Hydroxychloroquine$ (cutaneous)
- Infliximab$
- Isotretinoin+ (cutaneous)

- Methotrexate^
- Minocycline+ (cutaneous)
- Mycophenolate mofetil+ (cutaneous)
- Pentoxifylline$ (cutaneous)
- Pulse dye laser+, CO_2 laser+ (cutaneous)
- PUVA+ (cutaneous)
- Quinacrine+ (cutaneous)
- Steroids, oral (cutaneous$, pulmonary^, neurologic^), pulse (neuro-logic$, polyneuropathy+, hypopituitarism+), intralesional+, topical+
- Surgical excision+
- Tacrolimus, topical+ (cutaneous)
- Thalidomide$

SCABIES

▓ DEFINITION

Scabies is the term for infestation with the itch mite, *Sarcoptes scabiei* var. *humanus*. The disease is found worldwide, in all races and all age groups. It can be transmitted sexually as well as by nonsexual close skin-to-skin contact, especially within the family and at school. The hallmark of scabies is intractable pruritus, more severe at night. Variants are scabies incognito, in patients taking glucocorticoids; crusted (Norwegian) scabies, mainly seen in immunosuppressed patients; and bullous scabies, in children and adults, in whom it is almost indistinguishable from bullous pemphigoid.

Meinking TL. *N Engl J Med.* 1995; 333: 26.

▓ TREATMENT OPTIONS

- Ivermectin^
- Lindane*
- Permethrin*
- 5–10% sulfer in petrolatum base^
- Thiabendazole$

SCLERODERMA

■ DEFINITION

Scleroderma is a chronic disease of unknown etiology that affects the micro-vasculature and loose connective tissue and is characterized clinically by fi-brous deposition and obliteration of vessels in the skin, lungs, gastrointestinal tract, kidneys, and heart. The diffuse thickening and induration of the skin in the systemic form of scleroderma is accompanied by fibrosis and vascular obliteration of internal organs. Its course is often progressive and oc-casionally fatal. The limited form has a more restricted pattern of involve-ment and does not affect internal organs.

Marmont AM. *Annu Rev Med.* 2000; 51: 115.

■ TREATMENT OPTIONS

- Alprostadil^
- Angiotensin-converting enzyme inhibitors (renal)^
- Avoidance of cold (Raynaud's phenomenon)
- Azathioprine$
- Becaplermin$ (ulcers)
- Calcipotriene$ (cutaneous)
- Chlorambucil^
- Cimetidine+ (esophagitis)
- Colchicine$
- Cyclophosphamide$
- Cyclosporin^ (for linear scleroderma)+
- Diltiazem$ (calcinosis cutis, Raynaud's phenomenon)
- Epoprostenol (pulmonary)^
- Etanercept$
- Hydroxychloroquine+
- Iloprost^
- Infliximab+
- Interferon gamma$
- Methotrexate^
- Minocycline$ (cutaneous)
- Penicillamine^
- Pentoxifylline$
- Photopheresis$
- Proton pump inhibitors (gastrointestinal)$
- PUVA$
- Relaxin^

- Stanozolol^
- Thalidomide$
- UVA for acral sclerosis$
- Warfarin$

SEBORRHEIC DERMATITIS

DEFINITION

Seborrheic dermatitis is a common chronic papulosquamous dermatosis that is often associated with increased sebum production (seborrhea) of the scalp and the sebaceous follicle-rich areas of the face and trunk. The affected skin is pink, edematous, and covered with yellow-brown scales and crusts. The disease varies from mild to severe, including psoriasiform or pityriasiform patterns and erythroderma. Seborrheic dermatitis is one of the most common skin manifestations in patients with HIV infection.

Nakayama J. *Eur J Dermatol.* 2000; 10: 528.

TREATMENT OPTIONS

- Benzoyl peroxide^
- Calcipotriene^
- Coal tar*
- Itraconazole$
- Ketoconazole^ (topical and oral)
- Metronidazole^
- Pimecrolimus+
- Salicylic acid^
- Selenium sulfide*
- Sodium sulfacetamide*
- Steroids, oral* (severe), topical*
- Sulfur$
- Tacrolimus, topical$
- UVB$

SQUAMOUS CELL CARCINOMA

▨ DEFINITION

Cutaneous squamous cell carcinoma (SCC) is a malignant neoplasm derived from suprabasal epidermal keratinocytes. SCC probably evolves in most cases from precursor lesions of actinic keratosis and Bowen's disease (SCC in situ). SCC represents a broad spectrum of disease ranging from easily managed, superficially invasive cancer to highly infiltrative, metastasizing tumors that can result in death.

Weisberg NK. *J Am Acad Dermatol.* 2000; 43: 483.

▨ TREATMENT OPTIONS

Surgical treatment is the preferred modality.

- Acitretin$ (lowers risk of SCC in psoriatic patients treated with PUVA)
- Cidofovir, topical+
- CO_2 laser$
- Cryotherapy^
- Curettage and desiccation^
- Excision with margins
- Fluorouracil, topical$
- Imiquimod$ (erythroplasia of Querat+), invasive+
- Interferon alpha 2A$, 2B$
- Interferon gamma^ (Bowenoid papulosis)
- Mohs micrographic surgery
- Photodynamic therapy topical with ALA^, intravenous with verteporfin for Bowen's disease^
- Radiation^
- Tretinoin, topical$

STEVENS-JOHNSON SYNDROME

▨ DEFINITION

Stevens-Johnson syndrome is an acute mucocutaneous reaction composed of erosions of at least two mucosal surfaces with extensive superficial necrosis of the lips and mouth and a purulent conjunctivitis. The extent of skin involvement varies but is usually less than 10% and may involve atypical target-like lesions. Generalized lymphadenopathy is usually present, and hepatosplenomegaly may be observed. Stevens-Johnson syndrome has a protracted course of 4–6 weeks with significant morbidity and mortality (less than 2%).

Brett AS. *South Med J.* 2001; 94: 342.

▓ TREATMENT OPTIONS

- Acyclovir[+]
- Cyclophosphamide[+]
- Intravenous immunoglobulin[$], recurrent cases[+]
- Mycophenolate mofetil[+]
- Steroids, oral[*]
- Supportive care[^]

SWEET'S SYNDROME

▓ DEFINITION

Sweet's syndrome is characterized by fever, peripheral blood neutrophilia, and painful erythematous pseudovesicular plaques, occasionally bullous, that favor the face and upper extremities and contain dense neutrophilic dermal infiltrates. Associated conditions include infections, malignancies, inflammatory bowel disease, autoimmune disorders, certain medications, and pregnancy.

Cohen PR. *Am J Clin Dermatol.* 2002; 3: 117.

▓ TREATMENT OPTIONS

- Chlorambucil[+]
- Clofazimine[+]
- Colchicine[$]
- Cyclosporin[+]
- Dapsone[+]
- Hydroxyurea[+]
- Interferon alpha[+]
- Potassium iodide[+]
- Steroids, oral[$], pulse with chlorambucil[+], topical[+], intralesional[+]
- Thalidomide[+]

TOXIC EPIDERMAL NECROLYSIS

■ DEFINITION

Toxic epidermal necrolysis (TEN) is a rare, acute, life-threatening, rapidly evolving mucocutaneous reaction characterized by tenderness, erythema, necrosis, and extensive mucocutaneous exfoliation of the epidermis. TEN is almost always drug related, and the medications most frequently involved are sulfa drugs, nonsteroidal anti-inflammatory drugs, antibiotics, and anti-epileptics. TEN usually occurs 7–21 days after initiation of the responsible drug. The exfoliation is due to extensive death of keratinocytes via apoptosis mediated by the interaction of the death receptor-ligand pair Fas-FasL. The average mortality rate is 25–35% but can be higher. The risk of death can be accurately predicted by applying a severity-of-illness score (SCORTEN).

Viard I. *Science.* 1998; 282: 490.

■ CLASSIFICATION

	ERYTHEMA MULTIFORME MINOR	STEVENS JOHNSON SYNDROME	SJS/TEN OVERLAP	TEN WITH SPOTS	TEN
Detachment	<10%	<10%	10–30%	<30%	<10%
Typical targets	+	–	–	–	–
Atypical targets	Raised	Flat	Flat	Flat	Flat
Spots	–	+	+	+	–

Bastuji-Garin S. *Arch Dermatol.* 1993; 129: 92.

■ SCORTEN

- Age >40 years
- Presence of malignancy
- Pulse >120 bpm
- Glucose >252 meq/L
- Blood urea nitrogen >27 meq/L
- Bicarbonate <20 meq/L
- Body Surface Area >10%

These values are recorded within first 24 hours of hospital admission. Patient gets one point for each of the criteria present.

TOTAL CRITERIA	% RISK OF MORTALITY
0–1	3.2%
2	12.1%
3	35.3%
4	58.3%
5+	90%

Bastuji-Garin S. *J Invest Dermatol.* 2000; 115: 149.

TREATMENT OPTIONS

- Acetylcysteine[+]
- Cyclophosphamide[+]
- Cyclosporin[+]
- Immediate withdrawal of causative medication[$]
- Infliximab[+]
- Intravenous immunoglobulin[$]
- Pentoxifylline[+]
- Plasmapheresis[$]
- Steroids, oral[*], pulse[+]
- Supportive care[^]

URTICARIA

DEFINITION

Urticaria is a descriptive term for recurrent whealing of the skin and represents transient superficial dermal swelling. It is characterized by the rapidity of its fluctuation, with individual wheals, pink and pruritic, lasting no more than 24 h in most patients. There are several different causes of urticaria, including allergy, autoimmunity, drugs, dietary pseudoallergens, physical stimuli, and infections. The pathophysiologic events producing urticaria also vary. Many cases remain unexplained (idiopathic) even after extensive evaluation. Diagnosis is based on the history and supported by blood tests, skin tests, and skin biopsy.

Grattan CEH. *Br J Dermatol.* 2000; 143: 365.

TREATMENT OPTIONS

- Cetirizine (chronic)[*], (acute, cholinergic, cold, heat, solar)[^]
- Cetirizine and zafirlucast for cold urticaria[^]

- Cimetidine^ with H₁ blockers
- Colchicine⁺
- Cyproheptadine*, aquagenic⁺
- Danazol^ (chronic, cholinergic)
- Desloratadine* (chronic)
- Diphenhydramine^
- Doxepin^, cold^
- Epinephrine^$
- Fexofenadine* (chronic)
- Hydroxyzine^, cold^
- Interferon alpha 2A and 2B^$ (chronic)
- Intravenous immunoglobulin (chronic)^$, (delayed pressure⁺)
- Loratadine* (chronic)
- Mizolastine^
- Montelukast^
- Nifedipine^
- Photopheresis⁺ (solar)
- Ranitidine^
- Ranitidine^ with H₁ blockers
- Scopolamine⁺ (cholinergic)
- Stanozolol^ (chronic)
- Steroids, oral*, intramuscular^$, topical*
- Sulfasalazine⁺
- Thyroxine^$
- UVB^$, solar⁺

VASCULITIS

DEFINITION

Vasculitis refers to disease processes involving inflammation and fibrinoid necrosis of blood vessels. Involvement may be localized or diffuse, and vasculitis may be primary or secondary to a systemic disease. It may involve the arterial or venous system, or it may represent an overlap between the two. Small, medium, or large vessels may be involved. The best-characterized mechanism mediating vasculitis is the deposition of immune complexes in the walls of affected blood vessels.

Crissey JT. *Clin Dermatol.* 1999; 17: 493.

■ TREATMENT OPTIONS

- Azathioprine (leukocytoclastic$^\$$, Wegener's granulomatosis$^\$$, poly-arteritis nodosa$^\$$, Henoch-Schönlein purpura$^\wedge$)
- Cetirizine (urticarial$^+$)
- Chlorambucil (Wegener's granulomatosis$^+$, cutaneous polyarteritis nodosa$^+$)
- Colchicine (leukocytoclastic$^\$$, urticarial$^+$, polyarteritis nodosa$^+$)
- Cyclophosphamide (leukocytoclastic$^\wedge$, Wegener's$^\wedge$, polyarteritis nodosa$^\wedge$, cryoglobulinemia$^\$$, Henoch-Schönlein purpura)
- Danazol (livedoid$^\$$)
- Dapsone (leukocytoclastic$^\$$, urticarial$^\$$, polyarteritis nodosa$^\$$, Henoch-Schönlein purpura$^+$)
- Etanercept (Wegener's granulomatosis$^\wedge$)
- Hydroxychloroquine (urticarial$^+$)
- Intravenous immunoglobulin (livedoid$^+$, leukocytoclastic, cutaneous polyarteritis nodosa$^+$)
- Methotrexate (leukocytoclastic$^+$, cutaneous polyarteritis nodosa$^+$, giant-cell arteritis$^\wedge$)
- Mycophenolate mofetil (urticarial$^+$, Churg-Strauss syndrome$^+$)
- Nonsteroidal anti-inflammatory drugs (leukocytoclastic$^+$, urticarial$^+$, polyarteritis nodosa$^+$)
- Pentoxifylline (urticarial$^\$$, leukocytoclastic$^\$$, livedoid$^+$, cutaneous polyarteritis nodosa$^+$)
- Plasmapheresis (cryoglobulinemia$^+$)
- Rituximab (hypocomplementemic urticarial vasculitis$^+$)
- Stanozolol$^\wedge$
- Steroids, oral (urticarial$^\$$, polyarteritis nodosa$^\wedge$, Churg-Strauss syndrome$^\wedge$, leukocytoclastic$^\$$, giant-cell arteritis$^\wedge$, cryoglobulinemia$^\wedge$, Henoch-Schönlein purpura$^\wedge$), pulse with cyclophosphamide (urticarial$^+$, polyarteritis nodosa$^+$)
- Thalidomide (leukocytoclastic$^+$)

VITILIGO

■ DEFINITION

Vitiligo is an acquired idiopathic disorder characterized by circumscribed, depigmented macules. Functional melanocytes disappear from involved skin by a mechanism or mechanisms that have not yet been identified. Vitiligo carries a risk for ocular abnormalities, particular uveitis. The most severe form of uveitis is seen in the Vogt-Koyanagi-Harada syndrome. Two major forms of vitiligo are recognized: (1) unilateral (segmental) and (2) bilateral (vulgaris). Koebner phenomenon can be seen in vitiligo. Three hypotheses have been advanced to explain the pathogenesis of vitiligo: (1) neural, (2) self-destruct; and (3) autoimmune.

Halder RM. *Dermatol Clin.* 2000; 18: 79.

■ TREATMENT OPTIONS

- Excimer® laser$
- Fluorouracil, topical$
- Grafting followed by topical steroids^
- Monbenzyl ether of hydroquinone$ (total depigmentation)
- Pimecrolimus+
- Pseudocatalase^
- PUVA^, with calcipotriene^
- Q-switched ruby laser$
- Steroids, oral$, topical^, pulse$, intralesional^
- Tacrolimus, topical^
- UVA with phenylalanine oral^
- UVB narrow band^, with calcipotriene+

WARTS

■ DEFINITION

Warts, or verrucae, are benign proliferations of the skin and mucosa that result from infection with human papillomaviruses (HPV). These viruses do not produce acute signs or symptoms but induce slow-growing lesions that can remain subclinical for a long period of time. A subset of HPVs has been associated with the development of epithelial malignancies. The papillomavirus genome encodes only eight to nine proteins, which are separated into two groups: E (early) and L (late). Cutaneous variants include common warts (verruca vulgaris), flat warts (verruca plana), filiform warts (cutaneous horn), plantar (myrmecia) and palmar warts, mosaic warts, Butcher's warts, anogenital warts (condylomata acuminata), bowenoid papulosis, epidermodysplasia verruciformis (HPV-5 and -8), cystic warts (HPV-60), oral focal epithelial hyperplasia (Heck's disease, HPV 13), Buschke-Lowenstein giant condyloma (HPV-6 or -11), and oral florid papillomatosis (HPV-6 or -11).

Schiller JT. *Expert Opin Biol Ther.* 2001; 1: 571.

■ TREATMENT OPTIONS

- Bleomycin intralesional injections^ (verruca vulgaris)
- *Candida* antigen intralesional injections (flat warts+)
- Cidofovir in cream base for genital warts+, verruca vulgaris in HIV-positive patients+
- CO_2 laser$
- Cryotherapy^
- Electrosurgery^
- Excision^
- Fluorouracil cream$ (condylomata acuminata)
- Imiquimod (genital warts*, verruca vulgaris$)
- Photodynamic therapy with topical aminolevulinic acid (ALA) for genital warts$, verruca plana+, verruca vulgaris^
- Podofilox* (condylomata acuminata)
- Podophyllin* (condylomata acuminata)
- Trichloroacetic acid^

WOUND HEALING

■ DEFINITION

Cutaneous wounds can be categorized according to their depth. If only the epidermis is lost, the wound is called an erosion. When the wound involves structures in the dermis, it is termed an ulcer. Ulcers are divided into partial thickness (epidermis and varying parts of the dermis) and full thickness (epidermis, all of the dermis, and deeper structures). Wounds are also classified as acute and chronic. Acute wounds are differentiated into partial and full thickness. Chronic wounds are also classified according to their depth, as in pressure ulcers stages I to IV.

Romanelli M. *J Am Acad Dermatol.* 1995; 32: 188.

■ TREATMENT OPTIONS

- Bacitracin^
- Becaplermin (postsurgical abdominal dehiscence^, diabetic ulcers*, pressure ulcers^, chronic leg ulcers$, scleroderma ulcers$, ulcerated hemangioma+, ulcerated lichen planus+)
- Benzoyl peroxide (acute surgical wounds^, leg ulcers$, decubitus ulcers+, Mohs surgical wounds+)

- Iodosorb® and Iodoflex® (infected traumatic and surgical wounds*, wet ulcers*, venous ulcers*, decubitus ulcers*)
- Lidocaine, topical^ (pain relief)
- Metronidazole^ (malodor)
- Mupirocin^
- Pentoxifylline (venous^, arterial$, diabetic$)
- Silver sulfadiazine (burn*, ulcers^)

XEROSIS

▧ DEFINITION

Xerosis is a dry, rough, scaly quality of the skin that may result from both exogenous and endogenous causes. The most common cause of xerosis is aging. Other causes are dry climate, excessive exposure to water, alkali and detergents, marasmus and malnutrition, renal insufficiency and hemodialysis, and hereditary conditions such as ichthyosis vulgaris and atopy. Xerosis of aging is caused by a complex dysfunction of the horny layer, with decreased water-binding capacity due to decreased synthesis of "natural moisturizing factors," such as profilaggrin degradation products, urea, and other compounds.

Engelke M. *Br J Dermatol.* 1997; 137: 219.

▧ TREATMENT OPTIONS

- Ammonium lactate*
- Emollients^
- Salicylic acid^
- Urea^

Index

Abelcet (amphotericin B), 22–24
acanthosis nigricans, 347
Accutane (isotretinoin), 182–184
Achromycin (tetracycline), 299–302
Acinetobacter baumannii, 334
acitretin, 3–4
Aclovate (alclometasone dipropionate), 283–287
acne, 347–348
Acticin (permethrin), 249–250
Actimmune (interferon gamma), 175–177
actinic keratosis, 348–349
Actinomyces israelii, 334
acyclovir, 5–6
adalimumab, 7–8
adapalene, 8–9
albendazole, 9–11
Albenza (albendazole), 9–11
alclometasone dipropionate, 283–287
Aldara (imiquimod), 166–168
alefacept, 12–13
alitretinoin, 13–14
Alkeran (melphalan), 207–208
Allegra (fexofenadine), 127–128
alopecia, androgenic, 351
alopecia areata, 349–350
Altinac (tretinoin), 311–313
aluminum chloride, 14–15
AmBisome (amphotericin B), 22–24
amcinonide, 283–287
Amevive (alefacept), 12–13
amikacin, 16–19
Amikin IV (amikacin), 16–19
aminoglycosides, 16–19
amitriptyline, 19–21
AmLactin (ammonium lactate), 21–22
ammonium lactate, 21–22
amoxicillin, 239–243
amoxicillin clavulanate, 239–243
Amoxil (amoxicillin), 239–243

Amphicol (chloramphenicol), 72–74
Amphocin IV (amphotericin B), 22–24
Amphotec (amphotericin B), 22–24
amphotericin B, 22–24
ampicillin, 239–243
ampicillin sulbactam, 239–243
amyloidosis, 350
Ancef IM/IV (cefazolin), 53–55
Ancobon (flucytosine), 133–134
androgenic alopecia, 351
angioedema, 351–352
anthralin, 24–25
Antiminth (pyrantel), 257–258
aphthous stomatitis, 352–353
Aralen (chloroquine), 74–76
Aristocort (triamcinolone), 278–282
Aristocort (triamcinolone acetonide), 283–287
Aristospan (triamcinolone), 278–282
aspergillosis, 327–328
Atarax (hydroxyzine), 165–166
atopic dermatitis, 353–354
atorvastatin, 25–27
ATS (topical erythromycin), 118–119
Augmentin (amoxicillin clavulanate), 239–243
Avage (tazarotene), 295–297
Avelox (moxifloxacin), 145–148
Avita (tretinoin), 311–313
Azactam IV (aztreonam), 31–32
azathioprine, 27–29
azelaic acid, 29–30
Azelex (azelaic acid), 29–30
azithromycin, 198–202
aztreonam, 31–32

Bacillus anthracis, 334
bacitracin, topical, 32–34
bacterial infections, 334–339

Bacteroides fragilis, 334
Bactocill (oxacillin), 237–239
Bactrim (trimethoprim/sulfameth-
   oxazole), 287–291
Bactroban (mupirocin), 220–221
Barc (pyrethrin), 259
Bartonella henselae, 335
Bartonella quintana, 335
basal cell carcinoma, 354
BayGam IV (intravenous immuno-
   globulin), 177–179
BCNU (carmustine), 51–52
Beben (betamethasone), 278–282
becaplermin, 34–35
Behçet's disease, 355
Benadryl (diphenhydramine), 110–111
Benzac AC (benzoyl peroxide), 35–37
BenzaClin (topical clindamycin/benzoyl
   peroxide), 86–87
Benzagel (benzoyl peroxide), 35–37
benzathine penicillin, 234–237
benzoyl peroxide, 35–37
Beta-Lift (salicylic acid), 271–272
betamethasone, 278–282
betamethasone dipropionate, 283–287
betamethasone valerate, 283–287
Betatar (coal tar), 90–92
Betatrex (betamethasone valerate),
   283–287
bexarotene, 37–39
Biaxin (clarithromycin), 198–202
Bicillin (benzathine penicillin),
   234–237
Bicillin CR (procaine and benzathine
   penicillin), 234–237
Biltricide (praziquantel), 256–257
blastomycosis, 328
Blenoxane (bleomycin), 39–40
bleomycin, 39–40
Borrelia burgdorferi, 335
Brevoxyl (benzoyl peroxide), 35–37
bromhidrosis, 252
bullous dermatoses, 374
bullous lupus erythematosus, 375
bullous pemphigoid, 355–356
butenafine, 40–41

cadexomer iodine, 42–43
calcipotriene, 43–45
Cancidas IV (caspofungin), 52–53

candidiasis, 328–330
Canthacur (cantharidin), 45–46
cantharidin, 45–46
capsaicin, 46–47
Carac (fluorouracil), 148–150
carbapenems, 48–50
Carmol (urea), 318–319
carmustine, topical, 51–52
caspofungin, 52–53
Ceclor CD (cefaclor), 56–59
Ceclor (cefaclor), 56–59
Cedax IV (ceftibuten), 60–65
cefaclor, 56–59
cefadroxil, 53–55
cefazolin, 53–55
cefdinir, 60–65
cefepime, 65–67
cefixime, 60–65
Cefizox IV (ceftizoxime), 60–65
Cefobid IV/IM (cefoperazone), 60–65
cefoperazone, 60–65
Cefotan IV (cefotetan), 56–59
cefotaxime, 60–65
cefotetan, 56–59
cefoxitin, 56–59
cefpodoxime, 60–65
cefprozil, 56–59
ceftazidime, 60–65
ceftibuten, 60–65
Ceftin (cefuroxime), 56–59
ceftizoxime, 60–65
ceftriaxone, 60–65
cefuroxime, 56–59
Cefzil (cefprozil), 56–59
Celbenin (methicillin), 237–239
Celestone (betamethasone), 278–282
CellCept (mycophenolate mofetil),
   222–224
cephalexin, 53–55
cephalosporins
   first generation, 53–55
   fourth generation, 65–67
   second generation, 56–59
   third generation, 60–65
Ceptaz (ceftazidime), 60–65
Certain-Dri (aluminum chloride),
   14–15
cetirizine, 67–69
Chlamydia pneumoniae, 335
Chlamydia trachomatis, 335
chlorambucil, 70–71
chloramphenicol, 72–74

Chloromycetin IV (chloramphenicol), 72–74
chloroquine, 74–76
cholestyramine, 77–78
chromomycosis, 330
cicatricial pemphigoid, 356–357
ciclopirox, 78–80
cidofovir, 79–82
Cidomycin (gentamicin), 16–19
cimetidine, 82–84
Cipro (ciprofloxacin), 138–142
ciprofloxacin, 138–142
Claforan IM/IV (cefotaxime), 60–65
Clarinex (desloratadine), 109–110
Claripel (hydroquinone), 159–160
clarithromycin, 198–202
Claritin (loratadine), 197–198
Cleocin (clindamycin), 84–85
Cleocin T (topical clindamycin), 86–87
clindamycin, 84–85
clindamycin, topical, 86–87
Clindets (topical clindamycin), 86–87
clobetasol propionate, 283–287
Clobevate (betamethasone dipropionate), 283–287
clocortolone pivalate, 283–287
Cloderm (clocortolone pivalate), 283–287
clofazimine, 87–89
Clostridium difficile, 335
clotrimazole, 89–90
coal tar, 90–92
coccidiodomycosis, 330
colchicine, 92–93
Condylox (podofilox), 253–254
contact dermatitis, 357
Cordran (flurandrenolide), 283–287
Cortef (hydrocortisone), 278–282
cortisone, 278–282
Cortone (cortisone), 278–282
cryptococcosis, 331
Cubicin IV (daptomycin), 106–107
Cuprimine (penicillamine), 232–234
cutaneous T-cell lymphoma, 358–359
Cutivate (fluticasone propionate), 283–287
Cyclocort (amcinonide), 283–287
cyclophosphamide, 94–96
cyclosporin, 96–99
cyproheptadine, 100–101
cystitis, candidiasis, 330

cytomegalovirus retinitis, 80
Cytovene (ganciclovir), 154–156
Cytoxan (cyclophosphamide), 94–96

danazol, 102–103
Danocrine (danazol), 102–103
dapsone, 104–105
daptomycin, 106–107
Darier-White disease, 359–360
Decadron (dexamethasone), 278–282
Deltasone (prednisone), 278–282
delusions of parasitosis, 362
Denavir (penciclovir), 231–232
denileukin diftitox, 107–108
Denorex (coal tar), 90–92
Depo-Medrol (methylprednisolone), 278–282
Dermarest (salicylic acid), 271–272
dermatitis
    atopic, 353–354
    contact, 357
    herpetiformis, 360
    seborrheic, 399
dermatomyositis, 361
Dermatop (prednicarbate), 283–287
dermatophytes, 331–332
desloratadine, 109–110
desonide, 283–287
DesOwen (desonide), 283–287
desoximetasone, 283–287
dexamethasone, 278–282
Dexasone (dexamethasone), 278–282
Dexone (dexamethasone), 278–282
DHS (coal tar), 90–92
dicloxacillin, 237–239
Differin (adapalene), 8–9
diflorasone diacetate, 283–287
Diflucan (fluconazole), 131–133
diphenhydramine, 110–111
Diprolene (betamethasone dipropionate), 283–287
Diprosone (betamethasone dipropionate), 283–287
discoid lupus erythematosus, 375–376
Doak Tar (coal tar), 90–92
Doryx (doxycycline), 299–302
Dosepak (methylprednisolone), 278–282
Dovonex (calcipotriene), 43–45
doxepin, 112–114
doxycycline, 299–302

Dritho-Scalp (anthralin), 24–25
Drithocreme (anthralin), 24–25
Drysol (aluminum chloride), 14–15
Duac (topical clindamycin/benzoyl peroxide), 86–87
Duofilm (salicylic acid), 271–272
Duplex T (coal tar), 90–92
Duricef (cefadroxil), 53–55
Dynapen (dicloxacillin), 237–239
dysesthesia, 362

E-Mycin (erythromycin base), 198–202
econazole, 114–115
EES (erythromycin ethyl succinate), 198–202
efalizumab, 115–116
Efudex (fluorouracil), 148–150
Elavil (amitriptyline), 19–21
Eldopaque forte (hydroquinone), 159–160
Eldoquin forte (hydroquinone), 159–160
Elidel (pimecrolimus), 250–251
Elimite (permethrin), 249–250
Elocon (mometasone furoate), 283–287
Elta Tar (coal tar), 90–92
EMLA (lidocaine and prilocaine), 192–193
Enbrel (etanercept), 120–121
endocarditis, candidiasis, 329
enoxacin, 138–142
Enterobacter cloaca, 335
Enterococcus faecalis, 335
Enterococcus faecium, 335
epidermolysis bullosa, 362–363
epidermolysis bullosa acquisita, 363–364
epoetin alpha, 116–118
Epogen (epoetin alpha), 116–118
Ery-Tab (erythromycin base), 198–202
Eryc (erythromycin base), 198–202
Erygel (topical erythromycin), 118–119
EryPed (erythromycin ethyl succinate), 198–202
erythema multiforme, 364
Erythrocin (erythromycin stearate), 198–202

Erythrocin IV (erythromycin lactobionate), 198–202
erythromycin, topical, 118–119
erythromycin base, 198–202
erythromycin estolate, 198–202
erythromycin ethyl succinate, 198–202
erythromycin lactobionate, 198–202
erythromycin stearate, 198–202
Escherichia coli, 336
esophagitis, candidiasis, 329
etanercept, 120–121
ethambutol, 121–122
Exsel (selenium sulfide), 272–273
extracorporeal photochemotherapy (photophoresis), 123–124

famciclovir, 125–126
familial benign pemphigus, 367
Famvir (famciclovir), 125–126
fexofenadine, 127–128
filgrastim, 128–129
Finacea (azelaic acid), 29–30
finasteride, 130
Flagyl (metronidazole), 214–216
Florinef (fludrocortisone), 278–282
Florone (diflorasone diacetate), 283–287
Floxin (ofloxacin), 138–142
fluconazole, 131–133
flucytosine, 133–134
fludrocortisone, 278–282
fluocinolone acetonide, 135–136
fluocinonide, 283–287
fluoroquinolones
    first generation, 136–138
    fourth generation, 145–148
    second generation, 138–142
    third generation, 142–145
fluorouracil, 148–150
flurandrenolide, 283–287
fluticasone propionate, 283–287
foliaceus pemphigus, 383–384
Fortaz (ceftazidime), 60–65
foscarnet, 150–152
Foscavir (foscarnet), 150–152
Francisella tularensis, 336
Fungizone (amphotericin B), 22–24
Fusarium, 332

gabapentin, 152–154
Gammagard IV (intravenous immuno-globulin), 177–179
Gammar-P IV (intravenous immuno-globulin), 177–179
ganciclovir, 154–156
Gantanol (sulfamethoxazole), 287–291
Garamycin (gentamicin), 16–19, 156–157
Gardnerella vaginalis, 336
gatifloxacin, 145–148
gentamicin, 16–19, 156–157
Gentamytrex IV (gentamicin), 16–19
gonorrhea, 337
graft-versus-host disease, 365
granuloma annulare, 365–366
Gris-PEG, 157–159
Grisactin (griseofulvin), 157–159
griseofulvin, 157–159
Grover's disease, 366
GVHD. *See* graft-versus-host disease

Haemophilus ducreyi, 336
Haemophilus influenzae, 336
Hailey-Hailey disease, 367
halcinonide, 283–287
halobetasol, 283–287
Halog (halcinonide), 283–287
Head and Shoulders intensive treatment (selenium sulfide), 272–273
head lice. *See* pediculosis
Helicobacter pylori, 336
herpes gestationis, 368
Hexadrol (dexamethasone), 278–282
histoplasmosis, 333
Humira (adalimumab), 7–8
Hydrea (hydroxyurea), 163–164
hydrocortisone, 278–282, 283–287
hydrocortisone butyrate, 283–287
hydrocortisone valerate, 283–287
hydroquinone, 135–136, 159–160
hydroxychloroquine, 160–163
hydroxyurea, 163–164
hydroxyzine, 165–166
hypereosinophilic syndrome, 368–369
hypertrophic lupus erythematosus, 376
Hytone (hydrocortisone), 283–287

ichthyosis, 369–370
IgA pemphigus, 384–385
Ilosone (erythromycin estolate), 198–202
imipenem, 48–50
imiquimod, 166–168
immunoglobulin, intravenous, 177–179
Imuran (azathioprine), 27–29
infliximab, 168–170
interferon alpha 2A, 170–172
interferon alpha 2B, 172–175
interferon gamma, 175–177
intravenous immunoglobulin, 177–179
Intron (interferon alpha 2B), 172–175
Iodoflex (cadexomer iodine), 42–43
Iodosorb (cadexomer iodine), 42–43
isoniazid, 179–181, 340–342
isotretinoin, 182–184
itraconazole, 185–187
Iveegam IV (intravenous immuno-globulin), 177–179
ivermectin, 187–189

Kaposi's sarcoma, 370
Keflex (cephalexin), 53–55
Kefurox (cefuroxime), 56–59
Kefzol IM/IV (cefazolin), 53–55
keloid, 371
Kenalog (triamcinolone), 278–282
Kenalog (triamcinolone acetonide), 283–287
Kerasal (salicylic acid), 271–272
Kerasal (urea), 318–319
ketoconazole, 189–192
Klebsiella pneumoniae, 336

Lac Hydrin (ammonium lactate), 21–22
Lamisil (terbinafine), 297–299
Lamprene (clofazimine), 87–89
LCD (coal tar), 90–92
Legionella pneumophila, 336
Leukeran (chlorambucil), 70–71
Levaquin (levofloxacin), 142–145
levofloxacin, 142–145
lice. *See* pediculosis
lichen planus, 371–372

lichen sclerosus et atrophicus, 372–373
lichen simplex chronicus, 373
Lidex (fluocinonide), 283–287
lidocaine, topical, 192–193
lindane, 193–194
linear IgA bullous dermatosis, 374
linezolid, 195–196
Lipitor (atorvastatin), 25–27
lipodermatosclerosis, 374–375
Listeria monocytogenes, 337
LMX (topical lidocaine), 192–193
lobomycosis, 333
Locoid (hydrocortisone butyrate), 283–287
lomefloxacin, 138–142
Lorabid (loracarbef), 56–59
loracarbef, 56–59
loratadine, 197–198
Lotrimin AF (clotrimazole), 89–90
Lotrimin (clotrimazole), 89–90
lupus erythematosus, 375–377
Lustra (hydroquinone), 159–160
Luxiq (betamethasone valerate), 283–287
lymphomatoid papulosis, 377–378

macrolides, 198–202
magic mouthwash, 202–203
male pattern baldness, 351
Maxaquin (lomefloxacin), 138–142
Maxiflor (diflorasone diacetate), 283–287
Maxipime IM/IV (cefepime), 65–67
Maxivate (betamethasone dipropionate), 283–287
mebendazole, 203–205
mechlorethamine, topical, 205–206
Medotar (coal tar), 90–92
Medrol (methylprednisolone), 278–282
Mefoxin IV (cefoxitin), 56–59
Melanex (hydroquinone), 159–160
melanoma, 378–380
melphalan, 207–208
meningeal cryptococcosis, 331
meningitis, 331
Mentax (butenafine), 40–41
Mepacrine (quinacrine), 260–261
meropenem, 48–50
Merrem IV (meropenem), 48–50

methicillin, 237–239
methotrexate, 208–212
methoxsalen, 212–214
8-methoxypsoralen (8-MOP), 123–124
methylprednisolone, 278–282
Meticorten (prednisone), 278–282
Metreton (prednisone), 278–282
MetroCream (topical metronidazole), 216–217
MetroGel (topical metronidazole), 216–217
MetroLotion (topical metronidazole), 216–217
metronidazole, 214–216
metronidazole, topical, 216–217
Mezlin (mezlocillin), 243–247
mezlocillin, 243–247
Micanol (anthralin), 24–25
miconazole, 218–219
Minocin (minocycline), 299–302
minocycline, 299–302
minoxidil, 219–220
Mintezol (thiabendazole), 306–308
molluscum contagiosum, 380
mometasone furoate, 283–287
Monistat (miconazole), 218–219
8-MOP (8-methoxypsoralen), 123–124, 212–214
Moraxella catarrhalis, 337
Morganella morganii, 337
morphea, 381
moxifloxacin, 145–148
mucormycosis, 333
mupirocin, 220–221
Mustargen (topical mechlorethamine), 205–206
Myambutol (ethambutol), 121–122
Mycelex (clotrimazole), 89–90
Mycobacterium bovis, 342
Mycobacterium chelonae, 342
Mycobacterium fortuitum, 343
Mycobacterium genavense, 343
Mycobacterium gordonae, 343
Mycobacterium haemophilus, 343
Mycobacterium kansasii, 343
Mycobacterium leprae, 344
Mycobacterium marinum, 343
Mycobacterium scrofulaceum, 343
Mycobacterium tuberculosis, 340–342
Mycobacterium ulcerans, 343–344

Mycobacterium xenopi, 344
Mycobutin (rifabutin), 265–266
mycophenolate mofetil, 222–224
Mycoplasma pneumoniae, 337
Mycostatin (nystatin), 228–230

nafcillin, 237–239
naftifine, 224–225
Naftin (naftifine), 224–225
nalidixic acid, 136–138
Nallpen (nafcillin), 237–239
naloxone, 226–228
naltrexone, 227–228
Narcan (naloxone), 226–228
Nebcin (tobramycin), 16–19
necrobiosis lipoidica diabeticorum,
    381–382
NegGram (nalidixic acid), 136–138
Neisseria gonorrhoeae, 337
Neisseria meningitidis, 337
neomycin, 32–33
Neoral (cyclosporin), 96–99
Neosporin
    (bacitracin/neomycin/polymyxin),
    32–33
Neupogen (filgrastim), 128–129
Neurontin (gabapentin), 152–154
Neutrogena oil-free acne wash (salicylic
    acid), 271–272
Neutrogena oil-free sunblock (salicylic
    acid), 271–272
Nilstat (nystatin), 228–230
nitrogen mustard, topical, 205–206
Nizoral (ketoconazole), 189–192
norfloxacin, 138–142
Noritate (topical metronidazole),
    216–217
Noroxin (norfloxacin), 138–142
Novacet (sulfur/salicylic acid), 291–292
Nydrazid (isoniazid), 179–181
nystatin, 228–230
Nystop (nystatin), 228–230

ofloxacin, 138–142
Olux (clobetasol propionate), 283–287
Omnicef (cefdinir), 60–65

Omnipen (ampicillin), 239–243
Oncovin (vincristine), 323–325
Ontak (denileukin diftitox), 107–108
onychomycosis, 331–332
Orap (pimozide), 252–253
oxacillin, 237–239
oxiconazole, 230–231
Oxistat (oxiconazole), 230–231
Oxsoralen (methoxsalen), 212–214
Oxsoralen-Ultra (methoxsalen),
    212–214

Panglobulin IV (intravenous immuno-
    globulin), 177–179
panniculitis lupus erythematosus, 376
PanOxyl AQ (benzoyl peroxide), 35–37
PanOxyl (benzoyl peroxide), 35–37
Panretin (alitretinoin), 13–14
paracoccidioidomycosis, 333
paraneoplastic pemphigus, 382–383
parapsoriasis, small plaque, 383
Pasteurella multocida, 337
Pediapred (prednisolone), 278–282
pemphigoid gestationis, 368
pemphigus
    foliaceus, 383–384
    IgA, 384–385
    paraneoplastic, 382–383
    vulgaris, 385–386
penciclovir, 231–232
Penetrex (enoxacin), 138–142
penicillamine, 232–234
penicillin G aqueous, 234–237
penicillin VK, 234–237
penicillins
    first generation, 234–237
    fourth generation, 243–247
    second generation, 237–239
    third generation, 239–243
penicilliosis, 333
Penlac (ciclopirox), 78–80
Penn-Vee K (penicillin VK), 234–237
pentoxifylline, 247–249
Periactin (cyproheptadine), 100–101
Periostat (doxycycline), 299–302
peritonitis, candidiasis, 330
permethrin, 249–250
phaeohyphomycosis, 333

photochemotherapy, extracorporeal, 123–124

photopheresis (extracorporeal photo-chemotherapy), 123–124

pimecrolimus, 250–251

pimozide, 252–253

Pin X (pyrantel), 257–258

piperacillin, 243–247

Pipracil (piperacillin), 243–247

pityriasis lichenoides chronica, 386

pityriasis lichenoides et varioliformis acuta (PLEVA), 386

pityriasis rosea, 387

pityriasis rubra pilaris, 387–388

Plaquenil (hydroxychloroquine), 160–163

PLEVA. *See* pityriasis lichenoides et varioliformis acuta

Plexion (sodium sulfacetamide/sulfur), 275–276, 291–292

Podocon (podophyllin), 255–256

podofilox, 253–254

podophyllin, 255–256

Polygam IV (intravenous immuno-globulin), 177–179

polymyxin, 32–33

Polysporin (bacitracin/polymyxin), 32–33

Polytar (coal tar), 90–92

porphyria, 388–389

postherpetic neuralgia, 389

praziquantel, 256–257

Pred-Pak (prednisone), 278–282

prednicarbate, 283–287

prednisolone, 278–282

prednisone, 278–282

Prednisone Intensol (prednisone), 278–282

Prelone (prednisolone), 278–282

Prevalite (cholestyramine), 77–78

Primaxin IV/IM (imipenem/cilastin), 48–50

Principen (ampicillin), 239–243

procaine penicillin, 234–237

Procrit (epoetin alpha), 116–118

Prograf (tacrolimus), 292–295

Propecia (finasteride), 130

Proteus mirabilis, 337

Proteus vulgaris, 337

Protopic (tacrolimus), 292–295

Providencia stuartii, 338

Prudoxin (doxepin), 112–114

prurigo nodularis, 390

pruritic urticarial papules and plaques of pregnancy (PUPPP), 390–391

pruritus, 391–392

Pseudallescheria boydii, 333

Pseudomonas aeruginosa, 338

Psorcon (diflorasone diacetate), 283–287

psoriasis, 392–393

PUPPP. *See* pruritic urticarial papules and plaques of pregnancy

pyoderma gangrenosum, 394

pyrantel, 257–258

pyrethrin, 259

Questran (cholestyramine), 77–78

quinacrine, 260–261

quinupristin/dalfopristin, 261–263

ranitidine, 263–264

Raptiva (efalizumab), 115–116

Regranex (becaplermin), 34–35

Reiter's syndrome, 395

Remicade (infliximab), 168–170

Renova (tretinoin), 311–313

Retin A (tretinoin), 311–313

ReVia (naltrexone), 227–228

Rheumatrex (methotrexate), 208–212

Rickettsiae, 338

Rid (pyrethrin), 259

rifabutin, 265–266

Rifadin (rifampin), 266–268

Rifamate (isoniazid and rifampin), 179–181

rifampin, 266–268

Rifater (isoniazid, rifampin, and pyrazi-namide), 179–181

Rimactane (rifampin), 266–268

Risperdal (risperidone), 269–270

risperidone, 269–270

Rocephin IM/IV (ceftriaxone), 60–65

Roferon A (interferon alpha 2A), 170–172

Rogaine (minoxidil), 219–220

Rosac (sodium sulfacetamide/sulfur), 275–276, 291–292
rosacea, 395–396

salicylic acid, 271–272
Salmonella typhi, 338
Sandimmune (cyclosporin), 96–99
Sandoglobulin IV (intravenous immunoglobulin), 177–179
sarcoidosis, 396–397
scabies, 397
scleroderma, 398–399
seborrheic dermatitis, 399
Sebulex (salicylic acid/sulfur), 271–272, 291–292
selenium sulfide, 272–273
Selsun Blue (selenium sulfide), 272–273
Selsun (selenium sulfide), 272–273
Septra (trimethoprim/sulfamethoxazole), 287–291
Serratia marcescens, 338
Sezary's syndrome, 358
Shigella dysenteriae, 338
Silvadene (silver sulfadiazine), 274
silver sulfadiazine, 274
Sinequan (doxepin), 112–114
SLE. *See* systemic lupus erythematosus
sodium sulfacetamide, 275–276
Solaquin forte (hydroquinone), 159–160
Solu-Cortef (hydrocortisone), 278–282
Solu-Medrol (methylprednisolone), 278–282
Soriatane (acitretin), 3–4
sparfloxacin, 142–145
Spectazole (econazole), 114–115
Sporanox (itraconazole), 185–187
sporotrichosis, 333–334
squamous cell carcinoma, 400
stanozolol, 276–278
Staphcillin (methicillin), 237–239
Staphylococcus aureus, 338–339
Staphylococcus epidermidis, 339
Sterapred (prednisone), 278–282
steroids
  systemic, 278–282
  topical, 283–287
Stevens-Johnson syndrome, 400–401

stomatitis, 329
Streptococcus pneumoniae, 339
Streptococcus pyogenes, 339
Stromectol (ivermectin), 187–189
subacute lupus erythematosus, 377
Sulfacet-R (sodium sulfacetamide), 275–276
sulfadiazine, 287–291
Sulfadiazine (sulfadiazine), 287–291
sulfamethoxazole, 287–291
sulfonamides, 287–291
Sulfoxyl (benzoyl peroxide/sulfur), 291–292
sulfur, 291–292
Sulfur soap, 291–292
Sumycin (tetracycline), 299–302
Suprax (cefixime), 60–65
Sweet's syndrome, 401
Synalar (fluocinolone acetonide), 283–287
Synercid IV (quinupristin/dalfopristin), 261–263
systemic lupus erythematosus (SLE), 375–377

T-Sal (salicylic acid), 271–272
T-stat (topical erythromycin), 118–119
Tabloid (thioguanine), 308–310
tacrolimus, 292–295
Tagamet (cimetidine), 82–84
Targretin (bexarotene), 37–39
tazarotene, 295–297
Tazicef IM/IV (ceftazidime), 60–65
Tazidime (ceftazidime), 60–65
tazobactam, 243–247
Tazorac (tazarotene), 295–297
Temovate (clobetasol propionate), 283–287
Tequin (gatifloxacin), 145–148
terbinafine, 297–299
tetracyclines, 299–302
thalidomide, 303–306
Thalomid (thalidomide), 303–306
Theramycin (topical erythromycin), 118–119
thiabendazole, 306–308
thioguanine, 308–310
thrush, 329

Ticar (ticarcillin), 243–247
ticarcillin, 243–247
Timentin IV (ticarcillin/clavulanate), 243–247
Tinactin (tolnaftate), 310–311
Tinamed (salicylic acid), 271–272
tinea barbae, 158
tinea capitis, 332
tinea corporis, 332
tinea cruris, 332
tinea pedis, 332
tinea versicolor, 332
TOBI IV (tobramycin), 16–19
tobramycin, 16–19
tolnaftate, 310–311
Topicort (desoximetasone), 283–287
toxic epidermal necrolysis, 402–403
transient acantholytic dermatosis, 366
Trental (pentoxifylline), 247–249
tretinoin, 135–136, 311–313
Trexall (methotrexate), 208–212
Tri-Luma (fluocinolone acetonide, hydroquinone, tretinoin), 135–136
Tri Pak (azithromycin), 198–202
triamcinolone, 278–282
triamcinolone acetonide, 283–287
Triaz (benzoyl peroxide), 35–37
Tridesilon (desonide), 283–287
trifluridine, 313–314
trimethoprim/sulfamethoxazole, 287–291
Trimox (amoxicillin), 239–243
trovafloxacin, 145–148
Trovan (trovafloxacin), 145–148

Ultravate (halobetasol), 283–287
ultraviolet A-1, 315–316
ultraviolet B, 316–317
Unasyn (ampicillin sulbactam), 239–243
urea, 318–319
urticaria, 403–404
UVADEX (methoxsalen), 212–214

vaginitis, candidiasis, 329
valacyclovir, 319–321

Valisone (betamethasone valerate), 283–287
Valtrex, 319–321
Vancocin (vancomycin), 321–323
vancomycin, 321–323
Vantin (cefpodoxime), 60–65
vasculitis, 404–405
Vectrin (minocycline), 299–302
Veetids (penicillin VK), 234–237
Venoglobulin-S (intravenous immunoglobulin), 177–179
Vermox (mebendazole), 203–205
verruca vulgaris, 80
Vfend (voriconazole), 325–327
Vibramycin (doxycycline), 299–302
Vibrio cholerae, 339
vincristine, 323–325
Viroptic (trifluridine), 313–314
Vistide (cidofovir), 79–82
vitiligo, 405–406
voriconazole, 325–327

warts, 406–407
Westcort (hydrocortisone valerate), 283–287
Winpred (prednisone), 278–282
Winstrol (stanozolol), 276–278
wound healing, 407–408
Wycillin (procaine penicillin), 234–237

Xerac AC (aluminum chloride), 14–15
xerosis, 408
Xylocaine (topical lidocaine), 192–193

Yersinia enterocolitica, 339
Yersinia pestis, 339

Z Pak (azithromycin), 198–202
Zagam (sparfloxacin), 142–145
Zantac (ranitidine), 263–264
Zeasorb (miconazole), 218–219

Zetacet (sodium sulfacetamide/sulfur), 275–276, 291–292
Zetar (coal tar), 90–92
Zinacef IV/IM (cefuroxime), 56–59
Zithromax (azithromycin), 198–202
Zonalon (doxepin), 112–114
Zostrix (capsaicin), 46–47
Zosyn (piperacillin/tazobactam), 243–247
Zovirax (acyclovir), 5–6
Zyrtec (cetirizine), 67–69
Zyvox (linezolid), 195–196